PRAISE FOR *CBD*

"A magnificent approach to the use of medical cannabis in both humans and pets, not only for caregivers, patients, and their families, but also for skeptical physicians. This book is a must-read for anyone interested in discovering the real power of this millennial medicinal plant."

—DR. GISELA KUESTER, neurologist and epileptologist, clinical research director at Daya Foundation, Chile

"A clearly written and informative book on a complicated subject. Medical marijuana is not a panacea, and is not a substitute for the extraordinary skills of modern scientific medicine, but as this fine book shows, cannabis in its many forms is now an important part of the Western medical tradition."

—DALE PENDELL, author of *Pharmako/Poeia: Plant Powers, Poisons, and Herbcraft*

"*CBD: A Patient's Guide to Medicinal Cannabis* is a well-written guidebook to one of the most exciting compounds in cannabis medicine today. This book is comprehensive enough to be a useful reference to the layperson and expert alike, on matters relating to CBD as well as cannabis in general. Excellent job!"

—OWEN SHIBATA, MD

"CBD is a hot topic right now, but there's a tremendous amount of misinformation about how it works. This book clears up the confusion, and gives you expert guidance that could make a profound difference in your life."

—MAX SIMON, founder of Green Flower Media

"I love this book. It is both beautiful and practical, grounded in all the right qualities needed to make working with CBD easy and effective."

—UWE BLESCHING PHD, author of *Cannabis Health Index*

"This book will put patients and doctors on common ground when it comes to CBD. After reading it, patients will be ready to have an informed discussion with their doctor about how to use medical cannabis."

—SCOTT GIANNOTTI, founder of Cannabis and Hemp Association

"This comprehensive book combines scientific evidence with practical advice for specific health challenges and preventive measures. I highly recommend this guidebook for people who are considering CBD treatments, and for health care practitioners who want to learn more about CBD for their patients."

—SONDRA BARRETT, PhD, author of *Secrets of Your Cells: Discovering Your Body's Inner Intelligence* and *Ultimate Immunity: Supercharge Your Body's Natural Healing Powers*

"A testament to the source of Leonard Leinow's passionate stewardship of CBD-rich cannabis products, *CBD: A Patient's Guide to Medicinal Cannabis* reveals the scope and profundity of this game-changing component of medical marijuana."

—LAURIE VOLLEN, MD, MPH, founder of Naturally Healing MD

"Leonard Leinow's powerful advocacy for medicinal cannabis places us squarely on the cusp of accessing what is potentially the most incredibly diverse medicine that comes from one plant. We as individuals, families, therapists, doctors, and vets, need the power of informed choice to use this unparalleled plant appropriately—to heal ailments and save lives, to relieve pain and provide dignity in life passing."

—KIMBERLY CALL, CCHT, CMT, HHC, author of *Morning Rituals—How We Awaken* and *A Beautiful Passing*

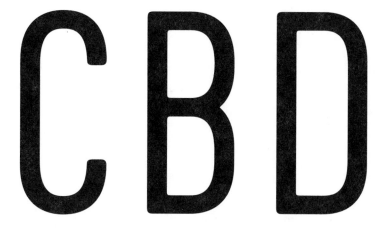

CBD

A PATIENT'S GUIDE
TO MEDICINAL CANNABIS

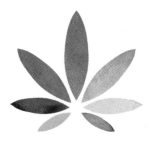

LEONARD LEINOW AND JULIANA BIRNBAUM

Foreword by Michael Moskowitz, MD

North Atlantic Books
Berkeley, California

Published by
North Atlantic Books
Berkeley, California

Cover design by Howie Severson
Interior design by Happenstance Type-O-Rama
Printed in the United States of America

CBD: A Patient's Guide to Medicinal Cannabis is sponsored and published by the Society for the Study of Native Arts and Sciences (dba North Atlantic Books), an educational nonprofit based in Berkeley, California, that collaborates with partners to develop cross-cultural perspectives, nurture holistic views of art, science, the humanities, and healing, and seed personal and global transformation by publishing work on the relationship of body, spirit, and nature.

MEDICAL DISCLAIMER: The following information is intended for general information purposes only. Individuals should always see their health care provider before administering any suggestions made in this book. Any application of the material set forth in the following pages is at the reader's discretion and is his or her sole responsibility.

North Atlantic Books' publications are available through most bookstores. For further information, visit our website at www.northatlanticbooks.com or call 800-733-3000.

Library of Congress Cataloging-in-Publication Data

Names: Leinow, Leonard, author. | Birnbaum, Juliana, 1974- author.
Title: CBD : a patient's guide to medicinal cannabis / Leonard
    Leinow and Juliana Birnbaum ; foreword by Michael H. Moskowitz, MD.
Description: Berkeley, California : North Atlantic Books, [2017] | Includes
    bibliographical references and index.
Identifiers: LCCN 2017006334| ISBN 9781623171834 (paperback) | ISBN
    9781623171841 (ebook)
Subjects: LCSH: Cannabis—Therapeutic use. | Marijuana—Therapeutic use. |
    BISAC: HEALTH & FITNESS / Herbal Medications. | MEDICAL / Alternative
    Medicine.
Classification: LCC SB295.C35 L45 2017 | DDC 615.7/827—dc23
LC record available at https://lccn.loc.gov/2017006334

3 4 5 6 7 8 9 VERSA 23 22 21 20 19 18
Printed on recycled paper

North Atlantic Books is committed to the protection of our environment.
We partner with FSC-certified printers using soy-based inks
and print on recycled paper whenever possible.

This book is dedicated to all beings whose health could benefit from the use of CBD and medical cannabis. We hope this guide will help light the way toward healing and wellness for each and every reader, their family, friends, and pets!

Lokah Samastah Sukhino Bhavantu

लोकाः समस्ताः सुखिनो भवन्तु

May all beings everywhere be happy and free, and may the
thoughts, words, and actions of my own life contribute in some
way to that happiness and to that freedom for all.

CONTENTS

PART I: A Patient's Primer on Cannabis and CBD

Part II: CBD for Health Concerns

Part III: Veterinary CBD

Part IV: Varieties of Cannabis

Part V: The Future Frontier of Cannabis-Based Medicine

ACKNOWLEDGMENTS

This book is a collection of facts, ideas, and data gathered by a magnificent team of experts, mentors, professional colleagues, family members, friends, and editors. Many of them are acknowledged in the main section of the book, and I could not have completed the book without their help and support. Special thanks to Juliana, my co-author, who inspired me to write this book and who brought together much of the research.

I am grateful to my very dedicated and loyal staff at our medical cannabis collective, Synergy Wellness, and at the Healing Essence CBD company. I want you all to know how much love and appreciation I have for your support, and for giving me the time that allowed me to write this book. I want to thank Dr. Michael Moskowitz for his tremendous contribution and encouragement, and his spectacular Forward to the book, and to Lion Goodman for his guidance, contributions, editing and friendship.

Special thanks to my wife, Terumi, for putting up with me. I know I can get a little crazy at times, so thank you for being the guiding light and grounding cord in my life. I offer my heartfelt thanks to the many teachers and mentors I have had throughout my life, especially Neem Karoli Baba, who continues to guide and inspire this venture.

To the members of Synergy Wellness Collective: It is an honor to be part of your healing process. Thank you for your support and your feedback about the efficacy of our products.

And to all those who have touched my life, and made it better, please know that I appreciate you, and your contribution, even though your name does not appear here.

Most of all, I want to acknowledge the Sacred Plant known as Cannabis. I have long felt your Spirit, and I appreciate your guidance along this path of exploration and healing. Thank you for partnering with me, and allowing me to be a pioneer in this new realm of nature-based medicine.

—Leonard Leinow

HOW TO BEST USE THIS BOOK

At first, most readers new to the use of CBD and medicinal cannabis will find the topic complicated and confusing, or even overwhelming, with too many options and with terminology that may not be familiar (see the glossary in the back of the book for definitions of some of the unfamiliar terms and abbreviations). This book is intended to be a user's guide to help shorten the time it takes to figure out a strategy and a protocol, including dosage guidelines. There is a lot of information here, maybe too much to start with. If you just want to find the treatment for a particular condition in the shortest time possible, here is the way to do that:

1. Medical condition—Go to Chapter 4 and find the health issue being treated in the alphabetized list (go to Part III if treating an animal). From there, you can find related research and information on the varieties of suggested cannabinoid products and in what forms they are commonly used (oral, inhaled, topical delivery methods, etc.). You can also find information on general dosage guidelines for the condition (micro, standard, or macro dosing). Then, go back to Chapter 3 to read about the specific delivery methods and skip ahead to Part IV to learn about the varieties or strains of high-CBD cannabis.

2. Dosage guidelines—Go to the section on dosage guidelines in Chapter 3. Though only one factor, the target dose, based on weight, can be estimated using the charts. Review the other factors that influence the dose (sensitivity, tolerance, etc.), and figure out a good target dose for the condition being treated. Dosage, which refers to both the quantity in a specific dose and the frequency with which you take the dose(s), is highly related to the severity of your condition and how your body reacts to the cannabinoid product. You will probably need to adjust your dosage until you achieve a result that works best for you.

3. Titration—After finding the appropriate type of cannabis, the method of delivery, and the target dose, decide on a schedule that will lead

from a starting micro dose up to a specific dose that works best for you. Remember to go slowly and be cautious with new substances. Each individual is unique, and finding out what strain and dose combination works best will be an experiential process of discovery. Try a little. See how it goes. Take detailed notes. Plan and adjust the dose, strain, or delivery method for the next dose.

4. Psychoactivity vs. non-psychoactivity—Some medical conditions recommend use of a spectrum of cannabinoids, such as various ratios of THC with CBD (see more on this "entourage" effect in Chapter 2). If it is recommended, decide if THC is appropriate for the particular patient, knowing psychoactivity may be a side effect. These protocols minimize or eliminate the high:

   a) Use CBD without THC or with a ratio of 20:1 CBD:THC, or higher.

   b) Use THC as a suppository.

   c) Use THC as a topical application (skin cream, salve, or balm).

   d) Use THC in the micro dosing range.

   e) Use THCA orally, the unheated raw plant.

   See Cautions, Side Effects, and Drug Interactions in Chapter 3 for contraindications.

5. If a term or section seems too technical, skip that section, and use it later as a reference if needed.

6. Relax and enjoy the process. Time and experience will prompt intelligent questions to accelerate the learning curve and facilitate decisions about future directions and doses.

FOREWORD

By Dr. Michael Moskowitz, MD, Bay Area Pain Clinic,
Sausalito, California

Here in Northern California, there is an extremely small artisanal medical cannabis clinic run by an elder and visionary named Leonard Leinow, a man dedicated to relieving the suffering of people. He currently has four thousand members who make up the membership base of the collective he named Synergy Wellness. To put this in perspective, most urban dispensaries in the state have tens of thousands, even up to 150,000 patients. He has organically grown and developed over thirteen high-cannabidiol (CBD) plant strains, with six strains at 10:1, 20:1 (2), 22:1, 24:1, and 25:1 CBD:THC. He has many other strains with different percentages of CBD:THC ratios ranging from approximately 4:1 to 1:1. He is a pioneer in the CBD world and makes tinctures and CBD oil out of all of his strains. He blends the tinctures and oils, combining them to achieve different ratios of phytocannabinoids and terpenoids. He also grows high-THC plants that he makes into tinctures and oils. He is constantly experimenting to improve his strains. He does not sell his products to other dispensaries and carefully tests his plants. He treats his plants as "sacred medicine," and his wife even sings to and blesses them with sacred Hawaiian hula ceremony as they grow.

Leonard uses the most sophisticated scientific and organic approaches to growing his plants and puts his patients' needs above his own. His motivation is helping others rather than making money. He constantly updates and refines his products and works on ways to use medical cannabis without the mind-altering effects, unless members wish it so. He reads the scientific literature about medical cannabis and figures out how to incorporate new findings with what he grows and how he makes various embodiments. He attends cannabis conferences and contests and stays focused upon producing the most medically valuable plants and products. He is open to new ideas and is willing to try the things that make sense to him. He talks to the patients who are members of his collective about their problems and comes up with individualized approaches that work through any issues they might be having. He is kind to everyone. He knows he is doing what he is supposed to do.

What he knows must be passed on to a younger generation of growers (who are mainly focused upon high-THC plants for recreational use) to help them understand that growing CBD-rich plants that do not make the user high will always be in demand for medical cannabis treatment. He knows that, for this treatment to grow and thrive, the public perception of medical cannabis users being stoned all the time must shift to an understanding of the usefulness of this treatment to help people remain highly functional and involved in their lives. Most importantly—and what makes him hesitant to retire—is that he knows that he has helped many people transform serious illness and despair into wellness and hope.

I was honored by the authors' invitation to submit a chapter on endo-cannabinoids and phytocannabinoids to this book and, subsequently, this foreword. I have been a physician since 1977 and am a pain medicine practitioner in San Rafael, California, a suburb of San Francisco. I am board-certified in both psychiatry and pain medicine, and work with people who have not had satisfactory treatment for their persistent pain disorders and who are referred into our practice for care. I am a lecturer on topics in pain medicine around the world. One of the topics I have spoken on is medical cannabis and pain medicine and have done so at the American Academy of Pain Medicine annual meetings, the 5th International Pain Skills Conference at Walter Reed Hospital, the 11th Annual Spine Symposium at University of California, San Francisco, and University of California, Davis as an assistant clinical professor. I developed a treatment program used around the world called neuroplastic transformation with my partner, Marla Golden, DO, and co-authored a book on this subject that has been sold in over fifty countries around the world. This approach emphasizes non-pharmaceutical and non-invasive approaches to treating persistent pain, by inducing the brain to reverse the process that causes this abnormal pain response in the first place.

I have been working with many of my patients to use medical cannabis to reduce their pain and their reliance on pain medications. I am currently following over three hundred of my patients in this treatment and have found it to be a highly successful addition to their treatment regimens. I met Leonard Leinow and Juliana Birnbaum through this work and always recommend that my patients start their treatment (and often continue it) with Synergy products because of the care taken there in growing, processing, researching, and transforming cannabis into medicine. This approach is nothing like standard pharmaceutical treatment, and, through my extensive research and clinical experience, it has become clear to me that this treatment causes basic and profound neuroplastic change, leading to symptom relief and, in some cases, cure.

Marijuana has been used as a recreational drug for over five thousand years. It has expanded its range from equatorial South America and the Kush regions of Asia to cultivation in every conceivable location around the world. It grows in lush, carefully tended acres of gardens, in elaborate indoor grow spaces, in closet-based, cardboard boxes, and in isolated ditches on the side of the road. One reason it has expanded its range so dramatically is that many people enjoy the psychotropic effects of "being stoned." That does not mean that medical use of the plant is a recent development—references to its use to treat various ailments goes back four to five thousand years. Its medical effects can be profound and are becoming increasingly documented in a recent spate of scientific articles published by outstanding researchers in top-quality, peer-reviewed scientific journals. These include *Nature, Science, British Journal of Pharmacology, The Lancet, Journal of the American Medical Association, Journal of Pain Medicine, Neuropharmacology, Journal of Mineral and Bone Research, Proceedings of the National Academy of Sciences,* and *Cell* (see the hundreds of these studies listed in the endnotes for a sense of the magnitude of this research). For readers unfamiliar with health science, these are the top journals in the world and are recognized as such by the scientific community. Simply put, and politics aside, marijuana is the single most medicinally valuable plant that has ever existed. Unfortunately, the problem is that policymakers, law enforcement, and the public associate its use with getting high or being stoned.

Enter the miracle of CBD, the one substance in cannabis that was bred out of the plant until recent times and the culmination of some of that research mentioned above. While we have known about CBD long before we discovered THC, it was incorrectly considered an inactive cannabinoid. Research from animal studies, basic pharmacology, and human studies have demonstrated the following properties of CBD: anti-cancer, anti-proliferative, anti-emetic (nausea and vomiting), anti-inflammatory, antibacterial, anti-diabetic, anti-psoriatic, anti-diarrheal, analgesic, bone stimulant, immunosuppressive, anti-ischemic, antispasmodic, vasorelaxant, cardio-protective, neuroprotective, anti-epileptic, antipsychotic, anxiolytic, and weight-loss promoting. For any scientist, lawmaker, or physician to deny this evidence is, in a word, unscientific. On the other hand, the relatively random way this treatment is conducted is just as unscientific. Into the breach is this gem of a book.

Leonard Leinow and Juliana Birnbaum have written a book that organizes medical cannabis treatment. While extolling the virtues of the "entourage" effects of the whole plant, this book emphasizes the importance of CBD. Leonard has grown high-CBD medical cannabis for over a decade and is truly a wizard. He keeps working on the ratio of CBD to THC that he wants with any individual strain, then clones his best plants to produce consistent results. An engineer by background, he meticulously grows each plant organically, moving them from clones to the vegetative state, to flowering and harvest. He combines science and art, searching out the strains he wants to develop, researching their genetics, and releasing them to the public only when he has stable cannabinoid ratios. He tests his plant strains then retests the tinctures, oils, and concentrates he makes from them. He talks with other growers about the value these CBD-rich strains bring to their work. He has talked to and advised thousands of patients using his products to treat a great variety of conditions, and, while he can't provide medical consults, he advises about strains, dosage, routes of administration, potency, and observed results. Juliana has worked with Leonard for two years. She has helped develop his clinic and brought her background as an anthropologist and investigative reporter to the task of assembling the latest research, gathering patient stories, and bringing Leonard's extensive knowledge to the page.

In the book that follows, the authors take information gathered through research and experience and lay out a way of using cannabis medically that has not been done before. They emphasize CBD-rich products but delve into history, scientific discoveries, our own built-in cannabinoid system, the plant-based cannabinoid system, and medical conditions that might be helped. They also discuss different forms of the medicine, dosage suggestions, and a description of the genetics, properties, and uses of specific CBD-rich strains of cannabis. It is an ambitious work and is highly successful in delivering understandable information to both inexperienced and experienced readers interested in pursuing the health benefits of medical cannabis. The breadth of this work is stunning. There is more information than any patient needs to absorb, but that is the beauty of this book. It is an excellent reference for patients, their caregivers, family members, physicians, the press, and anyone interested in this topic. This book is organized in a thoughtful way, reflecting the authors' experience fielding tens of thousands of questions from people inquiring about treatment with medical cannabis.

For the past year, the advice and knowledge of "the Wizard of Woodacre" has been just a phone call away for me to access help for my patients. Now it is available to the rest of the world, a once-hidden treasure trove of information that is finally accessible to the broader public. This authoritative guide to CBD takes the mystery out of cannabidiol while providing state-of-the-art knowledge and preserving the art, spirit, and soul of treatment with medical cannabis.

INTRODUCTION

By Leonard Leinow and Juliana Birnbaum

The plant known as hemp or cannabis is among the first ever to be used by people as medicine, with records of its use dating back to prehistory. Yet, the findings that it is the unique known source of a large number of powerful natural compounds known as phytocannabinoids are much more recent. Cannabidiol (CBD) is the most prevalent of these cannabinoids, of over a hundred currently identified. For many years, it was left by the wayside as scientists focused on the properties of what they assumed to be the "active ingredient": tetrahydrocannabinol or THC (the mind-altering component of the plant).[1]

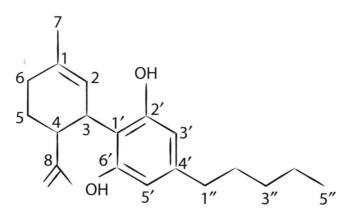

FIGURE 2: The Chemical Structure of Cannabidiol (CBD)

*Phyto*cannabinoids work in a similar way to chemical messengers called *endo*cannabinoids **found in our own bodies.** Despite only having been discovered by scientists in the mid-1990s (through research into the effects of cannabis), the endocannabinoid system probably originated millions of years ago in non-vertebrates and appears to help regulate many of our physical systems, from sleep to digestion. Endocannabinoids are considered neurochemicals that are found throughout the nervous system and are connected to our immune response and even our reproductive system. They, and the receptors they bind to, are found in virtually all animals—fish, reptiles, birds, mammals, and even earthworms!

THC, (Δ^9 THC to be exact), the better-known compound, works by binding **directly** to these endocannabinoid receptors in a similar way to that of anandamide, the neurochemical produced by the human body. On the other hand, CBD produces its profound anti-inflammatory, anti-anxiety, antipsychotic, antispasmodic, and analgesic effects by **indirectly** stimulating these same receptors through inhibition of the enzyme that metabolizes and destroys anandamide, allowing it to be more available to the body. While we attribute the healing effects to CBD, it is more accurate to say that CBD enables the body to heal itself through balancing the endocannabinoid system.

As this book goes to press, cannabis has been legalized to some degree in twenty-nine states and the District of Columbia, plus sixteen states that allow for the use of CBD only, for specific conditions. There are a few reasons behind this wave of change, one of the most important being that CBD does not produce the same euphoria or psychoactive "high" associated with THC.

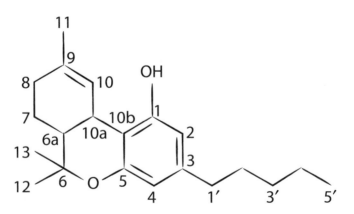

FIGURE 3: The Chemical Structure of Δ^9-Tetrahydrocannabinol (THC)

Cultural attitudes toward cannabis have shifted dramatically in the United States and other countries over the past decade. Patients who have found extraordinary results in treating cancer, ALS, Parkinson's, epilepsy, and a long list of serious diseases have become activists for the legalization of the plant. The growing body of science and research supporting CBD as a valid medicine with an extraordinary range of potential applications can simply no longer be ignored.

One of those applications is safe and effective pain relief. In states where cannabis has been legalized for medicinal or recreational use, deaths from overdoses of opiates have declined significantly.[2] Yes, that's the gist: CBD is saving lives that might be lost to overdose from pharmaceutical painkillers. And that's just one of its many benefits.

In 2008, I (Leonard Leinow) started Synergy Wellness, a small patient-centered business that grows, manufactures, and dispenses organic medical cannabis following California laws and regulations for membership-based collectives. Two years later, a doctor practicing complementary medicine recommended a patient to me who had lung cancer. Claudette was a seventy-one-year-old woman from Haiti with a tumor considered too large to operate on. She had tried chemotherapy, and it did not work. Radiation was not an option, given the tumor's size and location. Her oncologist had told her to put her affairs in order and gave her about six months to live.

She started taking a tincture of Harlequin, our first CBD-rich strain at Synergy Wellness, slowly working up to a target rate that gave her a total of 250 mg/day of combined CBD and THC. She was not undergoing any other physical, herbal, or pharmaceutical treatment during this time. However, she did have a very positive attitude and a robust spiritual practice that included lots of gratitude and prayers, which seemed to amplify her healing process.

After three months of treatment, her tumor shrank 50 percent in volume, which was determined by comparing MRI scans taken three months apart, before and after CBD treatment. The doctors were extremely surprised and said that the tumor was now small enough to remove surgically. Upon surgery, they found a small amount of cancer had spread to two lymph nodes, which was also removed. The client was now totally cancer free. She continued using CBD-rich tinctures at a much smaller maintenance dose after the operation. She continues to be cancer free six years later. Her maintenance dose is 40 mg daily of CBD+THC combination.

After witnessing the powerful effects of CBD on cancer, I decided that this was absolutely the direction for my work in the cannabis industry. Synergy Wellness has been a pioneer in this specialized field, searching for CBD-rich strains, propagating them locally using organic techniques, and making various medicinal products. My team has grown with the demand for high-CBD products, which are not available in many locations. We've had many cases of people being able to discontinue use of or greatly reduce reliance on pharmaceuticals that have debilitating side effects. Some members of our collective use CBD in addition to conventional medication; others have chosen to avoid pharmaceuticals or other medical procedures and are just using cannabis therapy to treat or manage their condition. Some credit our medicine with saving their lives when conventional treatment options have been exhausted. Many have told us our CBD tinctures allowed their child to be free of seizures and attend school for the first time. Others have used our products to treat serious illnesses in animals and have sent us photos of their healthy pets enjoying life (see Part III, contributed by veterinarian Gary Richter, for more on this).

While the results we've seen have been truly groundbreaking, a lot of misunderstanding persists around cannabis, including how to use CBD effectively. Medical schools are just now starting to include the endocannabinoid system in the curriculum. Most doctors have not had proper training in how to accurately recommend medical cannabis. Synergy Wellness now has more than four thousand members. We get calls every day, from patients looking for instructions and advice on using CBD to care for themselves, their children, or their pets. One of the most frequent comments we hear is that our patients do not want to "get high" and want to heal without the mind-altering effects of THC.

We decided it was time to bring the information we've collected directly to the thousands of people who could benefit profoundly from medical cannabis. This book is a guide for patients and caregivers to use CBD to treat common health disorders safely and effectively, including forms of delivery for the medicine, side effects, and dosage. *To find out how to treat a specific condition, consult the appropriate entry in the alphabetized list in Part II, then refer back to the page numbers specified to determine dosage by body weight and options for how to take the medicine.*

CBD is considered by expert scientists and physicians to have a wide scope of potential medical applications. Some of the factors that make it so exciting as a medical treatment are that 1) it has almost no side effects, 2) it has a very low risk of addiction, and 3) there is virtually no chance of a lethal overdose. These are serious benefits when compared to opiates and other pharmaceuticals prescribed for medical conditions.

Much more research needs to be done on the plant's potential medicinal benefits and effects, including its more than two hundred phytochemical compounds. Fortunately, progress is being made, as we report in Chapter 11. One thing that has become increasingly clear over the past decades of research on cannabis is that its effects on health are most available when the medicine is derived from the whole plant rather than isolates or synthetic versions of its components.[3]

Synergy and Plant Medicine

While science tends to focus on the classification and study of species one by one, the story of the evolution of life on planet Earth is one of profound interconnection. Human interaction with plants—our cultivation and consumption of them—has drastically altered and changed those plants over the long term. In the same way, the plants (and plant-derived medicines) have altered and changed us. Our bodies shift in response to them, and over time we evolve as a result. Our co-evolution with cannabis has had reciprocal benefits to both species.

Cannabis and people have been in a mutually beneficial relationship for millennia. Hemp (a variety of *Cannabis sativa* that is rich in CBD) may have been among the world's first cultivated crops. It has been confirmed as a common fiber for rope-making ten thousand years ago in ancient China. The earliest known record of its use as medicine was in 2737 BCE, when Emperor Shen Neng recommended a cannabis tea for the treatment of pain, arthritis, malaria, gout, and memory disorders. Its popularity spread throughout Asia, to India (where Ayurvedic texts included many uses for the plant), to the Middle East, and down the eastern coast of Africa. The ancient Egyptians are the first known civilization to have used it to reduce the growth of tumors. It was prescribed by ancient Greek and Roman physicians and is confirmed to have had innumerable ceremonial, recreational, medicinal, and therapeutic uses in Asia, Africa, Arabia, South America, and Central America.[4]

In 1937, political lobbyists colluded to scapegoat and eliminate cannabis and hemp as industrial crops in the United States (see Chapter 1 for more details on this topic). They represented the pharmaceutical, alcohol, tobacco, paper, cotton, synthetic fabric, and petroleum industries (hemp oil can fuel diesel engines). When they succeeded in banning both hemp and cannabis, most other countries followed suit with prohibitions of their own. This demonization of the plant caused research to stop. No scientist would risk his or her career looking for the benefits of an illegal drug.

Even though the plant was made illegal, an underground movement continued to grow and use cannabis. During the 1960s, I was introduced to cannabis while I was a senior engineering student at UCLA. At that time, the supply came from Mexico and was of mediocre quality, especially compared to today's standards. It had modest levels of THC and a significantly higher level of CBD than today's recreational products. I became a moderate user. It baffles me to this day that, during my senior year, I rarely went to classes, had little interest in my studies, and spent a lot of time using cannabis; yet I managed to get the best grades of my university career—good enough to get into UC Berkeley's Graduate School of Engineering. I minored in art and found cannabis helped open my creative talents and enhanced my intuitive abilities.

After completing my studies, I embarked on a spiritual quest. I went overland from Europe to Asia, traveling to thirty-five countries and visiting many places that produced cannabis. I landed in India where I lived for five years, studying music, yoga, and meditation. While in India, at the request of my teacher, I took a vow to abstain from using cannabis as part of my spiritual work. Ironically, I lived in Kulu Valley in the Himalayan mountains, where fifteen-foot cannabis indica plants were growing wild all around my house. I still loved the plant, felt a close relationship to it, and would watch the Sadhus (wandering holy men) come and make handmade hash from our plants for use in their own spiritual practices.

In the late 1970s, cannabis breeders in Amsterdam and Northern California were experimenting with methods that greatly magnified the potency of cannabis. Using selective breeding, they were able to find and propagate the specific plants that were higher in THC in order to increase the psychoactive effects (enjoyed by many but disliked by some). At the same time, because CBD is anti-psychoactive, the levels of CBD in many strains were bred downward to miniscule amounts. The combination of high THC and low CBD makes cannabis very potent for recreational purposes. In addition, they started growing cannabis as sensimilla (without seed), a technique that prevents the female flowers from being pollinated by male plants. Desperate to attract male pollen to fertilize their potential seeds, they produce large amounts of juicy, sticky resin, also known as pure "cannabis oil"—the strongest active ingredient in the plant and the substance responsible for its powerful effects. However, this "seedless" technology can be used to magnify the CBD as well as the THC levels.

Over the past twenty years, researchers began to circle back to the study of CBD as a separate cannabinoid. They discovered that it has promising results in the treatment of many medical disorders without the mind-altering effect of THC, and many researchers have called for more scientific clinical trials. The list of health issues that respond to CBD is quite long and includes seizures, autoimmune disorders, inflammation, pain, anxiety, stress, and cancer. We cover these specific ailments and others, with supporting studies and evidence along with suggested protocols for treatment, in Part II.

In the past decade, the number of these promising studies has grown exponentially. Yet CBD still lives in the shadows. Cannabis, and therein CBD, is still listed as a Schedule 1 drug by the United States Drug Enforcement Administration (though in March 2017 the DEA clarified that products derived from hemp are not illegal substances).[5] However, the highest quality CBD products are made from medical grade cannabis as we discuss in Chapter 7.

A Schedule 1 designation means that on a federal level, scientists have restricted access to the cannabis plant and limited funding to do research. It signifies that there is no accepted use for medical treatment and a high potential for addiction, which causes many legal barriers for doctors, researchers, growers, manufacturers, and distributors of CBD. Because of the Schedule 1 status, FDIC-insured banks cannot do business with or make loans to companies or individuals involved in the growing, manufacturing, or marketing of CBD. These businesses are forced to operate as "cash only," which not only heightens the security risk of doing business but also greatly hampers the growth of the industry. In addition, a Schedule 1 status prohibits insurance companies from reimbursing any claims for CBD as medicine, even if a doctor prescribes it. Furthermore, interstate commerce is prohibited, even if it is legal within the two states involved.

Despite all of these various factors dampening the growth of this emergent medicine, there has been huge groundswell of grassroots evolution within the industry, to a great extent because of the many positive benefits that CBD brings to people with medical issues. Many children suffering from severe forms of epilepsy have found CBD has given them a new life. The gratitude of their parents has touched me deeply. Many cancer patients have been told that they have exhausted conventional avenues for treatment and that they should go home and prepare for the end of life. After coming to Synergy Wellness, they have seen effective treatment for palliative care. Not only are many of these patients still alive, but a number of them are also currently cancer-free. People who have had crippling anxiety and autoimmune disorders are given a new lease on life. CBD is anti-stress medicine and it works on a cellular level. As a truly holistic remedy, healing takes place on the physical, mental, emotional, and spiritual levels. CBD has called to me to be a pioneer, an explorer, and a champion to help it emerge into the light of day. CBD has captured and opened my heart. Consequently, I have become dedicated to helping guide patients through uncertain, complicated terrain to health and wholeness.

An Ethnobotany of CBD-Rich Cannabis

When I (Juliana Birnbaum) applied to work at Synergy Wellness in 2015, I needed to find a local job but was somewhat skeptical about the concept of medical marijuana and assumed that most people were actually using it to, as they say, "get high." Not that I had a problem with that—as a person who likes to write, make music, hike, practice yoga, and dance, I had long found that cannabis helped me drop in quickly and deeply to creative work and sparked innovative thoughts and ideas. I had for many years intuitively felt that it was a safe and beneficial plant medicine, and that in small doses it helped with anxiety and depression. I used it for pain relief during my monthly cycle and in the early stages of labor during the otherwise un-medicated births of my two daughters. (It guided me to write a mantric poem that I used for strength during the most intense periods of my long first delivery.) My work as an assistant midwife and doula at nearly one hundred births in the San Francisco Bay Area had shown me that micro doses of cannabis could be effective in facilitating intervention and pharmaceutical-free births as well as healthy pregnancies in women with varying levels of *hyperemesis gravidarum*—extreme nausea and vomiting that endangers the unborn baby and causes dehydration and weight loss[6] (see Chapter 5 for more on women's health issues).

I spent my first few months as the new office manager at Synergy Wellness secretly looking for other jobs. After all, I had a graduate degree in cultural anthropology and a background as a reporter and editor. I had recently

published a book on the worldwide sustainable agriculture and design movement, so I was looking for what I considered more legitimate work connected
to writing, the environment, women's health, or social justice. And cannabis
still carries a stigma from its long history of carefully orchestrated propaganda
against its use—not the easiest job title to explain to other parents on the
playground.

Then I started to hear, firsthand, the stories of some of the Synergy Wellness members whose orders for medicine I was fulfilling each day. There was
the veteran treating his PTSD who told me he was trying our products after
six of his friends from the military committed suicide and he was determined
to go off the meds they were also on. There were the elderly patients, most
wary of getting high, but thrilled to be getting relief from arthritis or tremors
by using CBD without psychoactive effects. There were the parents who had
tried every other kind of drug to stop their baby's seizures and were now in
tears with me on the phone from across the country, telling me about seeing
their son laugh for the first time as a toddler or their daughter's new developmental milestone. There were the people who told me that, after using our
products, they got their first good night's sleep in years. There was the man
whose wife was in a wheelchair and was using our tinctures to address the
"phantom limb" pain from the nerves at the site of her amputated leg. And
then the cancer patients—I knew cannabis could help with chemo-related
nausea but had no idea of its powerfully anti-carcinogenic properties until I
heard some of our members' incredible stories of recovery.

I talked to medical professionals like Dr. Michael Moskowitz, the lead physician in a local pain clinic and extremely well loved by his patients. Moskowitz
has seen a major decrease in the need to prescribe opiates and other such
painkillers since directing people toward CBD therapy (we discuss this further
in Chapter 9). Could this medicine have saved the life of my beautiful friend
who lost her life at age thirty-five to an accidental overdose of pharmaceuticals,
just a few years after I'd been a bridesmaid at her wedding? I had to dig deeper.

The anthropologist in me realized that I was witnessing a little slice of a
major cultural sea change, a swing in the pendulum of public opinion in the
United States, after nearly a century of misinformation and corporate influence in health care. I saw that this shift is facilitating an exponential leap in
our scientific understanding of an ancient medicine and its potential to heal
modern disease. As I struggled to learn about CBD quickly enough to answer
the myriad questions I was being asked, I found connections to the research

I'd done for my last book, *Sustainable [R]evolution*. It focused on examples of sites worldwide that used regenerative design, also known as permaculture, to provide abundant food, water, and energy in their communities. Permaculture design is founded on the concept of *synergy:* cooperative interaction between the elements of a system.

Leonard named his company **Synergy Wellness** to emphasize how CBD works with our own physical systems to produce health: inspiring the body to heal itself. His work is about regenerative medicine, produced and grown locally and organically in a kind of "farm to patient" model. This approach encourages working holistically with natural systems in order to obtain an extraordinary result, one greater than the sum of the parts. Permaculture design focuses on the creation of diverse polycultures, where a combination of plants grown together creates resilience and abundance in a garden. By prioritizing biodiversity and growing high-CBD strains that had become close to lost in California cannabis agriculture, Leonard is part of a broader movement that is bringing this medicine back to the modern pharmacopoeia. It can be argued that he is part of the global "heirloom seed" network that is rescuing diverse plants from being lost to corporate monocropping.

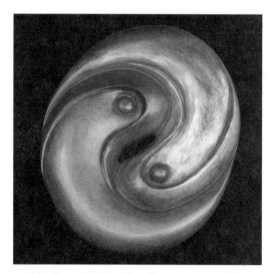

FIGURE 4: This bronze sculpture made by
Leonard illustrates the concept of synergy and
became the basis for the Synergy Wellness logo

"Cannabis is inherently polypharmaceutical," writes Dr. John McPartland, "and synergy arises from interactions between its multiple components."[7] Synergy is especially relevant to CBD and the way it interacts with the other active chemicals in cannabis; CBD and phyto-compounds called terpenes amplify the beneficial effects of cannabis while mitigating THC-induced anxiety. Also, as Dr. Moskowitz describes in Chapter 2, for many disorders the use of a wide spectrum of cannabinoids is of optimal benefit.

In recent scientific discoveries about the chemistry of cannabis, this key concept of synergy is called the "entourage" or "ensemble" effect. We understand now that CBD, THC, and other individual components work synergistically, so that the medicinal impact of the whole plant is far greater than that of the separate compounds.

Yet, as we explore in Chapter 11, since pharmaceuticals are based on the isolation of single molecules, and companies are not able to patent a whole plant, scientific research tends to focus on specific cannabinoids. I was floored to discover that a patent granting exclusive rights on the use of CBD and other cannabinoids to treat certain diseases was granted over a decade ago—to none other than a U.S. government agency. Patent 6630507, entitled "Cannabinoids as antioxidants and neuroprotectants," was awarded to the Department of Health and Human Services (HHS) in October 2003. Scientists forming part of the National Institutes of Health (NIH) filed it four years earlier, in 1999. It covers the use of nonpsychoactive cannabinoids to treat neurological diseases, such as Alzheimer's, Parkinson's, and stroke, and diseases caused by oxidative stress, such as heart attack, Crohn's disease, diabetes, and arthritis. In other words, the same government that is making it so difficult for patients to access this medicine is clearly aware of its efficacy and wants to control its distribution. Yet the bureaucratic red tape means that de-regulation is moving at a snail's pace for the multitudes of patients awaiting treatment options for life-threatening diseases.

Needless to say, I was called to help Leonard midwife this guidebook into being, in hopes that it would help the many patients seeking information and advice. It brings scientific evidence together with Leonard's wisdom and experience into a straightforward, research-based guide to wellness through CBD-rich cannabis. We, along with Dr. Moskowitz and the other contributors and professionals we consulted, believe that it is way past time for this medicine to get into the hands of people whose lives it has the potential to transform. It is our intention that this book will help that to happen, and that the legislation and education will catch up with the evidence and permit widespread medical use of this most mysterious and magical of healing plants.

PART I

A Patient's Primer on Cannabis and CBD

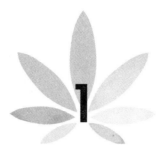

Cannabis as Medicine
through the Ages

A Highly Condensed History of Cannabis

While holding a special place in world history as a multidimensional plant that sparks opposing narratives, cannabis is quite simply a very common, adaptable, sun-loving weed that can be grown in many climates. Its origins have been traced 36 million years back to the Altai Mountains in the high plateau of Central Asia. From there it spread across the globe, going northward into China and Europe, where its use as a fiber became prevalent (although there is evidence that it was used as medicine there as well). It went south into India, the Middle East, and Africa, where its healing properties and psychoactive use caught on. Wherever the plant was introduced, it tended to stay, with a remarkable range of medicinal, dietary, and practical use by people in far-ranging cultures.

This kind of diverse use of a plant is a common indicator of the length of its relationship with humans. A characteristic of some of our oldest cultivated plants is that they serve multiple purposes, from fiber to food to medicine. In many parts of Eurasia, cannabis is self-sown, especially along river valleys where humans first tended to settle and change native environments. Known as a "camp-follower," the plant adapts quickly to newly cleared habitats and would often be among the first to colonize nitrogen-rich compost heaps created by people. As new uses were found for the plant, more direct cultivation took place in and around settlements. It went by literally hundreds of names and has a vast history—beyond the scope of this book—but was very commonly used in ancient Greek medicine. Its most popular scientific name is traced to Greece. Dioscorides referred it to in the first century AD[8] as kannabion (a familiar diminutive form translating to "little cannabis" or "dear cannabis," likely from the root *kanna* or *cane*).[9] Several different theories about the etymology of the word point to Sumerian or Sanskrit origins.[10] Some scholars claim that the plant is referred to in the Bible either as an "aromatic reed or cane" or as part of a "holy oil" made with several herbs and only permitted to be used to anoint members of the Aaronic priesthood.[11]

Over the centuries, people have selected and bred various types of cannabis for different purposes. As a non-medical product, hemp was widely used for its fiber production. When the thirteen U.S. colonies were getting established, farmers were required to produce crops consisting of at least 25 percent hemp. Sails and ropes were needed for trade ships. It was the common source of paper and clothes; the Declaration of Independence was written on hemp paper. Hemp was the backbone of the development of America and its founding fathers. Both George Washington and Thomas Jefferson were hemp farmers.

Although ethnobotanists and explorers describing their adventures would occasionally mention cannabis, Western physicians actually knew very little about it until the mid-nineteenth century. Credited with re-introducing cannabis to the modern world, Irish doctor William Brooke O'Shaughnessy read a groundbreaking paper to a group of students and scholars of the Medical and Physical Society of Calcutta in 1839. In addition to his pioneering work on cannabis therapy, O'Shaughnessy invented the modern treatment for cholera and made significant contributions to a number of fields, including underwater engineering!

O'Shaughnessy, who was an assistant surgeon and professor of chemistry at a prominent university in colonial India, conducted what were likely the first clinical trials of cannabis. He started with controlled experiments on mice, dogs, rabbits, and cats, and, when he was convinced of its safety, he made handmade extracts based on "native" recipes and gave them to some of his patients. His 1839 paper presented case studies of patients suffering from rheumatism, hydrophobia, cholera, and tetanus, as well as one involving an infant with seizures who responded well to cannabis therapy, reportedly going from near death to "the enjoyment of robust health" in a few days.[12] He cautioned other doctors to start with low doses, however, warning of a form of delirium "occasioned by continual Hemp inebriation." He concluded that these clinical studies have "led me to the belief that in Hemp the profession has gained an anti-convulsive remedy of the greatest value."[13] Between 1839 and 1900, more than one hundred articles appeared in scientific journals describing the medicinal properties of cannabinoids.[14]

Use of cannabis both as an intoxicant and for medicinal purposes became more and more common in Europe and across America from the 1850s to 1930s. Tinctures of "marihuana" or "cannabis extract" were often-used products with a reputation for effective pain relief sold by major pharmaceutical companies in the United States and Europe during this period.

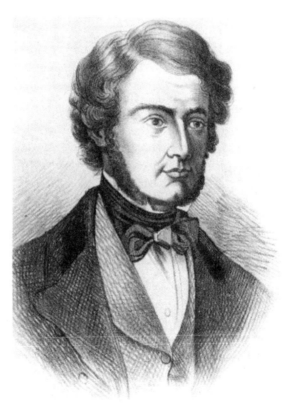

FIGURE 5: Irish physician William Brooke O'Shaughnessy
(1809–1889) is recognized as a founding father of
modern medical cannabis inquiry

The spelling "marihuana" is an anglicization of "marijuana," one of the more obscure Spanish slang words for the plant. It was purposely popularized during the anti-cannabis crusade of the 1920s and 1930s, headed in the media by press baron William Randolph Hearst in order to cement the connection between the plant and Mexicans. "By stigmatizing marijuana and the 'foreigners' who smoked it, Hearst succeeded in exacerbating anti-Mexican sentiment during the Great Depression, when many Anglos felt they were competing with brown-skinned migrants for scarce jobs," journalist and CBD activist Martin A. Lee wrote (see sidebar, Anslinger: The Archnemesis of Cannabis). Interestingly, the U.S. Drug Enforcement Agency insists on using the archaic "marihuana" in reference to cannabis products to this day, perhaps reflecting its anachronistic stance on the substance.

ANSLINGER: THE ARCHNEMESIS OF CANNABIS

ADAPTED FROM *SMOKE SIGNALS: A SOCIAL HISTORY OF MARIJUANA—
MEDICAL, RECREATIONAL AND SCIENTIFIC* BY MARTIN A. LEE

On August 11, 1930, Harry Jacob Anslinger became the director of the newly formed Federal Bureau of Narcotics (FBN) in Washington, DC. He was the godfather of America's war on drugs, and his influence on public policy would be felt long after death stiffened his fingers in 1975.

Anslinger didn't pay much attention to cannabis until 1934, when the FBN was floundering. Tax revenues plummeted during the Great Depression, the bureau's budget got slashed, and Harry's entire department was on the chopping block. Then he saw the light and realized that marijuana might just be the perfect hook to hang his hat on.

Anslinger understood that the likelihood of prohibitory legislation increased if the substance in question was associated with ethnic minorities. He eschewed references to benign-sounding *cannabis* and *hemp*, while calling for a federal ban on *marihuana*. Very few Americans knew that marijuana, the weed that some African Americans and Chicanos were smoking, was merely a weaker version of the concentrated cannabis medicines that everyone had been taking since childhood. By stigmatizing marijuana and the 'foreigners' who smoked it, Hearst succeeded in exacerbating anti-Mexican sentiment during the Great Depression, when many Anglos felt they were competing with brown-skinned migrants for scarce jobs.

To gain public support for his crusade, Anslinger depicted marijuana as a sinister substance that made Mexican and African American men lust after white women. His diatribes served as a not-so-subtle reminder to white women, who had only recently won the right to vote, that they still needed strong men to protect them from the "degenerate races." He never tired of telling new versions of the same morality tale. The film *Marijuana!* (1935) featured the lurid tag line "Weird orgies! Wild parties! Unleashed passions!" But when it came to ridiculous anti-marijuana propaganda, nothing could top Hot Fingers Pirielli, the bug-eyed piano player who pounds out jazz tunes in *Tell Your Children* (1936), better known by its later title *Reefer Madness*.

Although it bombed at the box office, *Reefer Madness* was destined to become a cult humor classic among American college students in later years. A vivid example of the national frenzy that set the stage for federal pot prohibition, this film epitomized the synchronicity among Washington, Hollywood, and mainstream media in the war against cannabis.

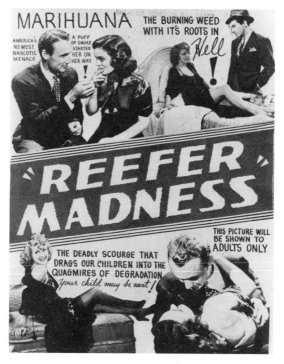

FIGURE 6: 1936: HULTON ARCHIVE/GETTY IMAGES

The intersection of cannabis prohibition and racism is apparent in the United States as well as England and other European nations. In 1937, when marijuana was officially criminalized in the United States, the propaganda used to support the ban emphasized its use by African Americans and Latinos and invented statistics about its relationship to crime. Through the next few American generations, use of the plant was illegal, and it continued to be associated with marginalized populations and those who chose to rebel against authority—namely the poets of the Beat generation and the counterculture of the 1960s (Martin A. Lee covers this and the decades that followed extensively in *Smoke Signals,* his social history of the plant, as described in the sidebar, Anslinger: The Archnemesis of Cannabis).

The Controlled Substances Act of 1970 classified marijuana along with heroin and LSD as a Schedule I drug, (i.e., having the relatively highest abuse potential and no accepted medical use). Most marijuana at that time came into the United States from Mexico, but in 1975 the Mexican government agreed to eradicate the crop by spraying it with the highly toxic herbicide *paraquat.* Colombia then became the number one international source. The "zero tolerance" climate of the Reagan and Bush administrations resulted in passage of strict laws and mandatory sentences for possession of marijuana and a crackdown on smuggling. The "war on drugs" thus brought with it a shift from reliance on imported supplies to domestic cultivation (particularly in Hawaii and California).

In 1973, Dr. Tod Mikuriya reprinted O'Shaughnessy's original paper as the lead article in *Marijuana: Medical Papers,* a book whose publication became a landmark in the contemporary medical marijuana movement. The previous year, the National Commission on Marihuana and Drug Abuse, appointed by President Nixon at the direction of Congress, considered laws regarding marijuana and determined that personal use of marijuana should be decriminalized. Nixon rejected the recommendation, but over the course of the 1970s eleven states decriminalized cannabis and most others reduced their penalties. Since then, there has been a general trend toward decriminalization and increased access for medical use on the state level.

The Re-emergence of CBD and Other Cannabinoids as Medicine

Cannabinol (CBN) was the first of the phytocannabinoids to be isolated at the end of the nineteenth century. CBN is now thought to be formed from THC during the storage of harvested cannabis. Its structure was illustrated in the early 1930s by R. S. Cahn, and its chemical synthesis was first achieved in 1940 in the laboratories of R. Adams in the United States and Lord Todd in the United Kingdom. A second component, cannabidiol (CBD), was first obtained from cannabis in the same year by Adams and his colleagues. THC was first extracted from cannabis in 1942 by Wollner, Matchett, Levine, and Loewe. Both THC and CBD are present in cannabis mainly as acids that are converted to non-acid form by adding heat, a process known as decarboxylation.[15]

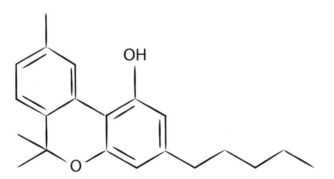

FIGURE 7: The Chemical Structure of Cannabinol (CBN)

It was in the laboratory of Dr. Raphael Mechoulam in Israel that the structure and stereochemistry of CBD was elucidated in 1963, and pure THC was isolated the following year. Research focus was first put on THC, as CBD was assumed to be a non-active precursor to THC. CBD is the most abundant phytocannabinoid found in all varieties of the plant, including hemp, and its immediate effects are more subtle. In the 1970s and 1980s, Mechoulam and his cohorts led numerous studies that showed the efficacy of both THC and CBD in treating seizure disorders and other health issues. Yet the legal prohibition of cannabis in the United States and many other countries meant that research was extremely limited. Still, it continued to some extent in laboratories in Europe, the United Kingdom, and Israel as well as some U.S. universities. Since the 1970s, the anti-cancer properties of both cannabinoids have been studied, with promising results.

In 1998, the British government contracted a company called GW Pharmaceuticals to grow cannabis for clinical trials. Dr. Geoffrey Guy, co-founder of GW, believed that CBD-rich plant varieties could create an effective medicine for numerous health issues, with little to no psychoactive effect. When he reported on his work that year at the International Cannabinoid Research Society, it was clear that CBD not only counteracted the psychoactivity of the THC in the plant but also conferred benefits of its own and merited being tested for effect on a long list of disorders.

In the past few decades, CBD became increasingly sought after in the United States when parents of children with seizure disorders began to find out about Mechoulam's work. In many cases, their children were not responding to conventional epilepsy medications. Catherine Jacobson, a neuroscientist, was one of them. After conventional pharmaceuticals failed, she learned of the research and was able to obtain some CBD-dominant plants and began making formulas administered as drops to her young son with epilepsy. His seizures diminished significantly, and her work to find the best medicine for him has led her to her current position as head of clinical research for Tilray, a Canadian company developing pharmaceutical-grade CBD medicines. She told a reporter that it is painful for her to think about "what might have happened if we had been able to do this [research] five years ago or six years ago—I know for a fact he would be a different kid today if he hadn't suffered all that brain damage."[16]

By the end of the first decade of the new millennium, many people in the United States were following the results of the continuing research abroad, but there was no way to test for CBD content of plants because no labs could perform the test. Many assumed that only trace amounts of CBD would be found in most domestic, popular recreational strains of cannabis. Finally, in 2009 analytic labs began testing cannabis for CBD content. About 1 in 600 samples was found to contain a significant amount of CBD, 4 percent or more, which equates to a 1:1 CBD:THC ratio or higher.[17]

Before long, several dozen labs in states with legalized medical cannabis were calibrating cannabinoid ratios and identifying the occasional CBD-rich strain. For data collection purposes, Project CBD defined "CBD-rich" as 4 percent or more CBD by dry weight.

"In addition to balanced strains with roughly equal amounts of CBD and THC (a cannabinoid ratio of 1:1), a handful of CBD-dominant strains—with 20-to-1 CBD:THC ratios or higher were discovered, fostering a cottage industry of CBD-rich concentrates, oil extracts, and other CBD-rich products," according to Project CBD, a major online source of information and research about cannabidiol.[18]

U.S. government agencies have been approving and funding studies related to CBD and seizures in children with treatment-resistant epilepsy since at least 2014.[19] That year, major network CNN aired *Weed,* the first of a series of documentaries about medical marijuana, which appears to have influenced a significant number of Americans regarding CBD in particular. The dramatic stories of children getting a chance at health and wellness, when previously they had been untreatable by current medications, made headlines and brought thousands of families to states that had legalized the medicine.

In the past few years, as the body of research and stories related to its use become publicized, CBD has become more widely known and accepted worldwide. Despite the legal gray area that cannabinoids continue to occupy in the United States (see more on legality in Chapter 10), there is currently more access to CBD products globally than ever before. The resource list in the back of this book provides a starting place for patients looking for local access to this medicine.

NOTE *For the purposes of this book, we define "CBD-dominant" strains as those with a ratio of 20:1 (CBD:THC) or higher. "CBD-rich" strains are defined as having a higher percentage of CBD than THC (i.e., 4:1, 8:1). "Balanced" strains have a ratio close to 1:1.*

NOTE *For updates to this chapter, visit www.CBD-book.com/Updates.*

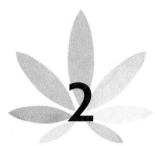

The Biology and Chemistry
of Cannabis and CBD

Understanding the way that the cannabis plant works within the animal body and brain requires a grasp of neuroscience. In 1970, the Nobel Prize for Medicine went to a small group of scientists who had made important discoveries in the study of neurotransmitters, and the Society of Neuroscience was founded. It was the nascent phase of an enormous inquiry, focused on the chemical messengers used by the brain to communicate information throughout the body. These messengers, called neurotransmitters, relay signals between nerve cells (neurons) to regulate the body's major systems. In other words, neurotransmitters are the messengers that relay information between neurons throughout the entirety of the nervous system, including the autonomic nervous system, the central nervous system, and the peripheral nervous system—from tiny receptors in the skin, to the spinal cord, to the brain itself.

Neuroreceptors are specialized protein molecules present in cell membranes and activated by a neurotransmitter, allowing communication through chemical signals. By 1973, researchers had identified receptor sites in the brain capable of binding with opioids, and the discovery of similar receptors for cannabis might have followed soon after. But efforts were, as Project CBD co-founder Martin A. Lee reported in a 2012 article, "circumscribed by the politicized agenda of the National Institute of Drug Abuse, which subsidized studies designed to prove the deleterious effects of cannabis while blocking inquiry into its potential benefits."[20]

CANNABINOID RECEPTOR CHART A

Endocannabinoid receptors influence, modulate or regulate the function of each of the cells, tissues, glands, organs and systems in which they are contained.

CB1 RECEPTORS ARE LOCATED IN THE CELLS OF THE:

Brain/CNS/Spinal cord (CB1)
Cortical regions (CB1): (neocortex, pyriform cortex, hippocampus, amygdala)
Cerebellum (CB1)
Brainstem (CB1)
Basal ganglia (CB1): globus pallidus, substantia nigra pars, reticulata
Olfactory bulb (CB1)
Thalamus (CB1)
Hypothalamus (Endocrine-brain link CB1)
Pituitary (CB1)

Thyroid (endocrine gland CB1)

CB1 and **CB2** RECEPTORS ARE LOCATED IN THE CELLS OF THE:

Eye (CB1 and CB2): Retinal pigment epithelial/RPE cells

Heart (CB1 and CB2)

Upper airways (of mammals CB1)
Liver (CB1): Kupffer cells (macrophage immune cells), Hepatocytes (liver cell), Hepatic stellate cells (fat storage cell)

Stomach (CB1 and CB2)

Pancreas (CB1 and CB2)

Adrenals (endocrine gland CB1)

Digestive tract (CB1 and CB2)

Ovaries (gonads and endocrine gland CB1)

Uterus (myometrium CB1)

Testes (gonads and endocrine gland CB1): Leydig cells; sperm cells

Bone (CB1 and CB2)

Prostate (CB1): Epithelial and smooth muscle cells

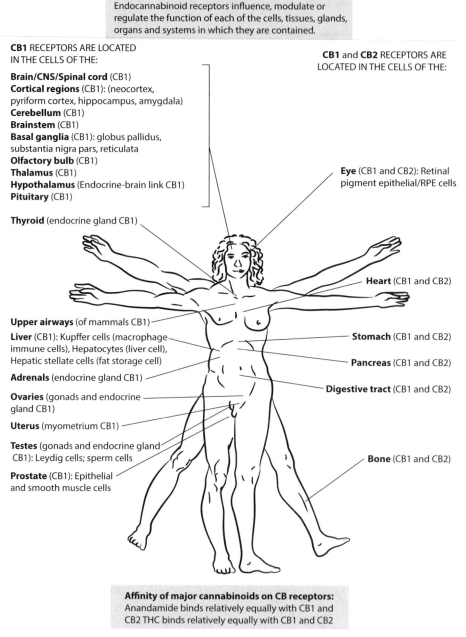

Affinity of major cannabinoids on CB receptors:
Anandamide binds relatively equally with CB1 and CB2 THC binds relatively equally with CB1 and CB2

FIGURE 8: Cannabinoid Receptor Chart

In 1992, Dr. Raphael Mechoulam (the same researcher who identified THC as the main psychoactive compound in cannabis thirty years prior) discovered that animal bodies naturally produce what he called endocannabinoids—chemical compounds similar to the plant phytocannabinoids present in hemp and cannabis.

Researchers have found the two main receptors in the body, CB1 and CB2, which respond similarly to both the endocannabinoids produced in the body and the plant-based ones when they are introduced. Receptor cells are part of a complex network of chemical messengers in the brain. Other such receptor systems utilize different neurotransmitters, such as serotonin, dopamine, GABA, histamine, or narcotic-like endorphins. Described in terms of a key fitting a lock, the cannabinoids fit in and activate the endocannabinoid system.

The Endocannabinoid System

By Dr. Michael Moskowitz,
Bay Area Pain Medical Associates

The endocannabinoid system, though relatively newly discovered, is extremely important and is responsible for two basic activities. The first is to modulate pleasure, energy, and well-being. The second is to slowly nudge the body back to health in the face of injury and disease. The complexity of how it accomplishes these tasks has generated an astonishing amount of research in the last several decades, culminating in a basic understanding of the scope of this system only within the last ten years. There is still a great deal to be discovered about it, and it is only beginning to be included in the curriculum at medical schools and incorporated into clinical practice. An informal 2014 survey of U.S. medical schools showed that only 13 percent of institutions covered it at all in their training of new doctors.[21]

In 1988 researchers discovered the cannabinoid-1 (CB1) receptor.[22] The cannabinoid-2 (CB2) receptor was uncovered about five years later.[23] One year before the CB2 receptor was discovered, a team headed by Raphael Mechoulam was tracking down the first endocannabinoid-signaling molecule, arachidonoyl ethanolamide (AEA). A few years later, they identified it and named it anandamide,[24] combining the Sanskrit word meaning bliss

15

(*ananda*) and the chemical name for a key part of the molecular structure of this compound (amide). Next, Mechoulam's group identified the second endocannabinoid-signaling molecule, 2-arachidonoyl glycerol (2-AG).[25] This discovery was followed by the search for and discovery of the enzymes responsible for synthesizing and breaking down AEA and 2-AG a little more than a decade ago, with the understanding of this whole system still unfolding to this day.[26]

Due to its part in restoring balance when illness or injury occurs, the endocannabinoid system plays a critical role in regulation of disease. Researchers Pacher and Kunos stated in a 2013 review article that "modulating Endocannabinoid System activity may have therapeutic potential in almost all diseases affecting humans, including obesity/metabolic syndrome, diabetes and diabetic complication, neurodegenerative, inflammatory, cardiovascular, liver, gastrointestinal, skin diseases, pain, psychiatric disorders, cachexia, cancer, chemotherapy induced nausea and vomiting, among many others."[27] The importance of this system to our survival and well-being cannot be overstated.

The current understanding of this system is that it consists of the following:

1. Two receptors
   - Cannabinoid-1 (CB1) receptor
   - Cannabinoid-2 (CB2) receptor
2. Two signaling molecules
   - arachidonoyl ethanolamide (AEA or anandamide)
   - 2-arachidonoyl glycerol (2-AG)
3. Five enzymes[28]
   - DAGL-α (for synthesis of 2-AG)
   - DAGL-β (for synthesis of 2-AG)
   - NAPE selective phospholipase-D (for synthesis of AEA)
   - MAGL (for breakdown of 2-AG
   - FAAH (for breakdown of AEA)

Additionally, several other possible ways that AEA is synthesized are currently being evaluated. It is also clear that this system is not confined to working solely within its own boundaries. Not surprisingly, it appears to interact robustly with several other non-cannabinoid systems in the body, to waccomplish its tasks of regulating disease and well-being, including the endorphin system, the immune system, and the vanilloid system (the system that is responsible for transforming pain from acute to chronic). In modifying these other systems, the endocannabinoid system regulates inflammation, pain, bone health, formation of new nerve cells, fat and sugar processing, mood, energy, brain health, and hormone balance.

The endocannabinoid system has several unique and remarkable actions. AEA and 2-AG are "on demand" substances. They exist as common, spare molecular parts until CB1 receptors or CB2 receptors increase in the central nervous system or in other organ systems in the body. When this occurs, the transmitters are constructed on demand, work within seconds, and disappear into spare parts again. They are gone almost as fast as they appear.

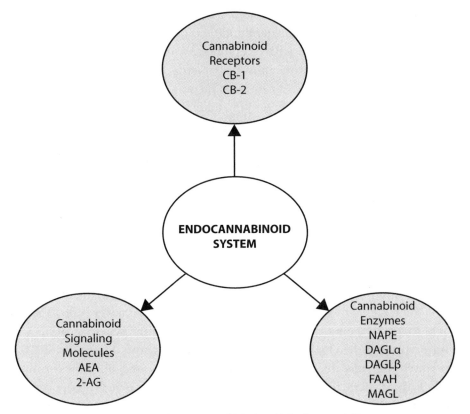

FIGURE 9: Courtesy of Michael Moskowitz MD

We have this system built into us that monitors the body's constant struggle between building itself up (anabolism) and breaking itself down (catabolism). When it detects too much of either, it appears, and almost as rapidly disappears, to nudge the body back to normal. This is a system that does not store up its main components but creates them on demand. It is the "ghost in the machine": responsible for rebalancing the most essential systems in the body to control pain, mood, inflammation, energy, wellness, and illness. It shifts its role from maintaining a balance between physical buildup and breakdown to fighting disease and injuries. The complex interplay of this system with other body and brain systems involves interaction of the endocannabinoids with endorphins,[29] hormones,[30] cytokines,[31] growth factors,[32] pleasure molecules,[33] immune cells,[34] connective tissue system,[35] bone metabolism,[36] nerve and glial cell inflammation,[37] cell regeneration,[38] and programmed cell death.[39] Needless to say, this is a system of immeasurable importance, and we are in the early stages of understanding the rich complexities at play.

The greatest number of CB1 receptors is located in the brain, while CB2 receptors are more numerous in the peripheral body.[40] AEA and 2-AG signaling molecules, regardless of location, activate both receptor types. CB1 receptors activated in the brain result in an experience of pain relief, anxiety relief, mood stabilization, well-being, and pleasure. When brain-based CB2 receptors are activated, local anti-inflammatory responses occur. This does far more than relieve pain, as it has become clear that chronic brain inflammation is involved in Alzheimer's disease, post-traumatic stress disorder, multiple sclerosis, Parkinson's disease, depression, autoimmune disorders, and cancer.

The CB2 receptors, while present in small quantities in the brain, are present in high quantity in the peripheral body in all tissue types but especially in the immune system. AEA and 2-AG function as activators of the immune system in the peripheral body more prominently than as neurotransmitters. The activity of AEA and 2-AG in the body is focused upon stopping inflammation. It also alerts the immune system to the presence of cancer cells, causing them to attack these cells. Cancer cells survive immune system surveillance and destruction by cloaking themselves from detection. Activation of CB2 receptors unmasks this cloaking. CB2 receptors located on bone-forming cells activate bone formation, when stimulated, reversing osteoporosis.[41] Activated CB1 receptors also affect the release of other neurotransmitters, including norepinephrine, serotonin, dopamine, orexin, histamine, GABA, and endorphins.[42,43] Since CB1 receptors are most frequently located in the autonomic nervous system, they affect many of the automatic functions in brain and body, resulting in fine-tuning of everything from breathing and heart rate to connective tissue health and metabolic rate.

In health and illness, CB1 and CB2 receptors have a profound effect upon the gut—the authors of a 2016 study concluded that virtually all major GI functions are controlled by the endocannabinoid system."[44] While CB1 receptor activation promotes increased blood lipid levels and liver fibrosis, CB2 receptors decrease blood lipid levels, fibrosis, and liver inflammation,[45] an example of how these receptors frequently have opposite effects in the body. Typically, this appears to happen in illness-related conditions rather than normal states.

Another example of this opposing behavior is the deterioration of heart health when CB1 receptors are activated during cardiac disease, while CB2 receptors promote cardiac health in such a case.[46] Within CB1 receptors, this behavior can also occur in muscle tissue, when activation of CB1 receptors may either promote or inhibit energy use, leading to muscle formation or destruction.[47]

The entire endocannabinoid system plays a critical role in male and female fertility, as well as implantation and embryo development (see more in Chapter 5).[48] CB1 and CB2 receptors are highly involved in suppressing skin inflammation and melanoma formation.[49] Activation of CB1 and CB2 receptors plays a role in how the brain develops in the growing embryo, which also affects the development of nerve cells that produce GABA and slows down excessive activity in the brain.[50] Furthermore, CB1 and CB2 receptors are involved in embryonic brain development, health, protection, and regulation of intellectual function of nerve cells.[51,52,53,54,55,56] The endocannabinoid system is also involved in new nerve cell formation in the adult brain, and the CB2 receptor is particularly important in this matter. Hence, the endocannabinoid system is highly involved in regulation of adult neuroplasticity throughout life.[57] CB1 and CB2 receptors, in both their complexity and their subtlety, have profound effects upon health, illness, and development.

The activity of AEA and 2-AG on the CB1 receptors also affects wellness and disease. AEA is specific to CB1 receptors and 2-AG to CB2 receptors, but they each activate both receptor types. These two signaling molecules even regulate each other's levels in the brain.[58] In the brain, they not only oppose inflammation but also are involved in the trimming away of old synapses to make way for creation of new ones. 2-AG blocks an animal model of multiple sclerosis[59] and causes bone breakdown and osteoporosis.[60] Combined with AEA and the CB1 receptor, 2-AG protects against neurodegenerative conditions, including Parkinson's disease, multiple sclerosis, and Alzheimer's disease and other dementias.[61] AEA-blocking CB1 receptors inside of nerve cells clears beta amyloid and the inflammation it creates to prevent nerve cell death, one of the major processes in Alzheimer's disease.[62]

Although AEA and 2-AG work on CB1 and CB2 receptors, they also influence processes in the body without working on these cannabinoid receptors. They attach to both nerve cells and glial cells in the brain and work deeply in the inflammatory system in the body on multiple aspects of inflammation.[63] AEA and 2-AG also promotes sleep[64] and blocks anxiety.[65] The endocannabinoid system is tumor suppressing in many types of cancer, including breast cancer, prostate cancer, ovarian cancer, thyroid cancer, endometrial carcinoma, liver cancer, colon carcinoma, bone cancer, glioma, glioblastoma, non-melanoma skin cancer, melanoma, leukemia, lymphoid tumors, and metastatic cancer.[66,67,68,69,70,71,72,73]

The endocannabinoid system also has enzymes that work on the raw material in the body to make AEA and 2-AG and subsequently break them down. Unfortunately, drugs that completely block these enzymes have had profound negative effects on the body, resulting in symptoms ranging from brain damage to death,[74] which demonstrates the complexity, richness, and importance of the endocannabinoid system to sustain life. Unlike the endocannabinoid system, drugs do not work in a pinpoint fashion. Their effects tend to be more global, and their activity on this profound system with such far-reaching effects is very risky.[75] "As might be predicted, a drug that blocks CB1 neuromodulation at synapses for the major stimulatory (in the case of glutamate) and inhibitory (in the case of GABA) transmitters throughout the brain would be likely to produce multiple 'off-target' effects."[76]

In summary, the endocannabinoid system is newly discovered and is an extremely important system to our survival. It maintains and restores balance in multiple ways throughout the body, which affects varied issues regarding health and disease. If injury or disease occurs, the system shifts from one that regulates well-being, pleasure, and energy to one that restores balance and normal functioning processes. The system simultaneously pinpoints its actions and is active throughout the body. It is present throughout the body and brain and appears and disappears in a matter of seconds. It affects conditions as varied as multiple forms of cancer, heart disease, osteoporosis, degenerative brain diseases, inflammation, pain, and mood.

Brain Regions in Which Cannabinoid Receptors Are Abundant

REGION	FUNCTION
Basal ganglia	Movement control
Cerebellum	Body-movement coordination
Hippocampus	Learning and memory, stress
Cerebral cortex	Higher cognitive function
Intrabulbar anterior	Link between cerebral hemispheres
Nucleus accumbens	Reward pathway

Adapted from a presentation by Raphael Mechoulam, *The Cannabinoids: Looking Back and Ahead*, at CannMed 2016.

Chemistry and Cannabis: A Tour of Its Active Compounds

Phytocannabinoids (CBD, THC, and Other Compounds)

While there has been controversy about using cannabis to treat health conditions, there is growing scientific acceptance that the plant has significant medicinal value. Phytocannabinoids are the name given to cannabinoids of a plant-based nature. These substances are unique to cannabis and occur in all varieties. Although THC is the well-known phytocannabinoid that is responsible for most of the psychotropic effect of cannabis, other phytocannabinoids exert their own profound effects. Phytocannabinoids are different from endocannabinoids, but they interact with that internal body system and also upon related non-cannabinoid systems in a similar manner. Unlike endocannabinoids, the phytocannabinoid system works all over the body all of the time it is present—so why are phytocannabinoids never lethal? Some feel it is because there are no endocannabinoid receptors in the brainstem, but this doesn't explain why synthetic drugs that block or enhance the endocannabinoid system have killed and caused severe psychiatric, cardiac, and brain damage. More likely, the complexity of this system matches up well with the complexity of our own system, and co-evolution of both systems has positively affected the genomes of each.

Cannabidiol (CBD) was among the first of the phytocannabinoids discovered and was incorrectly thought to be a non-active cannabinoid because researchers were looking for the psychoactive aspect of the plant. Not only did CBD lack this activity, but it also turned out to not be directly active on CB1 or CB2 receptors when they were discovered over sixty years later. Instead, CBD works indirectly, stimulating the body's endogenous cannabinoid system by blocking the FAAH enzyme responsible for breaking down anandamide. When more anandamide is present, there is greater CB1 activation and a more vital endocannabinoid system. CBD also binds to various other receptors in the brain, including serotonin 5HT1A (contributing to its antidepressant effect), TRPV1 (contributing to its anti-psychoactive effect), the nuclear receptor PPAR-gamma (regulates gene expression), and the orphan receptor GPR55 (contributing to its anti-cancer and osteoprotective effects), among others.[77]

At the time of this writing, 111 phytocannabinoids have been identified. Yet we know only some of the pharmacological effects of 10 percent of these. Research in the last decade around the world has exploded, with over six thousand papers on phytocannabinoids and endocannabinoids in PubMed peer-reviewed articles.[78] Table 2 lists a few of the phytocannabinoids and their currently identified pharmacologic activities.[79,80,81,82]

Pharmacology of Phytocannabinoids

PHYTOCANNABINOID	PHARMACOLOGICAL EFFECTS
Δ9-THC Δ9-Tetrahydrocannabinol	Anti-cancer, anti-proliferative, anti- and pro-inflammatory, anti-oxidant, analgesic, anxiolytic and anxiogenic, anti-epileptic, anti-emetic (nausea and vomiting), neuroprotective, euphoriant, hedonic, sleep promoting
CBD Cannabidiol	Anti-cancer, anti-proliferative, anti-emetic (nausea and vomiting), anti-inflammatory, antibacterial, anti-diabetic, anti-psoriatic, anti-diarrheal, analgesic, bone stimulant, immunosuppressive, anti-ischemic, antispasmodic, vasorelaxant, neuroprotective, anti-epileptic, antipsychotic, anxiolytic, transforms white fat into brown fat, increases anandamide activation of CB1 and CB2 receptors

PHYTOCANNABINOID	PHARMACOLOGICAL EFFECTS
Δ9-THCV Δ9-Tetrahydrocannabivarin	Appetite suppression, bone stimulant, anti-epileptic, anti-diabetic, anti-lipidemia
CBG Cannabigirol	Anti-proliferative, antibacterial
CBC Cannabichromene	Anti-inflammatory, analgesic, bone stimulant, anti-microbial, anti-proliferative, anti-fungal
CBDA Cannabidiolic acid	Anti-cancer, anti-proliferative, anti-emetic (nausea and vomiting), anti-inflammatory
Δ9-THCA Δ9-Tetrahydrocannabinolic acid	Anti-spasmodic, anti-proliferative, analgesic, pleasure, mild euphoria, well-being, anti-emetic (nausea and vomiting), anti-inflammatory, neuroprotective
CBDV Cannabidivarin	Bone stimulant
CBN Cannabinol	Analgesic, anti-inflammatory, anti-cancer

When looking at Table 2 it is clear that denying the medicinal value of phytocannabinoids is a political act, not a scientific determination. Phytocannabinoids play a complex, multilayered role in the body's endocannabinoid system. Plant cultivators have been developing high-THC strains of the plant, but they have also been developing low-THC and high-CBD strains. As can be seen in Table 2 THC does have therapeutic benefits. Too much, however, can cause anxiety, paranoia, and increased inflammation. The focus of medical treatment needs to be that of achieving the right dose of a balanced spectrum of cannabinoids tailored to the particular condition.

Careful titration of high-THC preparations, planning of medication delivery route and timing, customizing individual treatment, and balancing phytocannabinoid profiles can limit or eliminate the cannabis "high." The plant can be ingested in numerous ways and does not need to be smoked. Multiple plant strains have been bred for various purposes, and the phytocannabinoid profiles of these plants can be mixed and matched to create a treatment as varied as the endocannabinoid and phytocannabinoid systems.

We are born with DNA that determines our genetic makeup. As early as implantation of the fertilized egg, our genome changes, influenced by the uterine environment. Called an epigenetic change, it occurs on the surface of the genes throughout our lives. While we have consciously altered the genome of cannabis, it has changed the epigenetics of humans as well. Epigenetic changes are inheritable, and over five thousand years of use has led to changes in the human genome of users and non-users of cannabis alike.[83]

There are 421 identified chemical compounds in cannabis, over 100 of which are phytocannabinoids. Most of the testing of this system has been with refined THC and more recently refined CBD.[84] The non-cannabinoids in the plant include many compounds known as terpenoids (terpenes), phenols, and flavonoids, found throughout a broad range of plant species (see Chapter 2 for more on the medicinal effects of terpenes found in cannabis).[85] While phytocannabinoids are unique to cannabis, the interaction of the phytocannabinoids with these non-cannabinoid substances common throughout the plant world may augment the broad-based effects of cannabis on the body.[86]

Another feature of the phytocannabinoids is that they work better in the whole plant or as plant-based extracts than they do as isolated, refined, and synthesized products. Pure THC has psychotropic effects that are partially modified and significantly decreased in the face of high CBD levels.[87] For example, in treating the spasticity of multiple sclerosis, the 1:1 ratio of CBD to THC was more effective than either pure THC or pure CBD.[88] In a separate study, high THC in a plant extract reversed the actual disease progression of multiple sclerosis, but CBD in a plant extract did not do so.[89] In a meticulous study done in Israel in 2015, pure CBD was consistently shown to have a very narrow dose range, below which or above which it was ineffective for the treatment of pain and inflammation, while relieving pain and inflammation in the narrow dose range. CBD-enriched whole-plant extract, with very low levels of THC, cannabichromene (CBC), cannabigirol (CBG), cannabinol (CBN), and cannabidivarin (CBDV), improved as a pain reliever and anti-inflammatory as the dose was increased and was far more effective than pure CBD.[90] In effect, THC acts as a catalyst that makes CBD work better.

The lesson here is that different phytocannabinoids have different effects, and even trace amounts of phytocannabinoids have "entourage" effects that vary with different diseases or even with different aspects of the same disease.

Remembering that there are still over three hundred non-cannabinoid substances in the plant, their synergy can help with effects from anti-inflammatory activity to tolerability.

THC is the most potent analgesic,[91] and its main analgesic effects are due to activation of the CB1 receptor in the brain. It also decreases signaling from the sensory part of the brain to the emotional part of the brain, reducing pain by disconnecting the sensation of pain from its emotional impact upon the person.[92] This effect is extremely important because it is the emotional component of pain, depression, and anxiety that connects the chronic aspects of pain to the person's sense of self. THC is also anti-inflammatory in body and brain—THC attached to CB2 receptors in the brain and body produces an anti-inflammatory response. THC also works on several non-cannabinoid receptors to reduce pain and inflammation. This quiets down runaway nerve firing and transforms chronic pain back to normal pain.[93] Perhaps most important of all of THC's effects is that, like anandamide, it blocks the inflammatory effects of nerve cell accumulation of beta amyloid and clears the cell of inflammatory processes that usually destroy the cell within four days.[94]

High-THC medical cannabis has been effective for treating cancer chemotherapy side effects, including chemotherapy-induced peripheral nerve pain, inflammation, and vomiting. There is increasing evidence that THC itself destroys cancer cells, limits tumor growth, and unmasks the tumor to detection and destruction by the immune system.[95]

The Entourage Effect

Why would a chapter in a book about cannabidiol (CBD) start by focusing on THC? It is precisely because of the "entourage" effect of cannabis that makes it so effectively therapeutic. There are conditions that will respond to pure CBD, but, remembering that our own endocannabinoid system is complex, it makes sense that the highly compatible phytocannabinoid system exploits the complexities of our built-in processes. Contrary to the original idea that CBD was an inactive component of cannabis, it has many effects in common with THC and many unique effects as well. Even when there are similar effects, such as the anti-inflammatory properties of both THC and CBD, each accomplishes them in a different way, resulting in a more varied and robust response as a result of the two working together.

More impressively, several other phytocannabinoids are anti-inflammatory in nature, and each works differently from the other. CBD is the most potent anti-inflammatory phytocannabinoid and is second in its analgesic effects only to THC.

CBD plays a major role in the central nervous system and the immune system by activating and inhibiting non-cannabinoid receptors as well as enhancing the synthesis and activity of anandamide (AEA).[96] High-CBD cannabis blocks inflammatory processes in brain and body.[97] CBD lowers the psychotropic effects of THC without lowering blood or tissue levels of THC.[98] CBD promotes bone fusion and improves the collagen profile in healing bone and in the connective tissue system of the body while THC does not.[99] CBD also uniquely converts inflammatory, weight-promoting, and cardiac-damaging white fat into anti-inflammatory, weight-losing, and cardiac-protective brown fat.[100] CBD, not the other phytocannabinoids, also appears to protect against destruction of heart muscle caused by diabetes.[101]

Different from the unique effects of either CBD or THC is the synergy between them and some of the other phytocannabinoids. A good example is that of treating prostate cancer, the most common cancer other than skin cancer among men, second only to lung cancer in male cancer deaths. Without activating CB1 receptors, THC causes prostate cancer cells to implode. CBD, CBDA, THCA, CBN, and CBG all block prostate cancer cells from rapid growth, inhibiting tumor size and spread.[102] THC, CBD, and CBC strengthen the immune system and are all anti-inflammatory. Testosterone-independent prostate cancer cells, which are harder to treat, more likely to spread cancer, and more likely to be deadly, are sensitive to CBD.[103]

Neither THC nor CBD are present in the plant in any significant quantity until it is heated, which can be accomplished by smoking the plant, vaporizing it, or pre-cooking it in an oven before adding to edibles or liquids, a process known as decarboxylation. The raw plant contains (Δ^9 tetrahydrocannabinolic acid (THCA) and cannabidiolic acid (CBDA). As seen in Table 2 these cannabinoids have their own anti-inflammatory, anti-cancer, and analgesic properties. While the body does not convert THCA to THC, it does convert CBDA to CBD, with blood levels up to four times higher if the plant is consumed raw or the fresh leaves are juiced than if the plant is preheated. Using the raw plant provides another way of consumption of cannabis with markedly reduced risk of psychotropic effects and increased levels of CBD in blood and tissue (see more on juicing raw cannabis in Chapter 3).[104]

CBD-dominant cannabis is effective on its own for various forms of degenerative brain disorders, including multiple sclerosis, Parkinson's disease, ALS, and dementias. CBD reverses inflammation in the brain's immune system.[105]

A very small amount of CBD breaks down to THC in the body, an action that may explain its rare side effect of drowsiness. If this occurs, dosing can be shifted to the evening, with the result being improved sleep. In some patients, daytime drowsiness can still occur. In this case, switching to a different strain of high-CBD/low-THC cannabis can be helpful. It appears that THC, CBD, CBN, and CBC all help to improve symptoms and signs of psoriasis.[106] At very high doses, such strains may lower cortisol levels.[107]

Cannabichromene (CBC) is anti-inflammatory in its own unique way, blocking nitric oxide, which, in turn, blocks the release of the main pain neurotransmitter, substance-P. It also blocks one of the pain receptors, PPAR gamma.[108] CBC, THC, and CBD show antidepressant effects in animal studies, while cannabigerol (CBG) and cannabinol (CBN) do not.[109] CBN has analgesic and anti-inflammatory properties, as well as anti-cancer effects.[110] CBN is also good for aiding in sleep disorders.

One of the problems with medical cannabis as a treatment is the illegality of the plant due to the effects of THC and its desirability as a recreational drug. Side effects of high-THC cannabis (more pronounced in new users) are discussed in Chapter 3. These side effects do not necessarily mean THC must be eliminated from treatment, but, instead, focus can be put on limiting its psychotropic side effects and avoiding impairment (see more on strategies to limit impairment on p. 65).

The phytocannabinoid and endocannabinoid systems both exhibit the entourage effect of synergism among various components. Phytocannabinoids have no lethal dose in standardized testing. Cannabidiol has a wide spectrum of benefits, being superior, synergistic, and activity-modifying of other phytocannabinoids, endocannabinoids, and non-cannabinoids. It has no significant psychotropic effects and works best in concert with other phytocannabinoids. As a single phytochemical, it presents a huge number of potential treatment options with a wide variety of diseases and disease states.

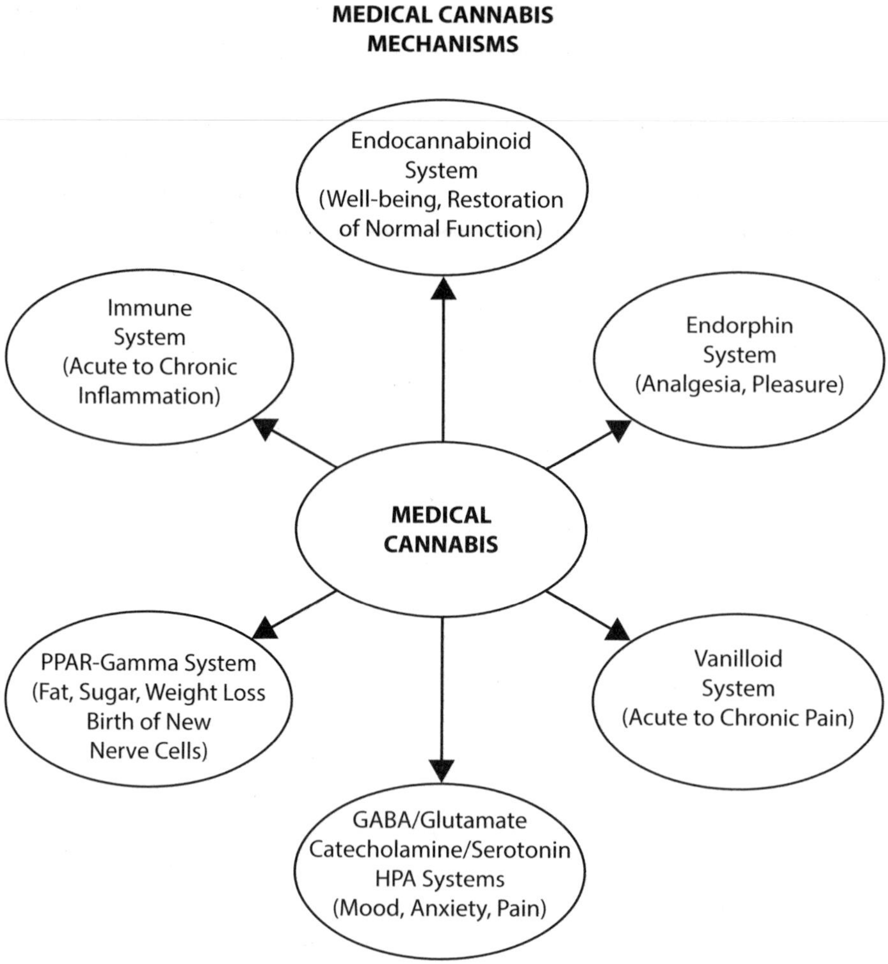

**MEDICAL CANNABIS
MECHANISMS**

FIGURE 10: Courtesy of Michael Moskowitz MD

The phytocannabinoid system enhances the endocannabinoid system and then works on that system to improve its function of restoring balance in the face of illness and injury. The science of understanding how these plant-based products work is rapidly unfolding. There are some problems with medical cannabis, including some side effects, unwanted effects, issues of abuse and misuse, and social disruption, but one only needs to listen to the disclaimers at the end of television ads for FDA-approved drugs to recognize that the risks of medical cannabis are far more acceptable than many pharmaceutical drugs. There are grave conditions, such as Alzheimer's disease, cancer, autoimmune problems, psychiatric disorders, and epilepsy that need new treatment approaches. If any other safe compound had similar effects on health as does medical cannabis, researchers, clinicians, pharmaceutical companies, and the government would be doing everything in their power and ability to fast-track them for public availability. Instead, the opposite has occurred.

To this day, research on these substances is still highly restricted. The bias of the national funding agencies toward finding research that supports prohibition and has negative hypotheses and results is evident in the concerted effort to keep debunked negative claims in the public eye on federal websites. Physicians are poorly informed about the science of the endocannabinoid and the phytocannabinoid systems. The moralistic and political decision making of the past must yield to rational approaches to exploring the full health potential of cannabis.

Terpenes

Reporting contributed by Sandeep Kumar

In addition to the cannabinoids, other molecules in the cannabis plant are biologically active (not to mention fragrant and flavorful). Terpenoids, known as terpenes, are very common chemical compounds in plants and animals that function as major biosynthetic cellular messengers. Many hormones, including estrogens, are terpenoids and share the same basic organic chemical structure.

All cannabinoids are chemically classified as terpenes, but they are unique to cannabis; this section will cover terpenes shared between cannabis and other plants.

Terpenes are oils secreted by the glandular hairs found most densely on the floral leaves and flowers of female plants. Their flavor and smell identify the particular strain along with their known health effects. Pine, grapefruit, lemon, and lavender are often used to describe the smell or taste of different varieties of cannabis.

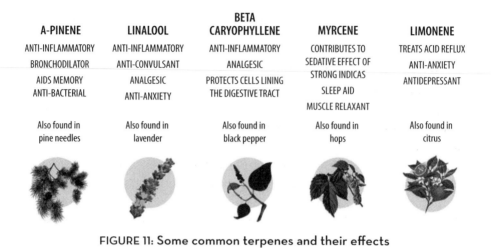

A-PINENE	LINALOOL	BETA CARYOPHYLLENE	MYRCENE	LIMONENE
ANTI-INFLAMMATORY	ANTI-INFLAMMATORY	ANTI-INFLAMMATORY	CONTRIBUTES TO SEDATIVE EFFECT OF STRONG INDICAS	TREATS ACID REFLUX
BRONCHODILATOR	ANTI-CONVULSANT	ANALGESIC		ANTI-ANXIETY
AIDS MEMORY	ANALGESIC	PROTECTS CELLS LINING THE DIGESTIVE TRACT	SLEEP AID	ANTIDEPRESSANT
ANTI-BACTERIAL	ANTI-ANXIETY		MUSCLE RELAXANT	
Also found in pine needles	Also found in lavender	Also found in black pepper	Also found in hops	Also found in citrus

FIGURE 11: Some common terpenes and their effects

Myrcene

The most common terpene produced by cannabis is myrcene (β-myrcene). In some cannabis varieties, myrcene comprises up to 60 percent of the essential oils.[111] Indica strains that have above 0.5 percent levels of myrcene can cause sedation.[112] Myrcene's aroma has been described as musky, earthy, and herbal, somewhat similar to cloves. Examples of plants whose oils contain myrcene include hops, citrus fruits, bay leaves, eucalyptus, wild thyme, lemongrass, as well as many other plants.[113]

Myrcene has specific medicinal properties. It works as a muscle relaxant and sedative. It has been known to lower the resistance across the blood-to-brain barrier, which allows it and many other chemicals to cross the barrier more quickly and easily. Myrcene allows the effects of cannabinoids like THC to take effect more quickly. Furthermore, myrcene can increase the saturation level of the CB1 receptor, which in turn can maximize the psychoactive effect of cannabis.[114]

Known as a potent analgesic, anti-inflammatory, antibiotic, and antimutagenic, myrcene blocks the action of cytochrome and other pro-mutagenic carcinogens.[115] A 2014 study revealed that myrcene acts as an inhibitor of gastric and duodenal ulcers and suggested it may be helpful in preventing peptic ulcer disease. Furthermore, myrcene's sedative and relaxing effects also make it ideal for the treatment of insomnia and pain.[116]

Limonene

Cannabis varieties high in limonene have strong citrusy odors like oranges, lemons, and limes and promote a general uplift in mood and attitude. A monocyclic monoterpenoid, limonene is one of two major compounds formed from pinene and is the major constituent in citrus fruit rinds, rosemary, juniper, and peppermint, as well as in several pine needle oils.[117]

Limonene is absorbed quickly in the bloodstream after inhalation. It aids in the absorption of other terpenes through the skin and other body tissue. Limonene is an ideal anti-fungal agent for ailments such as toenail fungus, suppressing the growth of many species of fungi and bacteria.[118] It may be beneficial in protecting against various cancers. Limonene reversed mammary tumors in mice and stimulated apoptosis—programmed cell death—in breast cancer. Furthermore, it has been found to help promote weight loss.[119]

Limonene is a natural insecticide that plants use to ward off predators, and, while its main use was in food and perfumes until a couple of decades ago, it is now best known as the primary active ingredient in citrus cleaner as it has very low toxicity or adverse effects.[120]

During testing on the effects of limonene, participants experienced an increase in attention, mental focus, well-being, and even sex drive. Limonene prevents the deterioration of the RAS gene, one of the factors that contributes to the development of tumors, and protects against aspergillus and carcinogens present in smoke.[121]

Beta-caryophyllene

With a peppery, woody, and/or spicy aroma, the sesquiterpene beta-caryophyllene is found in Thai basil, clove, cinnamon leaf, and black pepper, and in lavender in small quantities. Research indicates that beta-caryophyllene may be effective in cancer treatment plans. It is the only known terpene to interact with the endocannabinoid system. Studies show that beta-caryophyllene selectively binds to the CB2 receptor and that it is a functional CB2 agonist. Beta-caryophyllene is a functional non-psychoactive CB2 receptor ligand in foodstuff and a macrocyclic anti-inflammatory cannabinoid in cannabis.[122]

Researchers in 2012 suggested that beta-caryophyllene may be an excellent therapeutic agent to prevent nephrotoxicity (impacting the kidneys) caused by anti-cancer chemotherapy drugs such as cisplatin when delivered through a CB2 receptor pathway.[123] That same year, a study focused on the chemical composition and the pharmacological properties of essential oil isolated from black pepper, of which beta-caryophyllene is a main constituent. It was found to possess antioxidant, anti-inflammatory, and antinociceptive properties. Cannabis strains high in beta-caryophyllene, like Omrita RX, may be useful in treating pain related to arthritis and neuropathy.[124]

A 2013 study showed that the combination of phytocannabinoids, specifically cannabidiol (CBD) and beta-caryophyllene, administered orally appears to be a potential treatment for chronic pain.[125]

Pinene

Pinene is a bicyclic monoterpenoid, possessing aromas of pine and fir. Two structural isomers of pinene are found in nature—alpha-pinene and beta-pinene—and both are important components of pine resin. Alpha-pinene is nature's most prevalent terpenoid, found mostly in balsamic resin, pinewoods, and some citrus fruits, as well as many other conifers and non-coniferous plants. The two isomers constitute the main component of wood turpentine. Pinene is a principal monoterpene, important physiologically in both plants and animals, and tends to react with other chemicals, forming other terpenes, such as limonene, and other compounds.[126]

Pinene has been used as a local antiseptic and an anti-inflammatory expectorant.[127] It is also thought to be a bronchodilator.[128] The smoke of plants rich in pinene give the sensation of sucking more air, which can cause hyperventilation or sometimes cough.[129] Alpha-pinene is a natural compound that can be isolated from pine needle oil and has shown anti-cancer properties.[130] In Traditional Chinese Medicine, it has been used as an anti-cancer agent. THC effects may be diminished when combined with pinene.[131]

Pinene easily crosses the brain barrier to prevent the destruction of molecules responsible for the transmission of information, which results in memory improvement. Rosemary and sage have been considered beneficial over thousands of years of traditional medicine due in part to the presence of pinene in their makeup. Pinene counteracts the effects of THC and tends to improve concentration. Memory lapses tend to occur more often with the use of pure THC versus THC mixed with pinene.[132]

Terpineol

The three closely related monoterpenoids, alpha-terpineol, terpinen-4-ol, and 4-terpineol have aromas comparable to lilacs and flower blossoms. Often found in cannabis varieties also high in pinene, terpineol's fragrances are overpowered by other more redolent terpene. Alpha-terpineol is known to have calming, relaxing effects and exhibits antibiotic, antioxidant, and anti-malarial properties. It also has anti-tumor, anti-inflammatory, anxiolytic, and sedative properties.[133]

Linalool

Cannabis varieties high in the non-cyclic monoterpenoid linalool promote calming, relaxing effects. Linalool has floral and lavender undertones and for centuries has been used as a sleep aid. Linalool tends to diminish the anxiety pure THC can provoke, making it helpful in treating psychosis and anxiety.[134]

One study suggested that linalool may significantly reduce lung inflammation induced by cigarette smoke. It may block the carcinogenesis aggravated by benz[α]anthracene, a component of the tar generated by the combustion of tobacco.[135]

Linalool activates immune cells through specific receptors and/or pathways and may boost the immune system in general. Research has shown that the anti-inflammatory effect of linalool can contribute to the slowdown and reversal of Alzheimer's disease.[136]

The Environmental Protection Agency has approved its use as a pesticide, flavor agent, and scent. Linalool's vapors seem to be an effective insecticide to ward off fruit flies, fleas, and cockroaches.[137]

Delta-3-carene (Δ^3-carene)

The bicyclic monoterpene Δ^3-carene has a sweet, pungent odor. In higher concentrations, it can be a depressant for the central nervous system. It also has anti-inflammatory properties. Found naturally in many beneficial essential oils, including cypress oil, juniper berry oil, and fir needle, this terpene is used to dry out the body's excess fluids, such as tears, mucus, and sweat. Though nontoxic, it may cause irritation when inhaled. High concentrations in some strains may partially cause symptoms of coughing, itchy throat, and eye irritation when smoking cannabis. Δ^3 carene can be found in pine extract, bell pepper, basil oil, grapefruit and orange juices, and citrus peel oils from fruits like lemons, limes, mandarins, tangerines, oranges, and kumquats. Carene is a major component of turpentine.[138]

Terpinolene

A common terpene of sage and rosemary, terpinolene can be found in Monterey cypress oil. Used largely throughout the United States in soaps and perfumes, it is also a renowned insect repellent. With a piney aroma and hints of herbs and flora, terpinolene has a sweet flavor of orange and lemon citrus.[139]

A study on terpinolene found that it can reduce anxiety and act as a sleep aid.[140] Another study found that it significantly reduced the protein expression of AKT1 in K562 cells, inhibiting the cell proliferation involved in a variety of cancers.[141]

Phellandrene

Peppermint-scented, with a slight hint of citrus, phellandrene is perhaps the easiest terpene to identify in a laboratory setting. Pepper and dill oil are composed almost entirely of phellandrene, and it is the principal constituent in oil of ginger. Phellandrene has been used in Traditional Chinese Medicine to treat digestive disorders and is a primary compound in turmeric leaf oil, which is used to prevent and treat systemic fungal infections.[142]

Humulene

Humulene, a sesquiterpene, is found in *Cannabis sativa* strains, Vietnamese coriander, and hops, giving beer its distinct "hoppy" aroma. Humulene is considered an anti-tumor, antibacterial, anti-inflammatory, and anorectic (appetite suppressant). Commonly blended with beta-caryophyllene, humulene has been used for generations in Chinese medicine and is a major remedy for inflammation.[143]

Nerolidol

With woody and fresh bark aromas, nerolidol can be found in ginger and citronella. It has anti-fungal and antimalarial properties, producing a sedative effect.[144]

Alpha Bisabolol

Alpha bisabolol is found in chamomile and has long been used in the cosmetic industry. It has a floral aroma. Medicinal uses include the healing of wounds, and it can be used as a deodorizer. Alpha bisabolol has been effective in treating various kinds of inflammation. It is also analgesic, anti-microbial, antioxidant, antibacterial, and anti-irritant.

β-Elemene

β-elemene has a medium strength, sweet aroma. The concentrated form of β-elemene is isolated from rhizoma zedoariae, a type of ginger. It is a volatile terpene found in botanicals such as celery and mint, and it is prevalent in a variety of medicinal plants. It has strong anti-proliferative and anti-cancer effects against a broad spectrum of tumors.

α-Eudesmol

α-eudesmol has a sweet, woody odor. It has been shown to protect against brain injury after focal ischemia in rats. Recently, α-eudesmol has shown signs that it may become useful for the treatment of migraines.

Valencene

Valencene is a sesquiterpene that gets its name from the fruit in which it is most commonly found: Valencia oranges. Its citrusy, sweet aromas and flavors can be reminiscent of oranges, grapefruits, tangerines, and occasionally of fresh herbs or freshly cut wood. The fragrant terpene is responsible for familiar citrus aromas frequently found in a wide variety of cannabis strains. It is anti-inflammatory, anti-fungal, and insect repellent.

Full Spectrum, Whole-Plant Therapy

Considering this chapter's focus on the variety of phytocannabinoids and terpenes present in cannabis, be reminded that using the whole plant or products derived from the whole plant bring the most powerful and efficacious results.[145] The sum of all the components, working together, is greater than the parts—the synergistic entourage effect mentioned previously. Use the information provided to figure out which compounds (phytocannabinoids and terpenes) are most likely to be beneficial. Then, look for strains and whole-plant medicines that contain a large amount of the desired compounds. Another aspect to consider is the CBD:THC ratio for optimum benefit. CBD has been called the feminine aspect of cannabis and THC has been called the masculine. While THC works directly on the endocannabinoid receptors, CBD is indirectly balancing this system by allowing the body's own neurochemicals to be longer-acting. While both are important, they work better together. Finding the ideal ratio for a particular condition is a key part of this full-spectrum approach to cannabinoid therapy.

NOTE *For updates to this chapter, visit www.CBD-book.com/Updates.*

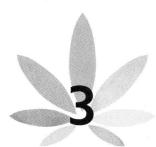

Ways to Take the Medicine

Using CBD-dominant medicine is easier in many ways than using cannabis that is higher in THC. The effect tends to be more body-centered and not mind altering—sometimes described as a "body high." The body feels more relaxed, the mood may improve, and the mind may feel calmer as a result, and most people are able to work, drive, and carry on with their normal routine without the "stoned" side effect. A small percentage of CBD users who are very sensitive to THC may notice mental/emotional effects that are more commonly associated with higher-THC cannabis. For this reason, first-time users should not operate automobiles or machinery until they become familiar with the effects and their own response to them.

A longstanding issue with the medical use of THC is that one person may feel relaxation and stress release, while another feels over-stimulated and anxious, while another feels energized and on-task. There are many factors that impact the effect, including the amount, strain, and form of the cannabis as well as the particular biochemistry, diet, history, emotional state of being, and experience level of the user.

Delivery Methods:
To Ingest, Inhale, or Use Topically?

The growing popularity of CBD has sparked an evolutionary revival in the use of cannabis as medicine. It has opened the door to a wide range of patients and health care practitioners who formerly had not considered cannabis part of the modern pharmacopeia. The more commonly known THC has an important status as a medicine, too, but the nature of CBD as a non-psychoactive compound allows greater access to the benefits of the plant's potent medicinal properties without the concern about potential impairment.

		ONSET	DURATION	BIOAVAILABILITY
	INHALATION Smoke or vaporize, medicine enters the bloodstream directly from the lungs.	immediate	2–4 hours	10–35%
	INGESTION With oral use, absorption is slow and erratic, resulting in maximal plasma concentrations usually after 60–120 minutes.	30 minutes–2 hours or more	6–8 hours	8–15%
	ORAL/MUCOSAL Tinctures, lozenges dissolved in the mouth (not swallowed). Medicine enters the bloodstream through the mucous membranes.	15–60 minutes	4–6 hours	6–20%

		ONSET	DURATION	BIOAVAILABILITY
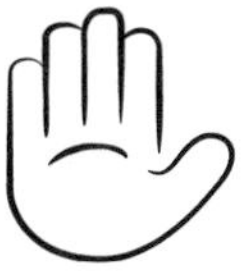	TOPICAL Applied to the skin for local relief, usually in a salve or balm. Only local effects. Medicine does not enter the bloodstream.	15 minutes (non-psychoactive)	2–4 hours	n/a
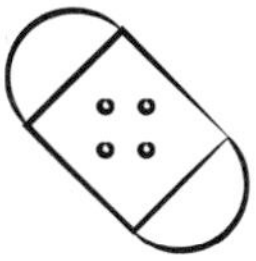	TRANSDERMAL Patch or gel, designed to be absorbed through the skin and into the bloodstream	15 minutes (possibly psychoactive)	12 hours (patch) 4 hours (gel)	100%

FIGURE 12

Unlike pharmaceutical drugs, which are delivered in specific doses, cannabinoid medicine is highly individualized. There are no researched standards of potency, delivery system, or dosage that physicians can consistently rely on. With cannabis, dosage can be as unique as the patient, and there are many possible ways to deliver the medicine into the patient's body in order to tap into CBD's health benefits. Cannabis can be smoked, vaporized, eaten in solid foods, taken as a liquid tincture, or rubbed on the skin as a topical. There are numerous ways to tap into the health benefits of CBD and other cannabinoids, with new technologies and innovations emerging daily.

While the classic "pot brownie" is not a thing of the past, options have become more sophisticated and varied, from raw to gourmet. As the end of the prohibition nears, the floodgates are opening and an enormous assortment of products is becoming available.

This array of options can be exciting and empowering, and also confusing and daunting, especially to the new user. By educating yourself thoroughly, you can understand your options and choose the proper form and dose of CBD medicine for yourself. Individual reactions to CBD medicine can vary greatly from person to person. The effects can change based on strain, dose, potency, how it is delivered, the time of day, the condition being treated, how much one has eaten and how recently, and the desired effect one wants (e.g., to wake up or go to sleep). Before you begin using CBD, consult with your health-care practitioner. To be safe, and to gain the optimum medicinal benefits, pay attention to your body and your own reaction, use your own intuition, experiment with different methods, and always remember this wise old saying: "Once you've ingested cannabis, you can always take more, but you can't take less." It is strongly recommended that you keep detailed records of your cannabis usage, addressing all of the parameters listed above that result in how each particular usage specifically affects you.

Oral and Edible CBD Products

Tinctures

Tinctures have been around for thousands of years. "Tincture" refers to an infusion of a plant in a liquid base—often alcohol—in which the plant has been soaked and brewed for days, weeks, or sometimes months. Tinctures have been used to administer a wide range of herbal plant medicines around the world. They are easy to use, they are long lasting, and you can make accurate dose measurements. Tinctures are concentrated liquids that usually come in small glass

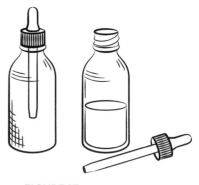

FIGURE 13: [MELNYK] © 123RF.COM

bottles, commonly in quantities of 0.5 oz, 1 oz, or 2 oz, with a dropper for measuring a specific number of drops.

A standard tincture dropper makes it easy to dose with consistency and accuracy. Tinctures are appropriate for micro and standard dose ranges. For alcohol tinctures, 25–30 drops = 1 milliliter (ml). The next measurement you need to know is the potency of the liquid, which is usually on the label in milligrams of CBD per milliliter of liquid (mg/ml). Potency for CBD is most often found in the range of 10–20 mg/ml, but it can be as high as 50 mg/ml. Therefore, always read the label and calculate the dosage carefully.

Once you know how many drops to take, you can shortcut the counting process by measuring out how many drops are in one quarter of a dropper, one half of a dropper, and three quarters of a dropper. Then, you can use the height of the liquid in the dropper as a good estimate, rather than counting out drops.

Tinctures can be taken in many ways, including:

1. Oral application (squirt into the back of the tongue and swallow)

2. Sublingual (place under the tongue and let it slowly get absorbed, swallowing the remainder)

3. In food or liquids

4. As capsules

The taste is comparable to other strong medicinal herbs, often described as bitter and pungent. Tinctures that use pure alcohol (190 proof) can be difficult to tolerate. It is not recommended to put strong alcohol mixtures directly on or under the tongue, as the alcohol can burn the membranes. If the tincture has been diluted for taste, it could then be appropriate to place directly on the tongue. For alcohol-based CBD tinctures, it is recommended to dilute the tinctures with an ounce of juice that is either bitter or sour, such as cranberry, grapefruit, lemon-ginger, or orange. Another option is to add it to hot water or tea (this allows a small amount, but not all of the alcohol, to evaporate off) for a few minutes before drinking. Many people use plain water for dilution, which also works well. However, there is often a taste left in the mouth. If this is the case, a "chaser" of additional water or juice may be used as a rinse. You can also mix it with solid foods, such as applesauce, bread, yogurt, pudding, or soup.

An oral dose typically takes thirty to sixty minutes to take effect. Once digested, the effects are long lasting, from six to eight hours. Given this timing, tinctures are often used three times a day, seven to eight hours apart. However, for severe conditions, some people use it six times a day. The objective of dosing is to have the medicine be just strong enough to feel it in the background, and not have it take over your focus of awareness. Alcohol-based tinctures are absorbed faster into the bloodstream than oil-based infusions. As with all edibles, the effects are faster and stronger when taken on an empty stomach. Alcohol-based tinctures have a shelf life of up to five years.

Oil Infusions

Oil infusions (also known as oil-based tinctures) are becoming more popular—because CBD is lipophilic (fat-loving), it is easily infused into oil. Oil infusions can be made with liquid coconut oil, olive oil, hemp oil, sunflower seed oil, or any other edible oil. Oil tinctures are best used directly under or on top of the tongue, because the mucous membranes of the mouth will absorb some of the tincture directly before it reaches the stomach (where stomach acids begin to break it apart). When counting drops, it can be easier to put it onto a spoon first. Dosing and usage is similar to alcohol tinctures, with some differences. Oil absorption takes slightly longer, approximately forty to seventy-five minutes, to take effect, but similarly lasts as long, approximately six to eight hours. If you find that your dose wears off in less time, you can increase the dose slightly. You can also increase the frequency to three or four times a day, while some users prefer taking it up to six times a day.

Doses are usually recommended in number of milligrams (mg). To find out how many mg of CBD or THC you are taking, multiply the volume (in milliliters, or ml) by the potency (mg per ml). The result is the number of mg.

Volume (in ml) × potency (in mg/ml) = dose (in mg)

Or, working backward, you can find the volume (number of drops you will be taking in ml) by dividing the recommended dose (in mg) by the potency (mg/ml). Then, divide the resulting ml by 0.85 to get the number of drops.

Calculation of an oil infusion dose is the same process as above; however, for oil infusions, 20 drops = 1 ml. For example, an infusion labeled "17.0 mg of CBD per ml" means every milliliter (20 drops) contains 17 mg of CBD, or 0.85 mg of CBD per drop. Thus, if you wanted to take 5 mg of CBD as your dose, you would divide 5 by 0.85 to get the number of drops you should take, which is 5.88, or, rounding up, 6 drops.

Most edible oils have a limited shelf life, and it is best to consume them within one year. If you keep oil-based infusions in the refrigerator, they will last longer, though they may solidify at cool temperatures.

While most people use CBD oils directly under or on top of the tongue, they can also be mixed with food. They do well placed in thick liquids such as blender drinks, soups, peanut or almond butter, honey, applesauce, or yogurt. Oil does not mix well with water or juices. Oil tinctures can also be used topically as well, such as on rashes, on sore muscles, or even on open wounds.

Glycerin Tinctures

Vegetable glycerin, also known as glycerol or glycerine, is a clear, syrupy, odorless liquid produced from plant lipids. It is produced using an extraction process called hydrolysis. The process includes the use of pressure, temperature, and water. Vegetable glycerin has many applications in the world including food, cosmetics, and alcohol-free herbal tinctures, including cannabis tinctures. As cannabis is lipid-soluble, glycerin is an effective way to create a botanical infusion.

Various glycerin-based cannabis tinctures are available and are a valid option for those who are intolerant to alcohol-based tinctures. This method of administration is easy to ingest orally, either straight or mixed with food or drink. When used sublingually, these tinctures are fast-acting, discreet, and easy to consume.[146]

It is worth mentioning that not all vegetable glycerin is made equally. Poor-quality vegetable glycerin can be made with genetically modified corn and soy or the by-products of industrial processing of biofuels, so choose organic whenever possible.

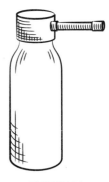

FIGURE 14:

[SEAMARTINI]
© 123RF.COM

Sublingual Uptake

Sublinguals take effect in thirty seconds to two minutes and last about as long as other ingested products, for about six to eight hours. Under the tongue and within the mouth, a large number of tiny blood vessels can absorb cannabinoids into the bloodstream before they are swallowed. Common examples of these types of medications include tinctures/infusions, dissolvable strips, oromucosal sprays, or medicated lozenges. Sublingual delivery is not only a convenient way to medicate, but intake through the oral mucosal membranes provides for rapid and effective absorption directly. Compared to other delivery methods, uptake through blood vessels and micro-capillaries in the mouth is one of the best ways to increase the bioavailability of cannabinoids. This "first-pass" of medication, as it is referred to, allows the medication to avoid having to pass through the digestive system and liver where it would be broken down, making it significantly less available to the bloodstream. Whenever you take any medication orally—that is, by swallowing pills or eating an edible—a small fraction of that medicine is metabolized in the liver before it even reaches systemic circulation (absorption into the bloodstream), thus decreasing the overall bioavailability of the medication.

Additionally, sublingual delivery provides rapid effects similar to smoking or vaporizing without exposing the lungs to heat, tar, or other by-products. It avoids dealing with the smell, smoky taste, dry mouth, and other issues such as throat irritation and coughing during administration.

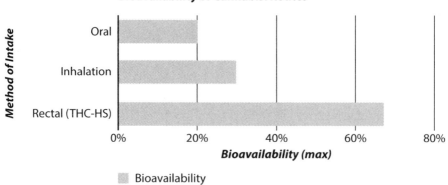

FIGURE 15: Bioavailability of Cannabis: Routes

CAPSULES

Cannabis capsules are a convenient and reliable form of medicinal cannabis. Concentrated oils, powders, and other concentrates are ensconced in either a soft gel or hardened shell, generally made from gelatin or vegetable starches or cellulose. Pre-measured dosing eliminates confusion or inaccurate dosage. Patients know exactly what they are getting every time. Generally, capsules can take thirty to ninety minutes to take effect, and are effective for six to eight hours. They can be taken two to three times a day for continuous medication effects. Capsules provide long-term effectiveness, particularly for longer-term treatments that require maintaining consistent levels of CBD in the body. While most people tolerate capsules well, a small percentage of people have difficulty digesting the capsules or the raw plant material, another area for self-experimentation.

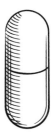

FIGURE 16:

[SEAMARTINI]
© 123RF.COM

Edibles

Administering medicine through food and snacks can be a delightful way to receive the benefits of CBD. Edibles are a fast-growing category in the emerging cannabis industry. They come in all shapes, sizes, and flavors, ranging from macaroons to muffins, gummy bears to lollipops, medicated trail mix and energy bars, chocolate and hot sauce—just to name a few of the sweet and savory edibles appearing on dispensary shelves.

Edibles can be made with raw-plant matter, oil infusions, butter, or any kind of extract. Because cannabis is lipophilic, as mentioned previously, it can be dissolved into fat and thus added to almost any food one can imagine. Some edibles are made from more concentrated forms of cannabis, including ethanol and CO_2-extracted cannabis. Every form has its own unique combination and ratios of CBD to other constituents. One of the difficulties with edibles is that it can be difficult to gauge the dose. Effective use of edibles requires accurate dosage, testing, and consistency. Because edibles have to go through the digestive system, it can take from one to three hours to feel the effects. Feeling misled, people often make the mistake of thinking that it isn't working, so they eat more than the ideal dose. Taking too much CBD does not usually cause adverse side effects; however, it can be temporarily uncomfortable and can last for eight hours or more. Another caution with edibles is that the increasingly flavorful and delicious food items can also tempt people into ingesting higher doses than necessary or desired. Edibles can also be attractive to children or pets, so be sure to keep them far away and locked up in a safe place.

LOZENGES

CBD-medicated lozenges provide a discreet and easy method for administering an oral dose of medicated soothing relief and relaxation. Lozenges (sucking candies) are oral doses that provide a fairly quick uptake of medicine, from twenty to forty minutes. They dissolve in minutes and provide a slow-to-medium release to buccal and mucous membranes in the mouth, delivering the medicine efficiently into the bloodstream. Check the

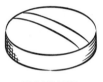

FIGURE 17:

[SEAMARTINI]
© 123RF.COM

labels carefully. Lozenges usually contain 10 to 20 mg of CBD. They are often available in sugar-free versions, or are honey based, and can contain other herbs (such as echinacea) or flavors that provide soothing effects for the throat.

Sublingual-Dissolvable CBD Strips

The sublingual dissolving strips (similar to breath strips) that contain CBD medicine are fast acting. They are convenient to carry and consume and are very discreet. There is no odor and they dissolve very quickly, within a few minutes. They provide effects in fifteen to thirty minutes and can last the typical six to eight hours. Because they do not go through the digestive system or liver, they have a high bioavailability. They are available in amounts of 5–40 mg of CBD per strip, and some companies offer them in various flavors. Placing the strip between the cheek and tongue will cause a slower onset and longer-lasting experience.

Concentrated CO_2 Oils

CO2 oils can be mixed with other carrier oils to make edibles or capsules (see more on how these concentrates are made on p. 52). CO2 oil is favored by patients needing a macro dose to treat their condition. The oil is extremely concentrated, often having a cannabinoid content of 50–75 percent. With this type of concentrate, dosing is often described as "equal in size to one grain of rice." This one-grain-of-rice size equals approximately 50 mg of CBD. This concentrate can come in a syringe dispenser for ease of use. This oil is very thick and viscous; it sticks like tar to anything it touches. Hence, the syringe allows easy application and placement without the need to touch it, and the applicator usually has measurement lines for accurate application. Unfortunately, small (micro) doses cannot be delivered this way, so it is best for application of doses 50 mg and larger. One favored way to take this medication is to put the desired dose in an empty capsule for easy oral consumption.

Raw Cannabis Juice

Let food be thy medicine and medicine be thy food.
—HIPPOCRATES, 431 BC (considered
the father of Western medicine)

The juice of raw cannabis leaves (which has not been heated) contains the acid forms of the cannabinoid. When cannabis is growing, it produces the acid form; CBD is CBDA and THC is THCA. When cannabis is dried and heated, in a process called decarboxylation, the heat converts it from the acid form to the typical form of CBD and THC. THCA is non-psychoactive, so you can consume large amounts of THCA without getting "high." CBDA and THCA have been shown to have anti-inflammatory, antioxidant, and neuroprotective qualities. It is full of beneficial enzymes and nutrients when used as a dietary food. Many people claim great benefits; however, there are significant challenges to its consumption. The juice of cannabis leaves has an extremely short shelf life—once the leaves have been pressed through an auger-type juicer, it should be consumed within four to twelve hours. It can be frozen, but some water must be added first because the fresh juice does not crystallize well. The other challenge is finding a good source of fresh leaves. William Courtney, MD, is a proponent of fresh cannabis juice and recommends adding it to other juices such as beet, green, or carrot juice. Many who use this method grow their own plants to juice.

Inhalable Products

Smoking Flowers (Buds)

Smoking cannabis is the traditional convention. It is a tried-and-true method that has been practiced throughout the ages. Inhalation has an immediate effect because the active molecules enter the bloodstream through the lungs, bypassing the digestive system. When looking to purchase flowers, look for high-CBD strains, many of which are available today, including Charlotte's Web, Harlequin, Sour Tsunami, Cannatonic, Remedy, Valentine X, and AC/DC. See Chapter 9 for information about specific strains.

There are countless devices and apparatuses that can be used to smoke CBD flowers and concentrates. Some require significant effort. Others offer convenience and minimal effort. Many of the modern smoking pens are discreet devices that look like regular pens.

METHODS OF SMOKING

Joints, marijuana cigarette. Cannabis cigarettes have traditionally been rolled in a thin paper made from materials such as hemp or rice paper. This is the most well-known method of smoking cannabis. Smoking cannabis can be a very fast way to administer CBD. However, the relatively strong odor from smoking cannabis is not very discreet and tends to stick to and linger on one's clothes and hair. Also, while the first or second "hit" of a joint tastes relatively clean, as you get to the end of the joint, the taste intensifies because the remaining cannabis acts like a concentrating filter for the smoke to get through.

It was once believed that smoking cannabis might contribute to cancer in the lungs or upper respiratory airways. Recent research indicates that it does not. A study published in the *International Journal of Cancer* showed that cannabis smokers did not have higher risk for lung cancer.[147] In fact, cannabis smokers often had a significantly lower rate of lung cancer than nonsmokers.

Pipes. Handheld pipes are another commonly used tool for smoking. Pipes come in many sizes and materials ranging from hand-blown glass, wood, metal, ceramic and stone. It is a simple matter to carve a single-use pipe from such materials since it requires only a bowl for the plant material and a chamber for air to flow through. Even a piece of tinfoil can be fashioned into a makeshift pipe. Small pipes are a very efficient method of smoking as one can use only a very small bud for a single use.

Water pipe, or bong. Water pipes, known as bongs or bubblers, are another popular way to smoke cannabis flowers or concentrates. Water pipes have been used across the world for at least 2,400 years. This device works by passing smoke through water and filtering and cooling the smoke before it is inhaled. Bongs are made from a wide variety of materials, including glass, acrylic, bamboo, metals, and ceramic. They come in a wide range of shapes, sizes, and cost. Some studies involving tobacco suggest water filtration can be an effective way of reducing exposure to the potential health risks associated with smoking by filtering out known toxicants from the by-products of burning plant material. When smoke is cooled, it is less of an irritant to the airways of the respiratory system. Bongs are relatively easy to use and maintain; however, they must be kept clean. Bong water can smell very bad very quickly. Bongs are generally kept at home because they are often not easy to transport.[148]

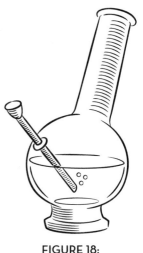

FIGURE 18:
[KERNELPANIC74] © 123RF.COM

Vaporizing

Vaporizing is the process of heating cannabis flowers, oils, or concentrates to a temperature below its combustion point, where it would burst into flame. Cannabinoids are thus released into the air without producing the potentially harmful by-products of smoke. Cannabis vaporization reduces noxious smoke and associated toxins (i.e., carcinogenic hydrocarbons), which are produced above the combustion point of around 450°F. Because vaporization can deliver doses of cannabinoids while reducing the user's intake of carcinogenic smoke, it is a preferred, and likely safer, method of cannabis administration than inhaling smoke.[149]

In the past few years, vaporizing cannabis has grown in popularity, both for the potential health benefits of vaping versus smoking and also for the discreet, convenient nature of portable vaporizers. There have been many advances in research and technology in the vaporizer industry. In addition, vapor does not have the intense smell of marijuana smoke (often no smell at all), and is therefore more discreet. Pure cannabis concentrates, when ingested or inhaled, can produce beneficial therapeutic effects in patients who are suffering from chronic obstructive pulmonary disease.[150]

The boiling point of CBD is between 320-356°F, depending on the pressure. The boiling point of Δ^9-THC is 315°F and Δ^8-THC is between 347-352°F. Some experts believe that the temperature "sweet spot" for vaporizing cannabis is around 338°F, although some cannabinoids begin to vaporize at even lower temperatures. Others prefer vaporizing at around 400°F to ensure that all the CBD is completely cooked. A joint can burn as hot as 2000°F or higher. Some vaporizers have a digital temperature control that can be adjusted to heat cannabis at lower temperatures and thereby maintain flavor profiles from terpenes, which can be burned up at higher temperatures. One advantage of higher temperatures is producing medicine good for sleep and insomnia.

Vaporizers generally use two types of heating elements:

1. Conduction—conduction heating works by transferring heat through direct contact (of the herb or oil) with an electrically heated surface. It can be difficult to regulate temperatures using conduction heating with vaporizers, but they have the advantage of being easy to construct and made portable and battery powered. Vape pens, and most portable vaporizers, are heated with conduction.

2. Convection—convection heating is more complex and works by passing heated air over the plant material evenly and efficiently. The heating element never comes in direct contact with the plant material. Desktop and home-use vaporizers use this method of heating, which is more easily controlled and ideal for maximizing the experience.

Pen vaporizers and vape pens. These digital electronic vaporizers are incredibly compact, easy to use, and cheaper than other types of vaporizers. "Direct draw" is a common feature of some vape pens. To initiate use, simply draw air through the mouthpiece. This action initiates the heating unit, and vapor flows directly from the heating element to the user. Other pen vaporizers have a button to press to engage the unit, and the button must be pressed continuously during the inhalation to vaporize the

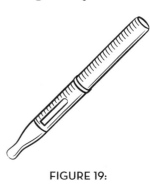

FIGURE 19:
[YLIVDESIGN] © 123RF.COM

material. Pen vaporizers are very discreet, compact, convenient, and odorless. They are generally very small and can easily be mistaken for a writing utensil or Sharpie. They utilize pre-loaded cartridges, which are quite economical, often lasting for three hundred inhalations, and usually have a built-in rechargeable lithium-ion battery. Depending on the type of oil used (providing there are no residual toxins or chemicals), there are no known adverse health impacts or side effects from vaporizing, except that you can take too much if you're not careful in how you inhale.

Portable/handheld. Portable vaporizers are slightly larger than vape pens, but are still relatively small compared to other devices. With this type of vaporizer, one can add different kinds of oils, concentrates, or flowers. They may come with various attachments for different types of plant materials. High-tech versions have advanced digital controls for regulating temperature.

Desktop/home use. These vaporizers are larger stationary units that require electricity. They often utilize convection heating, which optimizes the quality of vapor since the heat is evenly distributed and never comes in direct contact with the plant material.

Dabbing. Dabbing is a form of vaporization involving highly concentrated forms of cannabis. It is administered by using a specific type of water pipe with an extremely hot surface, which essentially "flash vaporizes" the concentrate. Dabbing is a more recent trend, typically used for high-THC concentrates to obtain the ultimate recreational "high." However, one can also "dab" CBD concentrates. If high doses required, it is a very strong and rapid way to medicate.

CONCENTRATES

Concentrates are becoming increasingly popular and exist in many forms, which can be ambiguous and confusing. They are also commonly referred to as cannabis extracts and are much more potent than flowers. Concentrates include a wide range of forms, referred to as kief, hash, wax, shatter, crumble, RSO, rosin, honey oil, sap, nectar, and others. The process involved in creating concentrates can be complex and can be potentially dangerous. There are a host of extraction methods, many employing high-tech processes that create a highly concentrated end product.

Alcohol extraction. A relatively low-tech process that uses high-proof alcohol or ethanol as a solvent to extract active ingredients in the plant. Alcohol is mixed into plant material and stored in a dark, cool place for several weeks. The plant material is then strained out of the alcohol, discarded, and the alcohol is used to make tinctures. The tincture solution is then subjected to low-pressure evaporation, and the resulting product is pure cannabis oil. Chlorophyll is not removed with this method, and the final oil has a dark green color.

RSO (Rick Simpson oil). This method was one of the first concentration methods and was popularized on the nternet. It is similar to alcohol extraction, using a solvent and then evaporating off the solvent. However, when Rick Simpson first started making his oil, he used some very toxic solvents, including naphtha, a petroleum distillate. Many different solvents can be used, such as hexane, pentane, or butane. Mr. Simpson claimed that his process removed these toxic substances completely, but that is a difficult task, especially without expert chemists to guide the process. We do not recommend using any product that could contain toxic residue from chemical processing. If you are not absolutely sure how it was made, avoid taking it into your body.

Supercritical fluid extraction. This method involves a sophisticated machine that separates one component from another by using carbon dioxide, creating a "supercritical" liquid state. This extraction process is nontoxic and has become the standard for safe, clean cannabis concentrates. The method uses the strange properties of gases that have been compressed beyond their "supercritical point." Carbon dioxide (CO_2) is the most frequently used gas because its critical point can be reached at around 90°F, cool enough that delicate terpenes and cannabinoids don't get deactivated.

Butane (BHO). Butane hash oil, commonly referred to as BHO, is a cannabis concentrate made by using butane as a solvent to remove cannabinoids. Many concentrates fall into this category, including wax, shatter, crumble, honey oil, and others. N-butane is highly flammable and can leave a toxic residual on the end product. BHO can be extremely hazardous. Unfortunately, because it is cheap and easily available, it has become popular. We do not recommend ingesting anything that could possibly have butane residue. Most "wax" products are made using butane.

CAUTION ABOUT BUYING CBD OIL
MADE FROM INDUSTRIAL HEMP

CBD oil extracted from industrial hemp is a thick tar-like substance that often needs to be thinned with a compound such as propylene glycol. A widespread additive found in CBD vape oil cartridges, propylene glycol might convert to formaldehyde, a known carcinogen, when heated and inhaled.[151]

Types of Concentrates

Kief. This is the least complicated of concentrates and is all-natural. Kief is a collection of the trichomes, the crystalline structures coating the outside surface of dried flowers. It can be captured using filtering screens and looks like a fine powder.

Hash. Hash has been made from cannabis plants around the world for centuries. In the United States, bubble hash using ice water is the most common method of producing non-solvent hash. The trichomes of the plant are frozen, isolated using various layers of filters, dried, and pressed. There are many other methods, including hand-rubbing the female flowers, which leaves a black tar on the hands and fingers that is then scraped off with a knife and rolled up into balls.

Rosin. Rosin is plant resin trichomes obtained by adding high pressure and heat to dried plant material. An industrial heat press can be used, or even a hair dryer for small batches. It's a relatively simple technique with a solvent-free, high-quality finished product.

CO2 oil. This oil is made from a supercritical extraction method. CO2 gas under high pressure and low temperature is a liquid that is used as a solvent to extract the cannabis oil. It requires very expensive machinery and is the primary method of commercial operations. Patients with medical conditions favor it as it is the purest and healthiest method of extraction. Usually, the waxes that remain after concentrating are removed by another process that involves ethanol, freezing, or the use of solvents. We do not recommend ingesting or smoking products that use solvents.

Topical/Transdermal/External Use of CBD Products

Salves/Lotions/Oils

Cannabis products can be applied topically to the body where they are absorbed transdermally (through the skin) for localized relief of pain, inflammation, muscle soreness, psoriasis, rashes, arthritis, and other conditions. Topicals come in the form of salves, balms, oils, and lotions. This form of cannabis medicine is non-psychoactive and the most non-invasive way to use cannabis therapeutically. Topical salves are useful for conditions that are within one inch of the surface of the skin. They do not penetrate to deeper areas and are great for a variety of skin conditions. For extreme medical conditions, such as skin cancer, pure cannabis oil concentrates like CO_2 extracts can be used.

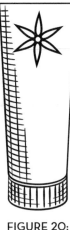
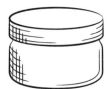

FIGURE 21:

[FOXROAR]
© 123RF.COM

FIGURE 20:

[YLIVDESIGN]
© 123RF.COM

Transdermal Patches

Transdermal patches are medicated adhesive patches that are placed on the skin and release small amounts of medication into the bloodstream over a long period of time. Patches are different from topicals because they can penetrate all seven epidermal layers of skin and reach the bloodstream. They have a systemic rather than localized effect, as opposed to most topicals. They provide a longer period of medication that can last from six to ten hours. Patches can be cut into smaller sizes if less medication is needed. Because they work systemically, THC patches do have psychoactive effects.

Suppositories

Suppositories have been used for centuries as a way to deliver medication to the colon where it can be absorbed directly, having bypassed the stomach and liver. It is an excellent way to obtain the health benefits of CBD, especially when oral intake is restricted. There is greater absorption and bioavailability when medication is delivered by way of rectal or vaginal tissues. Suppositories are especially useful for cancer patients with pelvic, rectal, colon, prostate, or ovarian cancer. In addition, most people report that they are able to take large doses of THC by suppositories without experiencing the psychoactive high from other delivery methods. It is recommended for cancer patients who need large doses of both CBD and THC and who want to minimize psychoactive side effects. Suppositories are best made from mixing concentrated cannabis oil with cocoa butter.

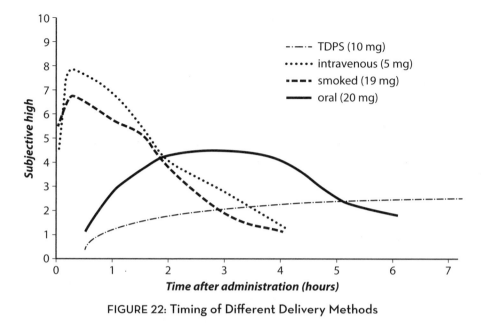

FIGURE 22: Timing of Different Delivery Methods

Pharmaceutical and Synthetic Versions of Cannabis

The following list provides some of the major pharmaceuticals related to cannabis that have been developed or are currently being developed.

Sativex (nabiximols) is a cannabis plant–based medicine from GW Pharmaceuticals that has been approved in twenty-four countries (excluding the United States), at press time, for multiple sclerosis and for muscle spasticity. The formula includes a 1:1 equal ratio of THC to CBD and comes as an oromucosal spray. It was approved and launched in the United Kingdom in 2010 as the first cannabis-based prescription medicine in the world. In the United States, Phase III clinical trials started in late 2006 for treatment of pain in cancer patients, and in 2011 a U.S. patent was granted for Sativex for cancer pain. In 2014 the FDA granted "fast track" designation to Sativex for the treatment of pain in patients with advanced cancer.[152]

Epidiolex (cannabidiol) is a plant-based, oral pharmaceutical formulation of pure CBD, made by GW Pharmaceuticals, which is in development for the treatment of a number of rare childhood-onset epilepsy disorders. GW has conducted extensive pre-clinical research of CBD for epilepsy since 2007. This research has shown that CBD has significant anti-epileptiform and anticonvulsant activity, using a variety of in vitro and in vivo models, and reduced seizures in various acute animal models of epilepsy. To date, GW has received orphan drug designation from the FDA for Epidiolex for the treatment of Dravet syndrome, LGS, tuberous sclerosis complex, and infantile spasms. Additionally, GW has received fast track designation from the FDA and orphan designation from the European Medicines Agency for Epidiolex for the treatment of Dravet syndrome. GW is currently evaluating additional clinical development programs in other orphan seizure disorders.

Dronabinol (trade name Marinol) is a synthetic version of THC manufactured by Solvay Pharmaceuticals. It was FDA-approved in the United States for nausea in 1985 and for appetite stimulation in 1992; it became a Schedule 3 drug in 1999.

It was approved in Denmark for multiple sclerosis in 2003. It is approved in Canada for AIDS-related cachexia (since 2000) and for nausea and vomiting associated with cancer chemotherapy (since 1988).

Nabilone (trade name Cesamet) is a synthetic cannabinoid pharmaceutical drug made by Valeant Pharmaceuticals, prescribed to treat nausea and vomiting as a side effect of chemotherapy and as an analgesic for neuropathic pain. It is a synthetic mimic of THC, the primary psychoactive compound that is naturally occurring in cannabis. Originally approved by the FDA for use in the United States in 1985, it was removed from the market until it was re-approved in 2006. It was approved in Canada in 1981, the United Kingdom and Australia in 1982, and Mexico in 2007. In 2006, the FDA approved safety-labeling revisions for nabilone to advise of warnings and precautions related to its use, such as its potential to affect the mental state of a patient.

Synthetic Cannabinoids

Synthetic cannabinoids refer to a growing number of man-made, mind-altering chemicals that are either sprayed on dried, shredded plant material so they can be smoked (herbal incense) or sold as liquids to be vaporized and inhaled in e-cigarettes and other devices (liquid incense).

These chemicals are called cannabinoids because they are related to chemicals found in the cannabis plant. Synthetic cannabinoids are sometimes misleadingly called "synthetic cannabis" (or "fake weed"), and they are often marketed as safe and legal alternatives, though they are neither. In fact, they may affect the brain much more powerfully than cannabis; their actual effects can be unpredictable and, in some cases, severe or even life-threatening.

Synthetic cannabinoids are included in a group of drugs called "new psychoactive substances" that have become newly available on the market and are intended to copy the effects of illegal drugs. Some of these substances may have been around for years but have re-entered the market in altered chemical forms or due to renewed popularity.

Manufacturers sell these herbal incense products in colorful foil packages and sell similar liquid incense products, like other e-cigarette fluids, in plastic bottles. They market these products under a wide variety of specific brand names; in past years, K2 and Spice were common. Hundreds of other brand names now exist, such as Joker, Black Mamba, Kush, and Kronic.

For several years, synthetic cannabinoid mixtures have been easy to buy in drug paraphernalia shops, novelty stores, gas stations, and through the internet. Because the chemicals used in them have a high potential for abuse and no medical benefit, authorities have made it illegal to sell, buy, or possess many of these chemicals.

Dosage Guidelines

Dosage is everything.

—PARACELSUS, sixteenth-century Swiss physician and chemist

Finding the correct dose of CBD for a particular patient is not an easy task, even for experts, because there are so many different factors that play an important part in the patient's experience:

- The medical condition or problem

- The condition's stage or intensity

- The patient's biology and metabolism and how they respond to CBD

- The patient's endocannabinoid system and how it functions and acclimates to CBD over time

- The patient's body weight

- The patient's sensitivity to cannabis—this is the most important factor

- The patient's body chemistry, including pharmaceuticals and foods ingested

- How more than one hundred different molecules may impact the body (largely unknown)

CBD is generally considered safe to consume (as long as it's clean and has no toxins); however, we use the "precautionary principle" in making recommendations. This principle serves as a guide to making wiser decisions in the face of uncertainty. It guides us to act cautiously in the face of the unknown—"do no harm" and prevent harm—while observing outcomes and making small adjustments over time.

"Titration" is a term borrowed from chemistry that means taking small steps over time in order to allow for adjustment slowly. This process lowers the risk of problems such as overdose, overwhelm, or over-reaction. We always recommend titration as the best way to introduce CBD to the body. It means starting off on the low side of a dosage range and adjusting upward slowly over time until the desired effect is reached. This cautious approach has served our patients well, and many experts now recommend it as a dosing protocol for medical cannabis.

Since there is a wide range of dosing possibilities, we have identified three dose ranges that are useful for different conditions: micro dose, standard dose, and macro (therapeutic) dose. These three ranges, combined with the patient's body weight, determine the recommended starter dose:

1. Micro doses are considered a low level of medication, in the range of 0.5 mg to 20 mg of CBD per dose per day (CBD/dose/day).

   - Micro doses can be effective for sleep, headache, mood disorders, nausea, PTSD, stress, and metabolic disorders.

2. Standard doses are the mid-range, between 10 mg to 100 mg of CBD/dose/day.

   • Standard doses have been shown to be effective for pain, inflammation, autoimmune disorders, Lyme disease, anxiety, depression, arthritis, some mental disorders, fibromyalgia, multiple sclerosis, inflammatory bowel syndrome, autism, and weight loss.

3. Macro (or therapeutic) doses are at the high range, between 50 mg and 800 mg of CBD/dose/day.

   • Doses at this level are often used to treat cancer, epilepsy, seizure disorders, liver disease, and other severe life-threatening conditions.

Here's how to use the tables:

1. First, decide whether you will be using the micro, standard, or macro dose protocol and then locate that table.

2. Find your body weight in the left column and read across the row.

3. We have provided five ranges of mg of CBD/dose/day in the micro and standard protocol, and ten ranges in the macro protocol.

4. The dose of CBD can be the total of CBD+THC. If you are taking a 1:1 product, and the chart says 20 mg, then you would be taking 10 mg of CBD plus 10 mg of THC per day.

5. If you are only taking one dose per day, then the number in the chart is your dose. If you are taking two doses per day, take half of the recommendation per dose. If taking three doses per day, take one third of the recommendation per dose. Take your doses seven to eight hours apart.

6. Begin at the lowest dose (the left column) and take your dose (see #5 to determine your dose if taking the medicine more than once a day) at least a half hour before a meal. This is your starting dose, not your target dose.

7. Continue this dosage for two to four days before increasing your dose. It is suggested that you record all parameters regarding your dosages and how they affect you so that you can make adjustments.

8. .Watch for any unpleasant or negative reactions. If you experience anything unpleasant or negative, cut your dose to half the amount and continue taking this dose for two to four days before increasing your dose.

9. Use the next dose level for another two to three days before increasing your dose. If you are not using the tables, increase your dose by 20 percent.

10. Continue this pattern, observing your body's reaction and any changes in your condition.

11. You may reach a dose level at which you experience a reduction in the benefit or an unpleasant or negative reaction. If this happens, step back to the previous dose and continue at that dose for at least four days. Then cautiously move up a step again. If your body responds positively to that level, continue at that dose. This is your target dose.

Continue to monitor and record your body's needs and wants. Adjust as necessary, upward or downward, whenever your body feedback—or your intuition—indicates that a change is needed.

Micro Dose

POUNDS (LBS)	.01 MG/LB/ DAY	.03 MG/LB/ DAY	.05 MG/LB/ DAY	.075 MG/LB/ DAY	0.1 MG/LB/ DAY
20	0.2	0.6	1	1.4	2
30	0.3	0.9	1.5	2.1	3
40	0.4	1.2	2	2.8	4
50	0.5	1.5	2.5	3.5	5
60	0.6	1.8	3	4.2	6
70	0.7	2.1	3.5	4.9	7
80	0.8	2.4	4	5.6	8

POUNDS (LBS)	.01 MG/LB/ DAY	.03 MG/LB/ DAY	.05 MG/LB/ DAY	.075 MG/LB/ DAY	0.1 MG/LB/ DAY
90	0.9	2.7	4.5	6.3	9
100	1	3	5	7	10
110	1.1	3.3	5.5	7.7	11
120	1.2	3.6	6	8.4	12
130	1.3	3.9	6.5	9.1	13
140	1.4	4.2	7	9.8	14
150	1.5	4.5	7.5	10.5	15
160	1.6	4.8	8	11.2	16
170	1.7	5.1	8.5	11.9	17
180	1.8	5.4	9	12.6	18
190	1.9	5.7	9.5	13.3	19
200	2	6	10	14	20
220	2.2	6.6	11	15.4	22
240	2.4	7.2	12	16.8	24

Standard Dose

POUNDS (LBS)	.15 MG/LB/ DAY	0.2 MG/LB/ DAY	0.3 MG/LB/ DAY	0.4 MG/LB/ DAY	0.5 MG/LB/ DAY
20	3	4	6	8	10
30	4.5	6	9	12	15
40	6	8	12	16	20

Standard Dose (cont.)

POUNDS (LBS)	.15 MG/LB/ DAY	0.2 MG/LB/ DAY	0.3 MG/LB/ DAY	0.4 MG/LB/ DAY	0.5 MG/LB/ DAY
50	7.5	10	15	20	25
60	9	12	18	24	30
70	10.5	14	21	28	35
80	12	16	24	32	40
90	13.5	18	27	36	45
100	15	20	30	40	50
110	16.5	22	33	44	55
120	18	24	36	48	60
130	19.5	26	39	52	65
140	21	28	42	56	70
150	22.5	30	45	60	75
160	24	32	48	64	80
170	25.5	34	51	68	85
180	27	36	54	72	90
190	28.5	38	57	76	95
200	30	40	60	80	100
220	33	44	66	88	110
240	36	48	72	96	120

Macro Dose

POUNDS (LBS)	.75 MG/ LB/ DAY	1.0 MG/ LB/ DAY	1.25 MG/ LB/ DAY	1.5 MG/ LB/ DAY	2.0 MG/ LB/ DAY	2.5 MG/ LB/ DAY	3 MG/ LB/ DAY	3.5 MG/ LB/ DAY	4.0 MG/ LB/ DAY	5.0 MG/ LB/ DAY
20	15	20	25	30	40	50	60	70	80	100
30	22.5	30	37.5	45	60	75	90	105	120	150
40	30	40	50	60	80	100	120	140	160	200
50	37.5	50	62.5	75	100	125	150	175	200	250
60	45	60	75	90	120	150	180	210	240	300
70	52.5	70	87.5	105	140	175	210	245	280	350
80	60	80	100	120	160	200	240	280	320	400
90	67.5	90	112.5	135	180	225	270	315	360	450
100	75	100	125	150	200	250	300	350	400	500
110	82.5	110	137.5	165	220	275	330	385	440	550
120	90	120	150	180	240	300	360	420	480	600
130	97.5	130	162.5	195	260	325	390	455	520	650
140	105	140	175	210	280	350	420	490	560	700
150	112.5	150	187.5	225	300	375	450	525	600	750
160	120	160	200	240	320	400	480	560	640	800
170	127.5	170	212.5	255	340	425	510	595	680	850
180	135	180	225	270	360	450	540	630	720	900
200	150	200	250	300	400	500	600	700	800	1000
220	165	220	275	330	440	550	660	770	880	1100
240	180	240	300	360	480	600	720	840	960	1200

General Dosage Guidelines for New Patients

- There is no such thing as a one-size-fits-all dosing recommendation.

- Consult your physician or health professional and listen closely to his or her recommendation. Discuss the information contained in this book and your own individual needs and preferences. This important decision should be a collaboration between the two of you.

- Decide the form in which you prefer to take your cannabis medication. Cannabis products are available in oils, tinctures, sprays, capsules, edibles, vaporizers, flowers, and other products. This topic is discussed in Chapter 3.

- Find your optimum ratio of CBD:THC. Cannabis products have varying amounts of the two most important cannabinoids, CBD and THC. They can be categorized by the ratio of CBD to THC (usually written as CBD:THC, but sometimes as THC:CBD). Find the proper combination to optimize your therapeutic use of cannabis. In Part II of this book, we discuss the current "best understanding" of optimal CBD:THC ratios to treat specific disorders. Find a product that contains the right balance for your condition. If you're not sure what to choose, start with very high-CBD products (which contain little or no mind-altering THC). You can always introduce THC later and see how you respond to it.

- Choose the strain or chemotype that is likely to give the best outcome. There are more than one thousand strains available. Look for lab results on any product that you're considering, and look especially for cannabinoid and terpene levels. Strains are sometimes identified as only "sativa" or "indica," which doesn't give enough information. Look for products that identify the potency of CBD and THC in mg/ml or percent. Strains and potency are discussed in detail in Part IV.

- Don't overdo it. In cannabis therapy, we often find that "less is more." If you are not getting the desired effects, even though you've tried raising your dose, try lowering your dose instead. This has helped many people find their "sweet spot," the best dose range for their particular condition and that period of time. Remember, the sweet spot can move over time. You have to continue to monitor yourself and adjust as necessary.

- Be aware of possible side effects and drug interactions. See more on this later in this chapter.

- Proceed cautiously, especially if you have a history of alcohol or drug abuse or mental illness, or are pregnant or breastfeeding.

WHEN HIGH DOSES ARE REQUIRED: OPTIONS FOR TITRATING UP THC WHILE MINIMIZING IMPAIRMENT

- For oral applications, start off with a lower dose of the 1:1 ratio and increase the dose every 3–4 days. The body has an ability to adjust and acclimate, and, after 4–6 weeks, patients will be able to tolerate very high doses without as many psychoactive side effects.

  or

- Start off with macro doses of CBD 20:1 for oral applications. The body is able to handle large amounts of CBD without psychoactive side effects. After the body builds a tolerance to CBD, slowly introduce THC, working up through a 4:1 and ultimately toward a 1:1 level.

  or

- Take lower doses of THC in the daytime when you might be driving or working. This can be accomplished with reduced doses or using high-ratio CBD products. Then, in the evening, before sleeping, use a stronger 1:1 ratio with more THC (generally indica or sedating-dominant strains are recommended).

  or

- Take high-dose 1:1 CBD:THC medicine as a rectal suppository, preferably 2–3 times a day. THC taken rectally at high doses does not cause psychoactive side effects for most people. Some approaches to treating cancer advocate this method, though more research is needed to address best practices for specific cancer types.

- Use large doses of the raw plant, high in THCA (as THCA shares many similarities with THC without producing any psychoactive impairment).

Tolerance

When a person uses cannabis over time—from a few months to a few years—the body gets acclimated to the medicine, and it can build up a tolerance. Many people find that they have to slowly raise their use level in order to maintain the same level of medicinal effect. Some people reach a "maximum effect," when increasing the dose does not increase the effect. Heavy use of cannabis desensitizes the CB1 receptors in the brain and nervous system. This can be a good thing for those fighting cancer or other diseases that require macro dose protocols, especially if they want to build up their tolerance to high levels of THC. For those who want to restore their earlier sensitivity, a few solutions are available:

- Take a tolerance break. Stop ingesting cannabis for a three days or a week, every three months or so. There should be no impact from this "tolerance fast" because cannabinoids are stored in the fat tissues, which the body utilizes when the outside supply is cut off. Once those stored supplies are used up, tolerance usually goes back down and the endocannabinoid system is "reset."

- Lower your dose level considerably and then slowly build it back up again.

- Switch strains. Each strain has a completely different cannabinoid profile. If you have several different strains that you rotate through, it's likely that you won't develop tolerance. This is often the best solution.*

The Biphasic Effect

The word *biphasic* simply means "two phases." Cannabis compounds have biphasic properties, which means that, as dose increases, the effects do not necessarily improve. In fact, a higher dose can actually produce the opposite effect. In general, small doses of cannabis tend to stimulate the body, and large doses tend to sedate it. Too much THC can amplify anxiety, paranoia, or mood disorders. Too much CBD could be less effective therapeutically than a moderate dose. "Less is more" is often the case with cannabis therapeutics.

---

*For more information about tolerance breaks, see www.whaxy.com/learn/cannabis-tolerance-break.

If a specific dose stops working, try lowering the dose, rather than increasing it, or changing the strain.

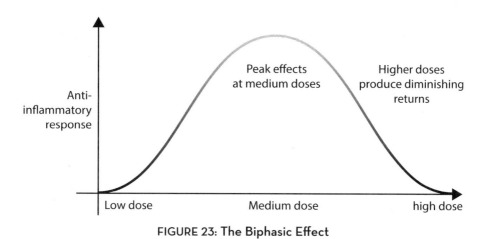

FIGURE 23: The Biphasic Effect

Cautions, Side Effects, and Drug Interactions

CBD has very few known adverse side effects at any dose. THC in high doses can make a person feel very weird for a while, but there are no known fatalities from overdosing on cannabis, as there are for many pharmaceutical drugs.

Many studies prove the effectiveness of CBD treatment of various conditions, and most conclude that it is safe and virtually free of side effects. A 2011 review paper concluded that, although further testing is needed, controlled cannabidiol administration appears to be relatively safe and nontoxic in humans and animals, without affecting food intake or physiological parameters like heart rate, body temperature, or blood pressure. According to the research review, high doses of up to 1,500 mg/day of CBD seem to be well tolerated in humans.[153]

Cannabis products containing THC, the compound responsible for the "high" associated with cannabis, have more contraindications and cautions associated with them. We will cover these below as well, since most products contain at least a small amount of THC, and some have higher ratios. It's important to note that, while most people do not experience the side effects associated with THC when taking CBD-dominant products (defined in this book as 20:1 ratio or higher), *some patients may be sensitive to small amounts.* For this reason, it is recommended to always start with a micro dose and go up from there until symptoms subside.

Keep in mind that all cannabinoids are **nontoxic, non-lethal medicine.** Researchers have failed to find a lethal acute dosage of cannabis and have found that the doses of long-term cannabis required to produce toxicity and death in animals were so high it would be nearly impossible for a human to consume such quantities via ingestion or inhalation.

Cautions and Side Effects

CBD and other plant cannabinoids can potentially interact with many pharmaceuticals, decreasing their effectiveness by inhibiting the activity of cytochrome P450, a family of liver enzymes. This key enzyme group metabolizes many commonly prescribed medications (see more in the Drug Interactions section in Chapter 3).

Most medications list a range of potential adverse side effects, and some of those lists are quite horrifying. The most commonly reported side effects of cannabis (mostly associated with high amounts of THC) are dizziness, dry mouth, nausea, fatigue, sleepiness, euphoria, depression, vomiting, diarrhea, disorientation, anxiety, confusion, impaired balance, impaired short-term memory, hallucination, and paranoia. Most people report that cannabis temporarily lowers body temperature slightly, though some report the contrary effect—we discuss more on this bidirectional quality of cannabinoids later in this section.

Cannabis strains that are high in THC can temporarily raise the heart rate for fifteen to twenty minutes. This condition, called tachycardia, subsides on its own, and does so faster when the patient stays calm. Indica strains appear to cause less tachycardia effects than sativa strains. CBD does not have this effect, and there is evidence that CBD is of benefit to patients with certain heart conditions. It is currently being studied for use in treating atherosclerosis, clogging of the arteries, which leads to cardiovascular disease.

Driving while using high-THC cannabis has been shown to significantly increase the risk of accidents, especially in new users. While CBD is not usually associated with these risks, it is advisable to avoid driving or using heavy machinery when starting the medication or adjusting the dose. Use caution when taking any cannabis medicine until you have sufficient experience with the medication that you feel comfortable engaging in activities.

Drinking alcohol while using cannabis-based products is **not** recommended. The combination of alcohol and cannabinoids can cause dizziness, drowsiness, and impaired judgment. In addition, cannabis products can increase the side effects of other drowsiness-causing drugs, including antidepressants, antihistamines, sedatives, pain relievers, anxiety medicines, seizure medicines, and muscle relaxants.

Some research shows that heavy chronic use of high-THC products can cause a short-term decrease in concentration levels, memory, and certain types of thinking and decision making. Most results showed that these effects are no longer significant after a few weeks of cessation, though some research demonstrated a long-term impact with adolescent onset of heavy use (see more on adolescent use later in this section).[154]

BIDIRECTIONAL EFFECT

Many of the adverse effects reported are curiously the same as the symptoms that can be relieved by cannabis. This interesting phenomenon, known as the bidirectional effect, is related to the function of the endocannabinoid system. Because its role is connected to the maintenance of homeostasis, or cellular balance, it has the capacity to influence physiology in opposite directions depending on dose, individual body chemistry, and other factors. For example, a small minority of individuals tends to report the opposite of the majority in terms of the effect of a particular cannabinoid on appetite, mood, body temperature, or sleep.

"By over stimulating the ECS [endocannabinoid system], patients can accidentally trigger or worsen the same symptoms cannabis would otherwise relieve when used correctly," reports Dustin Sulak, a licensed osteopathic physician with experience in cannabinoid medicine.[155]

For this reason, it is essential that you follow dosage recommendations from your physician, combined with suggestions in this book, and start any new cannabinoid-based product at micro dose levels to test for sensitivity.

POTENTIAL RISKS

When heavily and chronically smoked or vaporized, cannabis may cause irritation to the lungs and an increased risk of developing chronic bronchitis.

Cannabis smoke has *not* been definitively linked to cancer in humans, including those cancers associated with tobacco use. While it contains many of the same carcinogens as tobacco smoke, including greater concentrations of certain aromatic hydrocarbons such as benzopyrene, it is also high in cannabinoids that demonstrate anti-cancer properties. By contrast, nicotine promotes the development of cancer cells and their blood supply.

In addition, cannabinoids stimulate other biological activities and responses that may mitigate the carcinogenic effects of smoke, such as down-regulating the inflammatory arm of the immune system that is responsible for producing potentially carcinogenic free radicals.[156]

Cannabis vaporization limits respiratory toxins by heating cannabis to a temperature where cannabinoid vapors form but below the point of combustion where noxious smoke and associated toxins occur. See more on p. 49 regarding vaporization and choosing the safest products.

Dependence/addiction: Cannabis use does not carry the risk of physical addiction as most narcotics do. However, it has been shown that cannabis with high levels of THC has the potential for emotional or mental dependence.[157] It is likely (though not proven by research) that appropriate medical use within recommended dosage guidelines does not carry the risk of dependence.

High-THC products can cause withdrawal symptoms when abruptly stopped, including irritability, aggression, decreased appetite, anxiety, restlessness, and sleep difficulties. These symptoms emerge a few days after cannabis cessation and resolve in one to two weeks. Patients have compared the severity of cannabis withdrawal to caffeine withdrawal. CBD has not been associated with these risks according to the most recent research available at press time. In fact, CBD has been shown to be effective in treating nicotine, alcohol, and other drug addictions. Opponents of cannabis use the old propaganda claim that it is a "gateway drug" leading to addiction to harder drugs like methamphetamine and heroin. From our research and experience, CBD can function as a gateway *out of addiction,* not into it[158] (see more about addiction on p. 90).

Contraindications

While CBD products may have therapeutic value for the conditions described in this section, before using products containing more than a minimum amount of THC (approximately 5 mg), consult a physician if you have been diagnosed with or are at high risk of developing any of the following disorders:

- Schizophrenia, bipolar disorder, severe depression
- Heart disease, high blood pressure, angina, or arrhythmia
- Immune or autoimmune disorder

PREGNANCY AND BREASTFEEDING

See Chapter 5 for cautions and information regarding women's health issues.

YOUTH AND ADOLESCENCE

Caution is advised when using products containing THC to treat children, adolescents, and young adults. The effect of THC on the developing brain is different from its effect on the adult brain, and, though there are clearly cases where its use is medically necessary and justified, monitoring dose is essential, and a physician should be consulted before use. Products containing alternative cannabinoids to THC, such as CBD and THCA, are recommended for people under the age of twenty-two[159] (see specific health entries in Chapter 4 for details on treating young people with CBD-dominant products).

Adolescents who use THC are at higher risk for dependence than older users, and a number of studies have looked for correlations between use of high-THC marijuana and reduced academic performance or IQ scores. Some studies have found these links, especially with "heavy use" defined as five or more joints a week, though the effect on global intelligence was not measurable in the long term.[160] Two studies have cited decreased intellectual functioning and loss of brain volume in specific regions of the brain with daily cannabis use in adolescents and adults.[161,162] Despite being criticized for ignoring socioeconomic status and ongoing alcohol use and abuse, these studies have been cited in legislation in states that restrict medical cannabis use.

In a more recent study done at the University of Colorado in 2015, researchers matched both adult and adolescent daily cannabis users and non-users and screened for alcohol and tobacco use, depression, anxiety, impulsivity, sensation seeking, and education. They compared sophisticated brain imaging showing the brain volumes in areas cited as shrinking in the previous studies and found no difference in the structure, volume, or shape of any of the targeted regions or any other regions of the brain.[163] A 2016 study involving more than 2,200 students concluded that, when factors such as tobacco use are controlled, modest cannabis use in teenagers may have less cognitive impact than epidemiological surveys of previous cohorts have suggested.[164]

Other research has linked heavy use of high-THC cannabis in adolescents to a higher chance of developing schizophrenia.[165] The author of a 2016 study wrote: "Adolescence is a critical period of brain development, and the adolescent brain is particularly vulnerable. Health policy makers need to ensure that marijuana, especially marijuana strains with high THC levels, stays out of the hands of teenagers. In contrast, our findings suggest that adult use of marijuana does not pose substantial risk."[166]

OVERDOSING ON THC?

The most common type of accidental cannabis overdose is related to consuming cannabis edibles. It is reassuring to know that even incredibly high doses of cannabis do not produce brain damage, organ damage, or other types of physical toxicity, although they can cause delirium and hallucinations. These effects will pass, normally within three to eight hours. Use of a cytochrome P450 deactivator, such as CBD, or grapefruit, can reduce unwanted effects of a THC overdose. To ease your mind, in five thousand years of recorded history, there are no records of anyone dying from an overdose of cannabis or THC.

Drug Interactions

CBD, when ingested orally at sufficient doses, temporarily alters the activity of cytochrome P450, a family of liver enzymes. This potentially affects the body's metabolism of a wide range of compounds—even to 60 percent of commonly prescribed pharmaceuticals. The issue is that CBD is metabolized by cytochrome P450 enzymes, occupying the site of enzymatic activity and preventing it from metabolizing other compounds. Interestingly, components of grapefruit can have the same effect, leading some physicians to advise against consuming it when taking certain drugs.

"The extent to which cannabidiol behaves as a competitive inhibitor of cytochrome P450 depends on how tightly CBD binds to the active site of the metabolic enzyme before and after oxidation," writes Adrian Devitt-Lee, a researcher at Project CBD who has studied the topic of drug interactions extensively. "This can change greatly, depending on how—and how much— CBD is administered, the unique attributes of the individual taking this medication, and whether isolated CBD or a whole-plant remedy is used."[167] This means that patients ingesting CBD products should pay close attention to changes in blood levels of important drugs in their protocol and adjust dosage accordingly under a doctor's supervision.

Devitt-Lee points out that, in cancer treatment, the precise dosing of chemotherapy is extremely important, and the goal is often to reach the maximum dose that will not be catastrophically toxic. For patients using CBD, *the same dose of chemotherapy may produce higher blood concentrations of the chemo drugs.* If CBD inhibits the cytochrome-mediated metabolism of the chemotherapy and dosage adjustments aren't made, the chemotherapy agent could accumulate within the body to highly toxic levels.

That being said, adverse cannabinoid-drug interactions have rarely been reported among the many cancer patients who use cannabis to cope with the wrenching side effects of chemotherapy. It is possible that whole-plant cannabis, with its rich compensatory synergies, interacts differently from the isolated CBD that is administered in most research settings. As well, the cytoprotective effects of the cannabinoids may mitigate some of the chemotherapeutic toxicity.

In epilepsy patients, CBD has been shown to elevate the plasma levels and increase the long-term blood concentrations of clobazam, an anticonvulsant, and norclobazam, an active metabolite of this medication. A majority of these patients needed to have their dose of clobazam reduced due to side effects. A 2015 report concluded that CBD is safe and effective for treatment of refractory epilepsy in patients receiving clobazam, but emphasized the importance of monitoring blood levels for clobazam and norclobazam in patients using both CBD and clobazam.[168]

Other research has suggested that CBD can amplify the activity of certain cytochrome P450 enzymes. This evidence suggests that CBD can either increase or decrease the breakdown of other drugs, depending on the drug in question and the dosages used.[169]

"Drug interactions are especially important to consider when using life-saving or sense-saving drugs, drugs with narrow therapeutic windows, or medications with major adverse side effects," Devitt-Lee reports. "In particular, those patients who utilize high doses of CBD concentrates and isolates should keep these factors in mind when mixing remedies."[170]

Note that the list below does not necessarily contain every medication that could be affected by CBD, and not every medication in each of the categories listed will cause an interaction. For this reason, consult a medical professional before taking any combination of drugs at the same time, as alternative medications or dosage adjustments may be required. "If you are worried that your cytochrome P450 enzyme system may not be functioning properly," Devitt-Lee writes, "physicians can test the system to ensure that the medications you take are metabolizing as expected."[171]

Drugs that use the cytochrome P450 system include[172]:

- Steroids
- HMG CoA reductase inhibitors
- Calcium channel blockers
- Antihistamines
- Prokinetics
- HIV antivirals
- Immune modulators
- Benzodiazepines
- Anti-arrythmics
- Antibiotics
- Anesthetics
- Antipsychotics
- Antidepressants
- Anti-epileptics
- Beta blockers
- PPIs
- NSAIDs
- Angiotension II blockers
- Oral hypoglycemic agents
- Sulfonylureas

The Subjective-Intuitive Approach
to Medicinal Cannabis

Although it is always ideal to consult a doctor for diagnosis and guidance, the fact is that very few practitioners are skilled in the nuances of cannabis therapy, strain selection, CBD:THC ratio selection, and dose guidance (which are reasons we decided to write this book). In addition, each person has a distinct body weight and chemistry as well as a unique sensitivity or tolerance to cannabinoids. These factors combine with an individual's ever-changing dietary and pharmaceutical intake and hormone and emotional stress levels. One's total-body makeup is a moving target, and cannabis therapy can be subtly adjusted each time one medicates, in line with intuitive information about what is best at that moment.

Consult an experienced health care practitioner when possible; however, without tuning in to what the body is communicating, you risk giving power to someone who does not have the skill or knowledge to make informed decisions about what may be best for you. While many people may not feel confident in their own intuitive skills, it is our experience that cannabis helps open the door to this information, facilitating communication on all levels. The body is an intelligent and complex organism and has the ability to communicate what it needs to attain health, balance, and wholeness. See the Epilogue at the end of this book for a guided exercise in connecting to the medicine intuitively.

Each patient should listen to his or her own body's response to discover his or her own optimum delivery method, strain of cannabis medicine, and therapeutic window for dosing. A dose that is too small is suboptimal and may have no noticeable effect, while too much can actually increase the symptoms one is trying to treat. For example, cannabis can be used to reduce stress and anxiety, producing a state of calm relaxation. However, if too much is used, it can actually increase stress, causing more anxiety and the feeling of apprehension or even paranoia. This is the biphasic aspect of cannabis. Establishing one's own subjective-intuitive therapeutic window is governed by three things: the body's present endocannabinoid state of balance or deficiency, the cannabinoid profile in the medicine to be taken, and the form in which it is to be consumed.[173]

All life has consciousness, and all life is connected. This is the premise we operate on when crafting and offering our cannabis medicines at Synergy Wellness. In addition, we believe that the body is an intelligent organism, and it has the power to balance and heal itself. Our holistic view is that CBD allows and actually enhances the body's self-healing capacity. It accomplishes this marvel through the endocannabinoid system, facilitating balance in the physical, mental, emotional, and spiritual realms. Cannabis can help activate your ability to access your intuition and tap into your subjective (or Universal) knowledge base, so you can determine the specific dose and strain you need in this moment.

To illustrate this point, let's use pain as an example. Why is there pain in your body? Since the body is an intelligent and conscious organism, your body must be trying to communicate something to your awareness. It is trying to get your attention, saying, "Something is wrong, or out of balance. I need some help here." When it sends pain signals, it wants a response from you. If it does not get an adequate response, the signals get louder, and the pain gets worse. The Universe presents us with important lessons to learn. If we don't learn them adequately, the lessons get more intense, and so do the consequences.

Most doctors recommend a pharmaceutical approach to pain, employing opioid medication. Opioids accomplish pain control by deadening the pain receptors and dulling the pain signals traveling to the brain. This essentially, and temporarily, "kills the messenger." Your ability to detect the pain may stop, but there are often severe side effects. In many cases, opioids do not work very well, especially as your tolerance to the medication builds. Consequently, opioids are often overused, and long-term use is often addicting. There are times when an opioid is the perfect solution to the problem. They are not always bad. However, opioids do not actually heal the underlying cause of the problem. They treat the symptom of pain by cutting off the signal and message that something is wrong. They function as a tool to be used at certain times, but not as a foundation for the healing process.

Instead of shutting down the communication system of the body, as opioids do, cannabis actually increases cellular communication, bringing more awareness to the underlying cause of the problem. First, it takes the edge off the pain. It is an analgesic and antispasmodic, allowing the muscles to relax so the body doesn't contract in reaction to the pain. Second, it is anti-inflammatory, reducing swelling, which is often one of the causes of the pain. Third, it increases the overall healing process, allowing vital energy to reach the distressed area, relax the overall system, and enhance your awareness of health and wholeness.

Over fifty years ago, a foolish accident in college left me with a crushed vertebra, and multiple skiing accidents resulted in a severely compromised knee and a weak lower back. Twenty years ago, my orthopedic surgeon recommended a knee replacement to address the degeneration of my medial meniscus and the tear in my ACL. Instead, I used cannabis to manage the knee pain and avoid replacement surgery. In addition, cannabis stimulated my intuition, which guides me toward the best exercises for my condition and how to treat flare-ups of inflammation when they occur.

At seventy-four years of age, I am still able to ski, and I take weekly mountain bike rides that climb 1,000 feet up our local mountain, Mount Tamalpais, to the beautiful lakes near the top. Cannabis has allowed me to manage my health by listening to my body's intelligence. I do strengthening exercises to maintain my health, and, when an incident occurs that causes inflammation, my intuition guides me to the right actions immediately. At times, this includes the use of ice or a back or knee brace, and sometimes complete rest is indicated, using the sacred plant cannabis to heal the injury.

I have been privileged to participate in the healing journey of many patients. From this experience, I have learned that cannabis can be combined with other healing modalities, including Western medical approaches, and others that spring from the patient's own internal guidance system. Many people find that visualization of positive outcomes speeds their healing, reducing inflammation and increasing the flow of healing energy to the affected parts of the body. Where attention goes, energy flows. This can enhance the effect of any medication, and the body seems to respond more quickly.

Healing is a process that takes place on many levels at once—physical, mental, emotional, and spiritual. Practices such as meditation, Tai Chi, yoga, and deep breathing can help reduce stress and anxiety. Walking in nature, listening to music, and inspirational reading have healing effects. Love and joy are two of the greatest healing energies to bring to your healing process, and your intuition may guide you to a specific kind of medicine or a particular practitioner who can help you. All of these healing modalities work together in a synergistic way, which is one of the reasons our business name is Synergy Wellness.

I wish you well on your healing journey toward your optimum health. You have my best wishes and support as you walk your path.

LEONARD LEINOW

NOTE For updates to this chapter, visit www.CBD-book.com/Updates.

PART II

CBD for Health Concerns

The ancient doctors and healers across the globe who prescribed cannabis thousands of years ago did so because they witnessed its medical benefits firsthand. In the last half century, modern science has begun to shed light on the biological processes behind the healing, where plant and animal chemistry work in concert. The body of research on CBD, THC, and other cannabinoids has grown exponentially in the past decade. The following brings together the latest scientific studies and stories from patients and doctors with advice on treating specific symptoms. It also includes dosage suggestions and information on recommended types of cannabinoid-based medicines for the particular condition.

A 2016 opinion statement from the authors of a study on cannabinoids and gastrointestinal disorders summarizes the current climate and calls for action from the medical community to bring cannabis-based medicine into line with our current understanding of neurochemistry.

Despite the political and social controversy affiliated with it, the medical community must come to the realization that cannabinoids exist as a ubiquitous signaling system in many organ systems. Our understanding of cannabinoids and how they relate not only to homeostasis but also in disease states must be furthered through research, both clinically and in the laboratory.[174]

The words of these scientists convey the significance of the endocannabinoid system, first identified by Raphael Mechoulam in the mid-1990s and possibly one of the most important recent discoveries about the endogenous chemical transmitters involved in maintaining health. Endogenous (created naturally within the body) cannabinoids and their receptors are found not just in the brain but also in many organs as well as connective tissue, skin, glands, and immune cells (see much more on this in the section contributed by Dr. Michael Moskowitz on the endocannabinoid system in Chapter 2). The list of health concerns treatable by CBD is so long because these receptors are integral to so many bodily systems. This is also the reason cannabinoids can be used as a general preventative medicine, protecting the body against the damages of stress and aging.

CBD as Preventative Medicine

Cannabinoid therapy is connected to the part of the biological matrix where body and brain meet. Since CBD and other compounds in cannabis are so similar to the chemicals created by our own bodies, they are integrated better than many synthetic drugs. According to Bradley E. Alger, a leading scientist in the study of endocannabinoids with a PhD from Harvard in experimental psychology, "With complex actions in our immune system, nervous system, and virtually all of the body's organs, the endocannabinoids are literally a bridge between body and mind. By understanding this system, we begin to see a mechanism that could connect brain activity and states of physical health and disease."[175]

Reduced Risk of Diabetes and Obesity

Several studies have shown that regular cannabis users have a lower body mass index, smaller waist circumferences, and reduced risk of diabetes and obesity. One 2011 report published in the *American Journal of Epidemiology*, based on a survey of more than fifty-two thousand participants, concluded that rates of obesity are about one-third lower among cannabis users.[176] This is despite the findings that participants tend to consume more calories per day, an activity that is potentially related to THC's stimulation of ghrelin, a hormone that increases appetite but also increases the metabolism of carbohydrates. CBD on its own was shown in 2006 to lower the incidence of diabetes in lab rats,[177] and in 2015 an Israeli-American biopharmaceutical collective began stage 2 trials related to using CBD to treat diabetes.[178] Research has demonstrated that CBD helps the body convert white fat into weight-reducing brown fat, promoting normal insulin production and sugar metabolism.[179]

In studying over 4,600 test subjects, researchers found that current cannabis users had fasting insulin levels that were up to 16 percent lower than their non-using counterparts, higher levels of HDL cholesterol that protects against diabetes, and 17 percent lower levels of insulin resistance. Respondents who had used cannabis in their lifetime but were not current users showed similar but less pronounced associations, indicating that the protective effect of cannabis fades with time.[180]

Excess insulin promotes the conversion of sugars into stored fat and leads to weight gain and obesity. The research emerging about the interplay between cannabinoids and insulin regulation may lead to some major breakthroughs in the prevention of obesity and type 2 diabetes.

Better Cholesterol Profiles and Lowered Risk of Cardiovascular Disease

A 2013 study that measured data from 4,652 participants on the effect of cannabis on metabolic systems compared non-users to current and former users. It found that current users had higher blood levels of high-density lipoprotein (HDL-C) or "good cholesterol." The same year, an analysis of over seven hundred members of Canada's Inuit community found that, on average, regular cannabis users had increased levels of HDL-C and slightly lower levels of LDL-C ("bad cholesterol").

Linked to diet and lifestyle, atherosclerosis is common in developed Western nations and can lead to heart disease or stroke. It is a chronic inflammatory disorder involving the progressive depositing of atherosclerotic plaques (immune cells carrying oxidized LDL or low-density lipoproteins). A growing body of evidence suggests that endocannabinoid signaling plays a critical role in the pathology of atherogenesis.[181] The condition is now understood to be a physical response to injuries in the arterial walls' lining, caused by high blood pressure, infectious microbes, or excessive presence of an amino acid called homocysteine. Studies have demonstrated that inflammatory molecules stimulate the cycle leading to atherosclerotic lesions.[182] Existing treatments are moderately effective though carry numerous side effects. CB2 receptors triple in response to inflammation, allowing anandamide and 2-AG, the body's natural cannabinoids, to decrease inflammatory responses. The CB2 receptor is also stimulated by plant-based cannabinoids.[183]

A 2005 animal trial showed that low-dose oral cannabinoids slowed the progression of atherosclerosis. Researchers the following year wrote that the immunomodulatory capacity of cannabinoids was "well established" in science and suggested they had a broad therapeutic potential for a variety of conditions, including atherosclerosis.[184]

A 2007 animal study with CBD showed it had a cardio-protective effect during heart attacks,[185] and more details were published that year about the involvement of the CB1 and CB2 receptors in cardiovascular illness and health.[186]

Reduced Risk of Cancer

The use of CBD to treat cancer is discussed in Chapter 4, but could cannabidiol help prevent tumors and other cancers before they grow? A 2012 study showed that animals treated with CBD were significantly less likely to develop colon cancer after being induced with carcinogens in a laboratory.[187] Several studies had already shown that THC prevents tumors and reduces them, including one in 1996 on animal models that found that it decreased the incidence of both benign and hepatic adenoma tumors.[188] In 2015, scientists analyzed the medical records of over eighty-four thousand male patients in California and found that those who used cannabis, but not tobacco, had a rate of bladder cancer that was 45 percent below the norm.[189] Topical products can be used to treat and prevent skin cancers. Continuing research is focused on the best ratio of CBD to THC and the most effective dose level in cancer prevention and treatment.

Cannabinoids Help Maintain Brain Health and Create Resilience to Trauma and Degeneration

Cannabinoids are neuroprotective, meaning that they help maintain and regulate brain health. The effects appear to be related to several actions they have on the brain, including the removal of damaged cells and the improved efficiency of mitochondria.[190] CBD and other antioxidant compounds in cannabis also work to reduce glutamate toxicity. Extra glutamate, which stimulates nerve cells in the brain to fire, causes cells to become over-stimulated, ultimately leading to cell damage or death. Thus, cannabinoids help protect brain cells from damage, keeping the organ healthy and functioning properly. CBD has also been shown to have an anti-inflammatory effect on the brain.[191]

As the brain ages, the creation of new neurons slows down significantly. In order to maintain brain health and prevent degenerative diseases, new cells need to be continuously created. A 2008 study showed that low doses of CBD- and THC-like cannabinoids encouraged the creation of new nerve cells in animal models, even in aging brains.[192] CBD also helps prevent other nerve-related diseases like neuropathy and Alzheimer's disease.

Protects against Bone Disease and Broken Bones

Cannabinoids are facilitative of the process of bone metabolism—the cycle in which old bone material is replaced by new at a rate of about 10 percent per year, crucial to maintaining strong, healthy bones over time. CBD in particular has been shown to block an enzyme that destroys bone-building compounds in the body, reducing the risk of age-related bone diseases like osteoporosis and osteoarthritis. In both of those diseases, the body is no longer creating new bone and cartilage cells. CBD helps spur the process of new bone-cell formation, which is why it has been found to speed the healing of broken bones and, due to a stronger fracture callus, decrease the likelihood of re-fracturing the bone (bones are 35–50 percent stronger than those of non-treated subjects).[193]

Protects and Heals the Skin

The skin has the highest amount and concentration of CB2 receptors in the body. When applied topically as an infused lotion, serum, oil, or salve, the antioxidants in CBD (a more powerful antioxidant than vitamins E and C)[194] can repair damage from free radicals like UV rays and environmental pollutants. Cannabinoid receptors can be found in the skin and seem to be connected to the regulation of oil production in the sebaceous glands.[195] Cannabis-based topical products are being developed to treat related issues from acne to psoriasis and can promote faster healing of damaged skin. In fact, historical documents show that cannabis preparations have been used for wound healing in both animals and people in a range of cultures spanning the globe and going back thousands of years. The use of concentrated cannabis oils to treat skin cancer is gaining popularity with a number of well-documented cases of people curing both melanoma and carcinoma-type skin cancers with the topical application of CBD and THC products. Best known is the case of Rick Simpson, who cured his basal cell carcinoma with cannabis oil and now has a widely distributed line of products. Cannabis applied topically is not psychoactive.

Anti-inflammatory

Cannabinoids have been proven to have an anti-inflammatory effect in numerous studies.[196] CBD engages with the endocannabinoid system in many organs throughout the body, helping to reduce inflammation systemically. The therapeutic potential is impressively wide-ranging, as inflammation is involved in a broad spectrum of diseases.

NOTE *For updates to this chapter, visit www.CBD-book.com/Updates.*

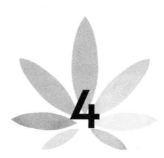

Alphabetized List of Health Issues

Note on the Cannabis Health Index Rating System

Simply put, the Cannabis Health Index (CHI) score is derived from an evidence-based rating system developed by Uwe Blesching that shows degrees of confidence in cannabis (in general, not broken down by specific cannabinoids such as CBD) as an effective treatment for a specific condition. It takes the type and caliber of the research study into account, which impacts the reliability of a study's conclusions. Each experiment is scored on a scale of 1 to 5 based on type of study, and then this number is multiplied by +1 (positive one) if the study concluded that medical use of cannabis was effective, or multiplied by -1 (negative one) if the study concluded it was ineffective as treatment for that disorder. Finally, all the ratings for individual studies included in the analysis of a disease are added together to create an overall CHI score. An overall high score means a large amount of high-caliber research has been done and that the probability of efficacy for that disorder is higher based on currently available evidence. However, the score reflects the amount of available published research to a much larger extent than it reflects the actual degree of efficacy to treat the particular disease.

Evidence-Based Ratings of Possible CHI Scores

STUDY DESIGN	EVIDENCE-BASED RATING OF POSSIBLE CHI SCORES
Double-blind, placebo-controlled, clinical, and crossover human trials	+/–5
Clinical human trials and cohort studies	+/–4
Reviews of relevant literature and studies and human case studies	+/–3
Animal studies	+/-2
Laboratory studies	+/–1

The ratings are on a scale of zero to five with zero indicating no observed therapeutic value and five indicating significant and demonstrably scientific therapeutic value. The CHI score is the total value points of each study divided by the number of studies conducted for that condition.

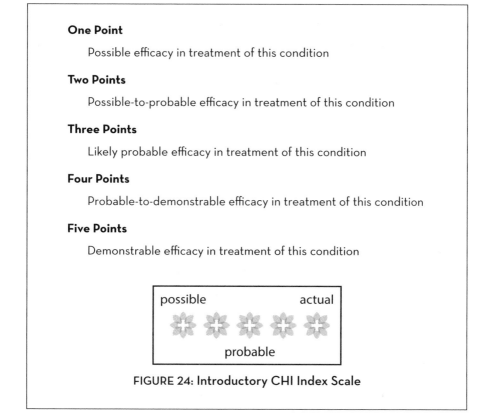

One Point

Possible efficacy in treatment of this condition

Two Points

Possible-to-probable efficacy in treatment of this condition

Three Points

Likely probable efficacy in treatment of this condition

Four Points

Probable-to-demonstrable efficacy in treatment of this condition

Five Points

Demonstrable efficacy in treatment of this condition

FIGURE 24: Introductory CHI Index Scale

ADHD
(Attention Deficit Hyperactivity Disorder)

ADHD (also known as ADD or hyperkinetic disorder) is characterized by difficulty focusing on tasks and excessive activity, and is the most commonly diagnosed developmental disorder in children and adolescents. It also affects 2–5 percent of adults. Controversy is related to both diagnosing and treating ADHD, which is often managed through a combination of behavioral therapy and pharmaceutical stimulants. ADHD patients are broken into subtypes: hyperactive-impulsive, predominantly inattentive, and combined.

ADHD is said to be a risk factor for addiction, including problematic high-THC cannabis use.[197] However, cannabis has been shown to reduce the symptoms of the disorder, and, when properly dosed and administered safely, CBD-dominant strains show promising results. While most people react to stimulants by becoming more energetic, ADHD brains have the opposite reaction—stimulants calm them down. Most other drugs for these disorders work by making dopamine more available in the brain, which helps to regulate behavior and focus attention. However, these drugs have negative side effects, especially when given to children, and the long-term benefits of their use are in question. More research is needed, but limited studies and anecdotal evidence suggest that the dopamine deficiency observed in ADHD patients can be balanced through cannabinoid therapy. High-CBD medicines may allow for more focus and concentration without the psychoactivity, although some studies have also shown benefit from THC for these patients, even enhancing their driving performance.[198]

Dr. David Bearman, a major figure in cannabis research, has forty years of experience working on substance abuse programs and was a member of Ronald Reagan's drug abuse task force. He has studied the relationship between the cannabinoid system and ADHD and discovered potential therapeutic value as cannabinoids interact with the brain's dopamine management systems.

"Cannabis appears to treat ADD and ADHD by increasing the availability of dopamine," Bearman states. "This then has the same effect but is a different mechanism of action than stimulants like Ritalin (methylphenidate) and Dexedrine amphetamine, which act by binding to the dopamine and interfering with the metabolic breakdown of dopamine."

"The most accepted theory about ADHD rests on the fact that about 70 percent of the brain's function is to regulate input to the other 30 percent," Bearman says. "Basically the brain is overwhelmed with too much information coming too fast. In ADHD, the brain is cluttered with and too aware of all the nuances of a person's daily experience."[199]

How to Take the Medicine: Dosage and Delivery

It is suggested that patients work with a health care practitioner experienced in recommending CBD or medicinal cannabis so that dosage and delivery methods can be developed and fine-tuned on an individual basis. At the same time, educated and aware patients can be their own highly informed health consultants (see p. 75 for information about the subjective-intuitive approach to using cannabis-based medicines).

For all orally administered medicines, refer to the dosage tables on pp. 61–63 for guidelines on CBD dosage by body weight. The dose level should be between the **micro and standard ranges.** Always start with the micro dose to test sensitivity and go up as needed within the dosing range by body weight until symptoms subside.

In treating ADHD in young people, it is recommended to use drops or edibles containing strains with a very high CBD:THC ratio such as 24:1. For children, CBD oil infusions, glycerin tinctures, sublingual products, or pure CO2–extracted concentrates are recommended (no alcohol tinctures). The oil can be given straight or mixed with yogurt or other food. Concentrates are more appropriate when higher doses are needed and can also be mixed with food, such as applesauce or nut butters, or made into capsules.

Adults can take any of the above, as well as alcohol-based tinctures, capsules, and other edibles.

More information about various forms of delivery (e.g., sublingual, edible, inhaled) for cannabinoid-based medication can be found starting on p. 38).

Varieties high in pinene and terpinolene, without high levels of myrcene, are suggested for ADHD. When hyperactivity is more of an issue, higher levels of myrcene and linalool may be calming.[200]

Effectiveness: Current Science—ADHD

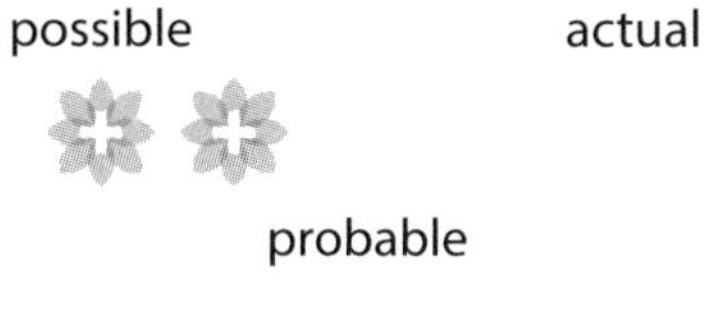

possible   actual

probable

FIGURE 25

The Cannabis Health Index (CHI) is an evidence-based scoring system for cannabis (in general, not just CBD) and its effectiveness on various health issues based on currently available research data. Refer to p. 86 for more on CHI scores, and check cannabishealthindex.com for updated information. Using this rubric, ADHD scored in the possible-to-probable range of efficacy for treatment based on the seven studies available at press time.

ADHD treatment with cannabis has emerged recently. While a number of studies look at the pros and cons of THC for the disorder in adults, few studies involving CBD only have been completed. A 2012 animal study showed that CBD significantly reduced hyperactivity and "deficits in social interaction."[201]

Patients with attention deficit–related disorders were broken into the sub-types in a 2014 study. Those characterized as having hyperactive-impulsive behavior were much more likely to "self medicate" by using cannabis. The findings indirectly support research linking relevant cannabinoid receptors to regulatory control.[202]

Addiction

Cannabidiol is thought to modulate various neuronal circuits involved in drug addiction. A number of studies suggest that CBD may have therapeutic properties that treat opioid, cocaine, and psycho-stimulant addiction, and some data suggest that it may be beneficial in nicotine addiction in humans. Further studies are clearly necessary to fully evaluate the potential of CBD as an intervention for addictive disorders.[203]

That being said, it is becoming evident that, in states where medical marijuana is legalized, the death rate from prescription opioids begins to measurably drop immediately—a trend that strengthens over time. Evidence reported in the *Journal of the American Medical Association* showed that states with a medical cannabis program had a 24.8 percent lower opioid overdose rate than states without one.[204] That itself is powerful evidence of the poten-tial for cannabis to treat addiction to pharmaceutical painkillers. In an active pain practice in the San Francisco Bay Area, over four hundred patients have been guided through medical cannabis treatment to reduce inflammatory and neuropathic pain, chronic anxiety, and opioid medication dependency, with excellent preliminary results in all three areas.[205] (See more on the opioid epidemic in Part V, and more on using CBD for pain relief in the entry on pain in this chapter.)

Results of a 2013 animal study using morphine suggest that cannabidiol interferes with brain reward mechanisms responsible for the expression of the acute reinforcing properties of opioids, indicating that cannabidiol may be clinically useful in "turning down the volume" of the rewarding effects of opioids.[206] Other studies have shown similarly promising results in relation to other drugs.

CBD can also be effective in treating withdrawal symptoms (e.g., anxiety, insomnia, migraine) from the overuse of high-THC cannabis, which could potentially cause the desensitization of CB1 receptors according to some preliminary studies. One case report concluded that CBD successfully attenuated all of those symptoms during the treatment period.[207]

"It is fair to say that CBD is the anti-gateway drug, as it is shown to treat symptoms of withdrawal from other kinds of drug abuse," writes Kenneth Stoller, MD. "CBD can be used in patients with nicotine, alcohol, high THC cannabis, and opioid addictions. It is synergistic with the pharmaceutical Baclofen in treating addictions, but because it won't make Big Pharma money, it is practically unknown in clinical practice."[208]

How to Take the Medicine: Dosage and Delivery

It is suggested that patients work with a health care practitioner experienced in recommending CBD or medicinal cannabis so that dosage and delivery methods can be developed and fine-tuned on an individual basis. At the same time, educated and aware patients can be their own highly informed health consultants (see p. 75 for more information about the subjective-intuitive approach to using cannabis-based medicines).

In using CBD to treat issues of addiction, it's important to assess the level of physical and psychological dependence, the underlying issues leading to the condition, and specific withdrawal symptoms. A person in the earlier stages of withdrawal may need to build up to the standard or macro dose of oral medication, and also use fast-acting delivery systems such as vaporization, smoking, or sublingual products for "trigger moments" or higher-stress situations. Later on in treatment, one may be able to titrate the dose down to the micro dose.

Withdrawal symptoms such as anxiety, insomnia, migraines, or loss of appetite can be referenced under their respective entries in this chapter for advice on best varieties and delivery methods. In considering terpene profiles that might be useful in reducing withdrawal and "trigger" symptoms, look for those that are calming, such as linalool and myrcene.

For all orally administered medicines, refer to the dosage tables on pp. 61–63 for guidelines on CBD dosage by body weight. Always start with the micro dose to test sensitivity and go up as needed within the dosing range by body weight until symptoms subside. In general, doses in the standard dosing range (10–50 mg) would be most effective. More information about various forms of delivery (e.g., sublingual, edible, inhaled) for cannabinoid-based medication can be found starting on p. 38.

Effectiveness: Current Science—Addiction

possible   actual

probable

FIGURE 26

The Cannabis Health Index (CHI) is an evidence-based scoring system for cannabis (in general, not just CBD) and its effectiveness on various health issues based on currently available research data. Refer to p. 86 for more on CHI scores, and check cannabishealthindex.com for updated information. At print time, for addiction to cocaine or crack, cannabis is rated likely probable (3 points). For treatment of alcohol, heroin, opioids, and nicotine addictions, the CHI scores were all in the range of possible-to-probable efficacy (2.5 points), and, for treatment of methamphetamine addiction, cannabis is currently in the range of possible efficacy (1.6 points).

The results of a 2009 animal study showed that CBD (5–20 mg/kg) had behavioral effects on addiction "triggers" by inhibiting cue-induced **heroin**-seeking behavior. It had a long-lasting effect, significant for over twenty-four hours and measurable even two weeks later. The authors wrote that their "findings highlight the unique contributions of distinct cannabis constituents to addiction vulnerability and suggest that CBD may be a potential treatment for heroin craving and relapse."[209]

In a 2013 study on **nicotine** addiction, twenty-four smokers randomly received either an inhaler of CBD or a placebo and were instructed, for one week, to use the inhaler when they felt the urge to smoke. Over the treatment week, placebo-treated smokers showed no differences in number of cigarettes smoked. In contrast, those treated with CBD significantly reduced the number of cigarettes smoked by about 40 percent during treatment. Results also indicated some maintenance of this effect at follow-up. These preliminary data, combined with the strong preclinical rationale for use of this compound, suggest CBD can be a potential treatment for nicotine addiction that warrants further exploration.[210] Several 2016 studies on rats showed a relationship between nicotine seeking and the endocannabinoid system and showed that phytocannabinoids could ease withdrawal.

A 2016 study showed that CBD was useful for reducing **methamphetamine**-induced psychosis, which adds another layer of benefits to the preliminary evidence that CBD affects reward pathways and helps reduce other withdrawal symptoms.[211]

ALS (Amyotrophic Lateral Sclerosis)*

Every ninety minutes someone is diagnosed with amyotrophic lateral sclerosis (ALS), a disease of the nerve cells in the brain and spinal cord that control voluntary muscle movement.[212] Also known as Lou Gehrig's disease, it can progress quickly and most people live just two to five years after the first signs of disease, though a small percentage live much longer. Currently there are few medical options for those with the disease—only one FDA-approved drug that slows progression a few months on average. The unmet need is very high, and the past few years have brought significant progress in both scientific understanding of ALS and public awareness, yet this has yet not translated into effective medical treatments.

CBD helps relieve muscle spasms and is an anti-inflammatory and a more powerful antioxidant than vitamins C or E. It has been shown to have beneficial effects on all diseases involving the mitochondrial and basal ganglia portions of the brain and has a neuroprotective effect that can prolong neuronal cell survival.[213] Other important cannabinoids for ALS sufferers include the anticonvulsant cannabinol (CBN), anti-inflammatory tetrahydrocannabivarin (THCV), anti-inflammatory and analgesic (pain killing) cannabichormene (CBC) that also promotes brain growth, and analgesic cannbicyclol (CBL).[214]

---

* Also see the entry on neurodegenerative disorders in this chapter for related information.

Properties of Marijuana Applicable to ALS Symptom Management

ALS SYMPTOM	MARIJUANA EFFECT
Pain	Nonopioid analgesia and anti-inflammatory
Spasticity	Muscle relaxant
Wasting	Appetite stimulant
Dyspnea	Bronchodilation
Drooling	Dry mouth
Depression	Euphoria
Dysautonomia	Vasodilation
Neuronal oxidation	Neuroprotective antioxidant

Adapted from Gregory T. Carter and Bill S. Rosen, "Marijuana in the Management of Amyotrophic Lateral Sclerosis." Retrieved from http://ajh.sagepub.com/content/18/4/264.abstract.

RS, a graduate of Harvard University and an avid cyclist, began experiencing the symptoms of ALS in 1998, specifically the loss of function in his right arm and problems swallowing. He used cannabis heavily for decades, which he believes slowed the progression of his disease, but in 2012 he began manufacturing his own cannabis oils, dosing himself with approximately a gram a day for sixty days. Within ten days of his regimen, he regained control of his right arm and was able to stop using opiates to manage his pain.

Another remarkable case comes from CJ who was diagnosed with ALS in 1986 and given less than five years to live. In the winter of 1989, she took a holiday in Florida, preparing for the end of her life, when she made a crucial discovery. While walking on the beach one night, she smoked a joint of Myakka Gold and felt her symptoms cease.[215] Though she never intended to become a cannabis activist, she has become one of the most outspoken as a result of the improvement in her symptoms that she has continued to experience and the decades she feels the treatment has added to her life.

How to Take the Medicine: Dosage and Delivery

It is suggested that patients work with a health-care practitioner experienced in recommending CBD or medicinal cannabis so that dosage and delivery methods can be developed and fine-tuned on an individual basis. At the same time, educated and aware patients can be their own highly informed health consultants (see p. 75 for information about the subjective-intuitive approach to using cannabis-based medicines).

For all orally administered medicines, refer to the dosage tables on pp. 61–63 for guidelines on CBD dosage by body weight. Always start with the micro dose to test sensitivity, and go up as needed within the dosing range by body weight until symptoms subside.

Dosage for ALS is generally in the macro/therapeutic range, with a suggested range of 1–2 mg/lb of cannabinoids per day. The most commonly suggested ratio is 1:1, as it is the most studied due to trials of the pharmaceutical Sativex, with its balanced ratio of CBD to THC. However, if a patient has difficulty tolerating medication with the higher amount of THC, ratios higher in CBD can be used during the day, with more THC added at night (generally, indica-dominant, or sedating, strains are recommended; see Chapter 7 for more on this).

When high doses are required, many patients use concentrated forms of cannabis oil and take it orally, either in capsule form or by adding it to food (nut butters seem to work well). The purest, most potent concentrates are made using a CO_2-extraction process. More information about various forms of delivery (e.g., sublingual, edible, inhaled) for cannabinoid-based medication can be found starting on p. 38.

For relief of immediate symptoms such as drooling, vaporized or smoked cannabis can be highly effective in quickly reducing saliva. This method is also favored to relieve pain immediately. The medication lasts one to three hours, whereas most ingested products take thirty to sixty minutes to take effect and last six to eight hours. Vaporizers that use a cartridge filled with the CO_2 concentrate are highly effective, and these are available in various ratios of CBD to THC. Herbal vaporizers with the whole plant are also an effective delivery method.

Effectiveness: Current Science—ALS

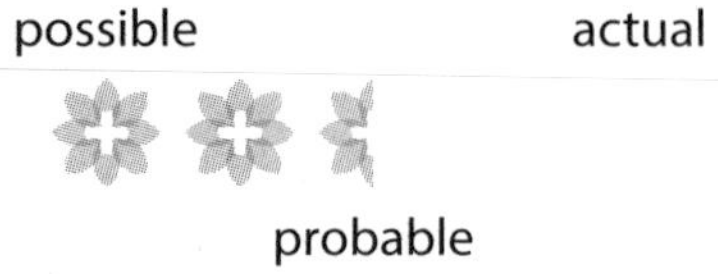

possible   actual

✻ ✻ ✻

probable

FIGURE 27

The Cannabis Health Index (CHI) is an evidence-based scoring system for cannabis (in general, not just CBD) and its effectiveness on various health issues based on currently available research data. Refer to p. 86 for more on CHI scores, and check cannabishealthindex.com for updated information. Using this rubric, ALS scored in the possible-to-probable range of efficacy for treatment based on twelve studies.

Research on ALS and cannabis is scarce, though there has been much discussion recently of its anecdotal effectiveness, and a number of articles in medical journals comment on successful case studies and the need for more work to be done. A 2010 research paper discussed the potential applications and referenced a previous animal trial in which cannabis slowed progression of the disease, calling for clinical trials and concluding, "it is reasonable to think that cannabis might significantly slow the progression of ALS, potentially extending life expectancy and substantially reducing the overall burden of the disease."[216] Further research showed that CBD in combination with THC lengthened life expectancy more than THC alone.[217]

One of the understood causes of the degeneration of motor neurons in the spines and central nervous systems of ALS sufferers is the lack of an enzyme called superoxide dismutase (SOD1), a powerful antioxidant that protects the body from damage caused by toxic free radicals. The antioxidant properties of CBD are, however, just one of its potentially beneficial agents when it comes to ALS. The authors of the 2010 article point out:

It appears that a number of abnormal physiological processes occur simultaneously in this devastating disease. Ideally, a multidrug regimen, including glutamate antagonists, antioxidants, a centrally acting anti-inflammatory agent, microglial cell modulators (including tumor necrosis factor alpha [TNF-α] inhibitors), an antiapoptotic agent, 1 or more neurotrophic growth factors, and a mitochondrial function-enhancing agent would be required to comprehensively address the known pathophysiology of ALS. Remarkably, cannabis appears to have activity in all of those areas.[218]

Alzheimer's Disease

Endocannabinoid signaling appears to be "essential to a number of molecular and cellular events important for learning and memory."[219] Characterized by a progressive mental deterioration that starts in middle or old age and linked to genetic, lifestyle, and environmental factors, Alzheimer's disease results in loss of memory, language, and cognitive skills. While indica strains of cannabis have been used historically to calm patients and help mediate symptoms of the illness, new science shows that the disease is strongly connected to the endocannabinoid system, and, with the re-emergence of CBD medicine, it is likely that cannabinoid-based treatments will become more standard. In fact, such treatments are showing promising results for a number of brain-related diseases, since cannabinoids protect against the destruction of neural circuits through several processes: neutralizing free radicals, reducing inflammation, improving function of mitochondria, clearing of beta amyloid, and clearing away of cellular debris.[220]

In 2004, scientists noted CBD's protective, anti-oxidative, and anti-apoptotic effects on the brain that result in a reduction of neurotoxicity caused by amyloid buildup.[221] Noting the synergistic potential of cannabis constituents like CBD and THC, researchers five years later wrote:

> The great therapeutic value of CBD, either given alone or in association with THC, derives from the consideration that it represents a rare, if not unique, compound that is capable of affording neuroprotection by the combination of different types of properties (e.g., anti-glutamatergic effects, anti-inflammatory action, and antioxidant effects) that almost cover all spectra of neurotoxic mechanisms that operate in neurodegenerative disorders (excitotoxicity, inflammatory events, oxidative injury, etc.).[222]

One of the characterizing pathological markers of Alzheimer's disease is the toxic buildup of plaque in the neural tissue and associated inflammation. In 2008, a study[223] found that THC slowed plaque overgrowth, a discovery that was confirmed in later studies.[224,225] Furthermore, the researchers discovered it blocks inflammation, which damages neurons in the brain.

"It is reasonable to conclude that there is a therapeutic potential of cannabinoids for the treatment of Alzheimer's disease," wrote Dr. David Schubert, a senior researcher on the study.[226]

How to Take the Medicine: Dosage and Delivery

It is suggested that patients work with a health care practitioner experienced in recommending CBD or medicinal cannabis so that dosage and delivery methods can be developed and fine-tuned on an individual basis. At the same time, educated and aware patients can be their own highly informed health consultants (see p. 75 for information about the subjective-intuitive approach to using cannabis-based medicines).

For all orally administered medicines, refer to the dosage tables on pp. 61–63 for guidelines on CBD dosage by body weight. Always start with the micro dose to test sensitivity and go up as needed within the dosing range by body weight until symptoms subside. Patients with Alzheimer's disease should be cautious when titrating up to a target **standard or macro dosing range** to ensure minimal psychoactive effects. Varieties that are high in myrcene have a more relaxing effect.

That being said, products made with sedating, indica-dominant varieties that are higher in THC can be helpful for sleep issues (see the entry on sleep disorders in this chapter for more information). A maximum range of 5–10 mg of THC per dose is suggested. Avoid products containing sativa-dominant strains as they can promote hyperactivity and dissociation. For safety reasons, smoked or vaporized products are not recommended for patients with advanced dementia.

When high doses are required, many patients use concentrated forms of cannabis oil and take it orally, either in capsule form or by adding to food (nut butters seem to work well). The purest, most potent concentrates are made using a CO_2-extraction process. More information about various forms of delivery (e.g., sublingual, edible, transdermal) for cannabinoid-based medication can be found starting on p. 38.

Effectiveness: Current Science—Alzheimer's

possible   actual

probable

FIGURE 28

The Cannabis Health Index (CHI) is an evidence-based scoring system for cannabis (in general, not just CBD) and its effectiveness on various health issues based on currently available research data. Refer to p. 86 for more on CHI scores, and check cannabishealthindex.com for updated information. For treatment of Alzheimer's disease, it is rated in the possible-to-probable range based on twenty-five studies (2.5 points).

Beyond the antioxidant, anti-inflammatory, and neuroprotective effects of cannabinoids, several studies showed that they also play a role in the growth of neural tissue in the hippocampus, the area of the brain associated with memory.[227,228]

Several findings in 2014 indicate that the activation of both CB1 and CB2 receptors by natural or synthetic agonists, causing action at non-psychoactive doses, have beneficial effects in experimental models by reducing the harmful β-amyloid peptide action and tau phosphorylation, as well as by promoting the brain's intrinsic repair mechanisms. "Endocannabinoid signaling has been demonstrated to modulate numerous concomitant pathological processes," the authors of one study wrote, "including neuroinflammation, excitotoxicity, mitochondrial dysfunction, and oxidative stress."[229] That same year, an Australian trial[230] showed that CBD treatment reversed cognitive deficits in the study of mice and suggested that it had therapeutic potential for these impairments.[231]

A study in 2016 of eleven Alzheimer's patients with THC showed a significant reduction in the severity of symptoms, including delusions, agitation, aggression, and insomnia.[232]

Antibiotic-Resistant Bacterial Infections

Antibiotic-resistant bacteria are now one of the top health concerns of the world. Common infections that have long been easily treatable can become life-threatening in the presence of these "super-bugs" that have developed resistance to commonly used antibiotics. Methicillin-resistant *Staphylococcus aureus* (MRSA), for example, a staph bacteria common in hospitals, is responsible for many thousands of related deaths each year. People with weakened immune systems are most at risk, but healthy individuals can also become infected when exposed to the bacteria. In 2014, President Obama issued an executive order and budgeted funds for the establishment of a special task force devoted to the issue, one that would develop an action plan for stopping the fast spread of antibiotic-resistant bacteria like MRSA.

Cannabis has been used successfully and studied periodically through the centuries in the treatment of other bacterial infections responsible for global epidemics, such as tuberculosis and gonorrhea. Research back in 1976 showed THC and CBD were both effective against staph and strep infections.[233] Since then, a major study done on the effects of cannabinoids on multidrug-resistant bacteria in 2008 found that all five cannabinoids studied (THC, CBD, CBG, CBC, and CBN) were potent against bacteria. The most effective application was a topical antiseptic directly on affected areas, but oral CBD products can be used as systemic antibacterial agents.[234]

Additionally, pinene was shown to be as effective against MRSA as vancomycin and other agents. Pinene also has the ability to increase skin permeability, a large barrier against uptake of phytocannabinoids. Investigating CBD/CBG-based extracts with pinene may prove fruitful in battling MRSA and other treatment-resistant bacteria.[235]

"The most practical application of cannabinoids would be as topical agents to treat ulcers and wounds in a hospital environment, decreasing the burden of antibiotics," said Giovanni Appendino, a professor at Italy's Piemonte Orientale University and co-author of the 2008 study.[236]

How to Take the Medicine: Dosage and Delivery

It is suggested that patients work with a health care practitioner experienced in recommending CBD or medicinal cannabis so that dosage and delivery methods can be developed and fine-tuned on an individual basis. At the same time, educated and aware patients can be their own highly informed health consultants (see p. 75 for information about the subjective-intuitive approach to using cannabis-based medicines).

Applied to the skin, topical products can be made using CBD-dominant cannabis or other strains. This method is used when bacterial infections affect the skin or a wound site. Topical products containing THC affect the cells near application but do not cross the blood-brain barrier, and, therefore, are not psychoactive. These products may be available as oils, ointments, sprays, or other forms, and with varying ratios of CBD and THC (a ratio of 1:1 is often recommended as ideal for skin application). The skin has the highest amount and concentration of CB2 receptors in the body. According to the 2008 study referenced earlier in this section, products containing any of the major cannabinoids can be effective against an antibiotic-resistant infection.

For all orally administered medicines, refer to the dosage tables on pp. 61–63 for guidelines on CBD dosage by body weight. Always start with the micro dose to test sensitivity and go up as needed within the dosing range by body weight until symptoms subside. More information about various forms of delivery (e.g., sublingual, oral, inhaled) for cannabinoid-based medication can be found starting on p. 38).

Effectiveness: Current Science—Antibiotic

possible   actual

probable

FIGURE 29

The Cannabis Health Index (CHI) is an evidence-based scoring system for cannabis (in general, not just CBD) and its effectiveness on various health issues based on currently available research data. Refer to p. 86 for more on CHI scores, and check cannabishealthindex.com for updated information. Based on three studies, for treatment of MRSA, cannabis rates as possibly effective.

The endocannabinoid system is involved in the process of healing and the formation of scar tissue on the skin. A 2010 study in China found that CB1 receptors increased at the site of skin injuries starting from six hours post-injury, peaking at five days, and returning to baseline by fourteen days.[237]

Anxiety and Stress

The oral use of cannabis to treat anxiety appears in a Vedic text dated around 2000 BCE,[238] and it is one of the most common uses of the plant across various cultures. While THC can increase anxiety in some patients, it lowers it in others. However, CBD has been shown to consistently reduce anxiety when present in higher concentrations in the cannabis plant. On its own, CBD has been shown in a number of animal and human studies to lessen anxiety. The stress-reducing effect appears to be related to activity in both the limbic and paralimbic brain areas.

A 2012 research review assessed a number of international studies and concluded that CBD has been shown to reduce anxiety, and in particular social anxiety, in multiple studies and called for more clinical trials.[239] Two years later, researchers in an animal study related to stress and the endocannabinoid system wrote that augmentation of the endocannabinoid system might be an effective strategy to mitigate behavioral and physical consequences of stress.[240]

These findings appear to support that the anxiolytic effect of chronic CBD administration in stressed mice depends on its proneurogenic action in the adult hippocampus by facilitating endocannabinoid-mediated signaling.[241]

How to Take the Medicine: Dosage and Delivery

It is suggested that patients work with a health care practitioner experienced in recommending CBD or medicinal cannabis so that dosage and delivery methods can be developed and fine-tuned on an individual basis. At the same time, educated and aware patients can be their own highly informed health consultants (see p. 75 for information about the subjective-intuitive approach to using cannabis-based medicines).

CBD products with a ratio of 20:1 or higher are recommended and administered as drops, capsules, or edibles. High-CBD cannabinoids can be very effective in reducing chronic anxiety, treating temporary stress, and protecting the body from the physiological effects of both. Varieties high in linalool, a terpene shared with lavender, are known to be effective for relieving anxiety. In particular, the strain AC/DC is very effective.

For all orally administered medicines, refer to the dosage tables on pp. 61–63 for guidelines on CBD dosage by body weight. Always start with the micro dose to test sensitivity and go up as needed within the dosing range, before going to the next, until symptoms subside. The **micro to standard dose** is usually recommended to treat anxiety and stress.

For relief of immediate symptoms, as in a panic or anxiety attack, vaporizing or smoking work well. The medication lasts one to three hours, whereas most ingested products take thirty to sixty minutes before taking effect and last six to eight hours. Vaporizers that use a cartridge filled with the CO_2 concentrate are highly effective, and these are available in various ratios of CBD to THC. Herbal vaporizers that use the whole plant are also an effective delivery method. Sublingual sprays or tinctures taken as liquid drops take effect quickly and last longer than inhaled products. More information about various forms of delivery (e.g., sublingual, oral, inhaled) for cannabinoid-based medication can be found starting on p. 38).

Effectiveness: Current Science—Anxiety

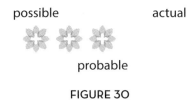

FIGURE 30

The Cannabis Health Index (CHI) is an evidence-based scoring system for cannabis (in general, not just CBD) and its effectiveness on various health issues based on currently available research data. Refer to p. 86 for more on CHI scores, and check cannabishealthindex.com for updated information. Using this rubric and based on eleven studies, cannabis rated in the possible-to-probable range of efficacy for treatment of anxiety.

Arthritis

Osteoarthritis, also known as degenerative joint disease, is the inflammation of a joint connecting two bones that develops gradually over many years. Initially, it presents as an occasional mild ache in the joints that progresses into chronic pain, stiffness, and swelling. Arthritis has become the leading cause of disability in the United States, with more than 46 million people suffering various forms of physical difficulty. It is most common in older adults.

Rheumatoid arthritis, however, is an autoimmune disease that can affect people at any age, even children. The immune system attacks synovial membranes in the joints, causing inflammation similar to that of osteoarthritis. Rheumatoid arthritis negatively impacts more than the joints, reaching all organ systems due to the extensive damage it can cause to blood vessels. More on using CBD for this type of arthritis can be found in this chapter in the entry for autoimmune disorders.

A 2001 study demonstrated that cannabinoid receptors are involved in the nervous system response linked to arthritis and concluded that "these novel targets may be advantageous for the treatment of inflammatory pain."[242] Research results suggest treatment with cannabinoids can also be effective for other types of inflammatory joint diseases such as gout.

JS had severe arthritis and fibromyalgia with constant pain in the knees. She started massaging CBD oil into her painful knees twice a day. In less than a week, she was nearly pain free. "I can even go up and down steps and not be in agony," she reported. "I'm also using the vapor pen twice a day. CBD works better than the prescription pain cream I was using! I feel like this product has given me my life back."

How to Take the Medicine: Dosage and Delivery

It is suggested that patients work with a health care practitioner experienced in recommending CBD or medicinal cannabis so that dosage and delivery methods can be developed and fine-tuned on an individual basis. At the same time, educated and aware patients can be their own highly informed health consultants (see p. 75 for information about the subjective-intuitive approach to using cannabis-based medicines).

Applied to the skin, topical products can be made using CBD-dominant cannabis or other strains. Topical products containing THC affect the cells near application but do not cross the blood-brain barrier, and, therefore, are not psychoactive. These products may be available as oils, ointments, sprays, or other forms, and with varying ratios of CBD and THC (a ratio of 1:1 is often recommended as ideal for skin application). The skin has the largest amount and concentration of CB2 receptors in the body.

CBD-dominant products (4:1 ratio of CBD:THC), taken sublingually or as drops, capsules, or edibles, have been most effective in reducing chronic pain from arthritis. For all orally administered medicines, refer to the dosage tables on pp. 61–63 for guidelines on CBD dosage by body weight. Always start with the micro dose to test sensitivity and go up as needed within the dosing range by body weight until symptoms subside. The micro to standard dose is usually recommended to treat arthritis. If the total amount of THC is causing unwanted side effects, then either lower the dose or switch to a higher ratio 20:1 CBD:THC product. Strains high in cannabichromene (CBC), noted for its anti-inflammatory effects, may be especially helpful for arthritis. Cannabis varieties high in terpenes such as linalool, myrcene, and limonene may add synergistic effects.[243]

For relief of acute pain, vaporizing or smoking work well. The medication effect is immediate and lasts one to three hours, whereas most ingested products take thirty to sixty minutes before taking effect (faster on an empty stomach) and last six to eight hours. Vaporizers that use a cartridge filled with the CO_2 concentrate are highly effective, and these are available in various ratios of CBD to THC. Herbal vaporizers that use the whole plant are also an effective delivery method. More information about various forms of delivery (e.g., sublingual, transdermal, inhaled) for cannabinoid-based medication can be found starting on p. 38.

A 2016 study showed success in the treatment of arthritis pain in animals through the application of a CBD-only gel transdermally. The study concluded that "topical CBD application has therapeutic potential for relief of arthritis pain-related behaviors and inflammation without evident side-effects."[244]

Effectiveness: Current Science—Arthritis

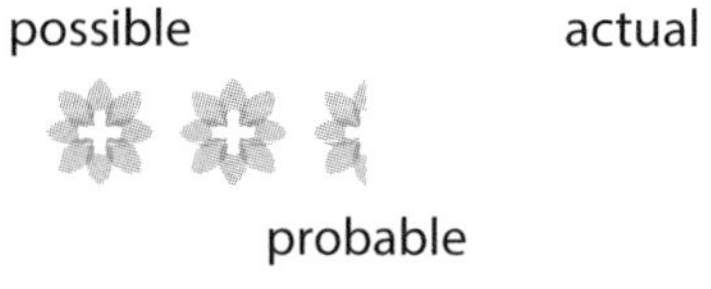

possible   actual

probable

FIGURE 31

The Cannabis Health Index (CHI) is an evidence-based scoring system for cannabis (in general, not just CBD) and its effectiveness on various health issues based on currently available research data. Refer to p. 86 for more on CHI scores, and check cannabishealthindex.com for updated information. Using this rubric, cannabis rated in the possible-to-probable range of efficacy for treating arthritis based on four studies.

In an animal study conducted in 2000, CBD was orally administered after the onset of clinical symptoms at a dose of 25 mg/kg, and in both models of arthritis the treatment effectively blocked progression.[245] In a 2006 trial using Sativex, a cannabis-derived pharmaceutical, a "significant analgesic effect was observed and disease activity was significantly suppressed following treatment."[246]

Additional relevant information can be found in the entry for pain in this chapter.

Asthma

Asthma is a chronic respiratory disease affecting up to 300 million people worldwide. Airways contract both spontaneously and in response to a wide range of environmental factors and endogenous stimuli. Children and elders are most vulnerable to asthma, but it can affect people at all ages with symptoms ranging from mild to life threatening. The hyper responsiveness of the airways is accompanied by inflammation—something that cannabinoids can be very effective at reducing.[247] The conventional treatment of asthma remains problematic and often involves a combination of drugs with varying side effects.

Research has shown that both CB1 and CB2 receptors are present in bronchial tissue and are involved in lung protection. The activation of CB1 receptors on nerve endings in the lungs creates a bronchodilator effect by acting on the airway's smooth muscle, and research has suggested this may be beneficial in airway hyper reactivity and asthma.[248] Several studies, dating back to the 1970s, suggest that targeting cannabinoid receptors could be a novel preventative therapeutic strategy in asthmatic patients.[249]

Evidence is mounting that asthma may be triggered by bacterial or viral infections, such as *Streptococcus,* in early childhood that leave the immune system more vulnerable to allergens. The resulting development of treatment strategies involving antibiotics, however, has led to antibiotic-resistant super-bugs. Cannabinoids have been shown to have a broad-spectrum bactericidal effect (see p. 99 for more on this).

Because airways contract and narrow during asthma attacks, the antispasmodic action of cannabinoids may also play a role in bronchodilation. In the past several years, cannabinoid inhaler systems have entered the market as these treatments for asthma become better researched and recognized.

How to Take the Medicine: Dosage and Delivery

It is suggested that patients work with a health care practitioner experienced in recommending CBD or medicinal cannabis so that dosage and delivery methods can be developed and fine-tuned on an individual basis. At the same time, educated and aware patients can be their own highly informed health consultants (see p. 75 for information about the subjective-intuitive approach to using cannabis-based medicines).

It has been known for many years that smoked cannabis is a bronchodilator and can be useful in treating asthma. Usually, asthma is a problem with bronchospasms (wheezes) and increased mucous production in the smaller airways of our lungs. There is a large component of anxiety associated with asthma, as who would not be scared when it is difficult to breathe. More anxiety causes worsening bronchospasms, which causes more anxiety. Typical inhalers contain adrenergic (adrenaline-like) stimulants, which work well but tend to heighten anxiety. It would be nice to have more alternatives to treat bronchospasms. Since richer levels of THC can cause increased anxiety, using CBD seems like a reasonable thing to try.

Last week a patient came into our office having obtained some CBD-rich tincture at a local collective that he felt was helping his asthma. He was off his Advair inhaler for a week and wanted to be "checked." We administered a baseline spirometry test and then repeated the test fifteen minutes after the patient had taken three drops of his CBD-rich tincture. The test showed the patient's forced expiratory volume and peak expiratory flow rate had doubled. This would generally be considered a great response to a typical bronchodilator! Taking CBD by any method does result in decreased airway resistance. So, how about taking it by inhalation without smoke? Now there are vape pens available that have CBD oil inside them. In general, a couple of puffs will give the patient 6–8 mg of whole-plant CBD plus some THC directly into the lungs.

ALLAN FRANKEL, MD

For relief of immediate symptoms of asthma, sublingual drops and oromucosal sprays work well, as does vaporizing with a high-quality CBD-concentrated oil without additives. The medication lasts one to three hours, whereas most ingested products take thirty to sixty minutes before taking effect (faster on an empty stomach) and last six to eight hours. The most effective vaporizers and inhalers use a cartridge filled with the CO_2 concentrate. Sublinguals also take effect quickly and last longer than inhaled products.

Effectiveness: Current Science—Asthma

possible   actual

probable

FIGURE 32

The Cannabis Health Index (CHI) is an evidence-based scoring system for cannabis (in general, not just CBD) and its effectiveness on various health issues based on currently available research data. Refer to p. 86 for more on CHI scores, and check cannabishealthindex.com for updated information. Using this rubric and based on eleven studies, cannabinoids rate in the possible-to-probable range of efficacy for asthma.

A number of studies in the 1970s showed the bronchodilatory effect of cannabis and compared it to other drugs used for asthma.[250,251] A 1978 study showed that THC produced bronchodilation in asthmatic patients and that the rate of onset, magnitude, and duration of the bronchodilator effect was dose-related.[252] More recently, a 2015 animal study reported that CBD has few side effects and represents a "potential new drug to modulate inflammatory response in asthma."[253]

Autism Spectrum Disorder

Autism is a complex neurobehavioral disorder with a wide spectrum of severity, from minor to requiring institutional care. It is characterized by impairments in social, language, and communication skills and is frequently complicated by rigid, repetitive behaviors. The current estimation is that about 1 percent of children in the United States have some form of autism, it is five times more likely to affect boys than girls, and the number of cases appears to be rising sharply. A 2013 study comparing autistic children to non-autistic subjects showed a difference in CB2 receptors and indicated neurotransmitters in particular as potential therapeutic targets for autism.[254]

Though research is still extremely limited, CBD is showing promising results in the treatment of the behavioral symptoms of autism, including violent outbursts, hyperactivity, repetitive behaviors, and hypersensitivity to physical sensations. Because current treatments are so limited and the disorder can be so serious, many parents of autistic children are exploring alternative therapies such as cannabinoids. Of note, CBD treatment is better documented for autism accompanied by seizures, which occurs in up to 30 percent of cases (see the Seizure Disorders entry later in this chapter for more information).

A 2013 study found an unexpected link between a protein implicated in autism and a signaling system that previously had not been considered particularly important for autism. Senior author Dr. Thomas Südhof of Stanford University wrote that the findings opened up a new area of research and "may suggest novel strategies for understanding the underlying causes of complex brain disorders."[255] The results indicated that targeting components of the endocannabinoid signaling system may help reverse autism symptoms. A clinical study with CBD on 120 autistic children and young adults was launched in Israel in 2016.[256]

KS, a child with autism so severe he wasn't able to speak, started speaking his first words after the use of a cannabinoid spray twice daily, according to Dr. Giovanni Martinez, a clinical psychologist in Puerto Rico. "He started using the product three weeks ago. He was a full non-verbal patient. He only made sounds. The only change in his treatments was the use of CBD." The parents pursued the treatment on their own. Dr. Martinez has also been doing his own research on CBD and shared it with the parents. "I'm very impressed with the language he has acquired," said Dr. Martinez. Dr. Martinez noted that, when KS couldn't communicate, his behavior became bad as he acted out due to his frustrations, but by opening up his communication abilities his conduct has improved. "He laughs every time he hears his voice," said Dr. Martinez.[257]

How to Take the Medicine: Dosage and Delivery

It is suggested that patients work with a health-care practitioner experienced in recommending CBD or medicinal cannabis so that dosage and delivery methods can be developed and fine-tuned on an individual basis. At the same time, educated and aware patients can be their own highly informed health consultants (see p. 75 for information about the subjective-intuitive approach to using cannabis-based medicines).

For pediatric autism, a starting dose similar to that for epilepsy, about 1 mg/kg per day every eight hours, is recommended. Increase in increments of 0.5–1 mg/kg/day every two weeks. The average dose for epilepsy is 5–8 mg/kg/day (2.5–4 mg/lb/day), but the amount needed for treating symptoms of autism varies according to the severity of the disorder. It is recommended to break the dose up into three doses taken every seven to eight hours, preferably between meals.

Refer to the dosage tables on pp. 61–63 for guidelines on CBD dosage by body weight. Always start with the micro dose to test sensitivity and go up as needed within the dosing range by body weight until symptoms subside.

For children, CBD-only oil infusions, glycerin tinctures, sublingual products, or pure CO2-extracted concentrates are recommended (no alcohol tinctures). The oil can be given straight or mixed with yogurt or other food. Concentrates can also be mixed with food such as nut butters or made into capsules or suppositories. If symptoms are not reduced or eliminated, blends that add a small amount of THC are sometimes effective.

Adults can take any of the above, as well as alcohol-based tinctures, capsules, and other edibles. For more immediate symptoms, vaporizing or smoking work well. The medication effect is immediate and lasts one to three hours, whereas most ingested products take thirty to sixty minutes before taking effect (faster on an empty stomach) and last six to eight hours. Vaporizers that use a cartridge filled with the CO2 concentrate are highly effective, and these are available in various ratios of CBD to THC. Herbal vaporizers that use the whole plant are also an effective delivery method. More information about various forms of delivery (e.g., sublingual, transdermal, inhaled) for cannabinoid-based medication can be found starting on p. 38.

Effectiveness: Current Science—Autism

possible   actual

probable

FIGURE 33

The Cannabis Health Index (CHI) is an evidence-based scoring system for cannabis (in general, not just CBD) and its effectiveness on various health issues based on currently available research data. Refer to p. 86 for more on CHI scores, and check cannabishealthindex.com for updated information. Using this rubric and based on two studies, cannabis rated in the possible-to-probable range of efficacy.

Authors of a 2011 animal study related to autistic behavior wrote that it was "tempting to suggest" cannabinoids for "irritability, tantrums and self-injurious behavior associated with autistic individuals."[258]

A 2015 article on endocannabinoid signaling (referred to as "eCB signaling" in the following extract) in autism called it a piece of the puzzle bringing together four features of autism: 1) social reward responsivity; 2) neural development; 3) circadian rhythm; and 4) anxiety-related symptoms.

Therefore . . . any potential therapeutic approach is unlikely to involve a simple choice between activation versus inhibition of the eCB system to target specific features related to autism. Any such approach will need to be precisely tuned to the developmental timeline and to the specific pathogenetic underpinnings of autism in the single patient. Our understanding of eCB signaling in autism is still in its infancy compared with other disorders of the central nervous system or of peripheral tissues, where eCB-based therapies have already reached preclinical and clinical phases. However, research in this field is rapidly evolving, and novel drugs able to hit specifically a distinct element of the eCB system are developed at a surprising speed.[259]

Autoimmune Disorders

Autoimmune disorders refer to problems with the body's immune system response. In an autoimmune reaction, antibodies and immune cells target the system's own healthy tissues by mistake, signaling the body to attack them in almost any part of the body—the heart, brain, nerves, muscles, skin, eyes, joints, lungs, kidneys, glands, digestive tract, and blood vessels can be affected by these disorders.

Autoimmune disorders typically cause inflammation, with the site depending on what part of the body is targeted. Sometimes inflammation manifests in several sites. The cause of autoimmune disorders is unknown and likely a combination of factors both genetic and exogenous. Common autoimmune disorders include Addison's disease, celiac disease, Graves' disease, Hashimoto's thyroiditis, multiple sclerosis, rheumatoid arthritis, lupus erythematosus, and diabetes. Lyme disease, the inflammatory disorder caused by a tick bite, can cause serious autoimmune symptoms.

Cannabinoids have been shown to be effective in treating disorders involving over activation of immune response and the associated oxidative stress.[260] Cannabinoid receptors (CB1 and CB2) are found on the cells of the immune system. Cannabinoids like THC and CBD trigger these receptors, which stimulates immunoregulation as cytokine and chemokine production is down-regulated and t-regulatory cells are up-regulated. Cannabinoids can help with the pain caused by chronic autoimmune diseases, both through their

At the age of forty-four, psychologist Constance Finley became very ill with an undiagnosed autoimmune disease and was housebound for ten years. During her struggle, she came close to death as a result of the pharmaceutical drug Adalimumab used to treat her condition. Out of complete desperation, she began researching alternative medicines that could help her chronic pain and inflammation and discovered cannabis as a potential option. Though extremely hesitant at first, she tried cannabis and it immediately helped with her pain and insomnia. Her results were so remarkable that Constance decided to study cannabis cultivation and spent years perfecting her infused oil recipes and ratios. She now markets her own medicines made by her team at her home laboratory.[261]

analgesic properties and by reducing the inflammation that often causes the pain. THC and CBD act on CB1 and CB2 receptors, which have been shown to be involved in the mediation of pain associated with inflammation.[262]

How to Take the Medicine: Dosage and Delivery

It is suggested that patients work with a health care practitioner experienced in recommending CBD or medicinal cannabis so that dosage and delivery methods can be developed and fine-tuned on an individual basis. At the same time, educated and aware patients can be their own highly informed health consultants (see p. 75 for information about the subjective-intuitive approach to using cannabis-based medicines).

It is difficult to generalize treatment for chronic autoimmune disorders because they affect the body in such varied ways, but a baseline dose **(micro to standard)** of CBD is recommended to reduce inflammation and address immune hyper response. For all orally administered medicines, refer to the dosage tables on pp. 61–63 for guidelines on CBD dosage by body weight. Always start with the micro dose to test sensitivity and go up as needed within the dosing range by body weight until symptoms subside.

For relief of immediate symptoms, sublingual drops and oromucosal sprays work well, as does vaporizing with high-quality CBD-concentrated oil without additives. The medication effect is immediate and lasts one to three hours, whereas most ingested products take thirty to sixty minutes before taking effect (faster on an empty stomach) and last six to eight hours. Vaporizers that use a cartridge filled with the CO_2 concentrate are highly effective, and these are available in various ratios of CBD to THC. Herbal vaporizers that use the whole plant are also an effective delivery method. More information about various forms of delivery (e.g., sublingual, transdermal, inhaled) for cannabinoid-based medication can be found starting on p. 38.

Effectiveness: Current Science—Autoimmune

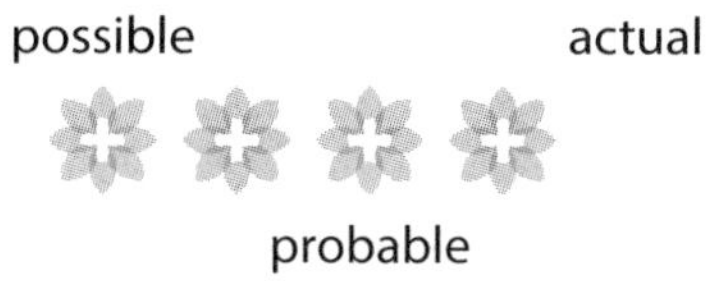

possible   actual

probable

FIGURE 34

The Cannabis Health Index (CHI) is an evidence-based scoring system for cannabis (in general, not just CBD) and its effectiveness on various health issues based on currently available research data. Refer to p. 86 for more on CHI scores, and check cannabishealthindex.com for updated information. Treatment of autoimmune disorders with cannabinoids was not generally scored, but treatment of some of the diseases included in this category was scored individually. Graves' disease treatment with cannabis was rated in the probable-to-demonstrable range of efficacy (4 points) based on one 2016 study related to autoimmunity. Crohn's disease treatment rated as likely probable (3.3 points), and diabetes treatment scored in the possible-to-probable range. (See entries in this chapter on inflammatory bowel syndromes and diseases, diabetes, and arthritis.)

A University of South Carolina animal study in 2014 showed that the suppression of immune response by THC could be a useful treatment for autoimmune disease. Cannabinoids can change critical histones and suppress inflammation by activating the cannabinoid receptors, CB2, on immune cells. Though this study only looked at THC, CBD is also known to help the immune system. It is thought that CBD works by improving the ability of the immune system to recognize the difference between normal internal body functions and foreign entities, keeping the body from attacking itself.[263]

Cancer

Cannabinoids are known to have palliative effects in oncology, including relief of chemotherapy-related nausea and vomiting, appetite stimulation, pain relief, mood elevation, and sleep in cancer patients (see the separate entries for nausea and vomiting, eating disorders, pain, depression, and sleep disorders in this chapter for information on treating these symptoms).

Evidence has been accumulating over the past decades that cannabinoids also have beneficial effects beyond palliative care, entering the "domain of disease modulation."[264] Better quality research is needed, but the direct anticancer effects that have been demonstrated so far include tumor-shrinking properties, inhibition of the growth of new cancer cells, and prevention of metastases. Researchers have demonstrated regression of a number of different cancer types.

Authors of a 2013 evidence review on CBD and cancer wrote that "cannabinoids possess anti-proliferative and pro-apoptotic effects and they are known to interfere with tumor neovascularization, cancer cell migration, adhesion, invasion and metastasization. However the clinical use of Δ^9 THC and additional cannabinoid agonists is often limited by their unwanted psychoactive side effects, and for this reason interest in non-psychoactive cannabinoid compounds...such as cannabidiol (CBD), has substantially increased in recent years."[265]

A number of studies limited to THC and CBD as synthetic cannabinoids showed anti-cancer effects. A Japanese study using THC determined that it had anti-inflammatory effects and reduced the growth of tumors in mice.[266]

Another study found that CBD may prevent cancer caused by smoking tobacco, linked to cytochrome P450, family 1, member A1 (CYP1A1). CYP1A1 is a protein found in humans. This protein is harmless at low levels but has been shown to be cancerous in high amounts. CBD was shown to bind to the protein and was able to keep it from increasing. It controlled CYP1A1 at a normal, healthy level, exerting a preventative effect on cancer caused by smoking.[267]

Using cannabis as a therapy to reduce cancer activity and tumor size does require high doses of cannabis medicine. THC is very effective in shrinking the tumor size,[268] and CBD is very effective in stopping the proliferation of new cancer cells.[269] While both THC and CBD are effective anti-cancer agents, the combination of CBD and THC together has exhibited even greater efficacy for healing. There is a true synergistic relationship between CBD and THC; the whole is greater than the sum of the parts. There is evidence that a combination of the various cannabinoids and terpenes found in products derived from the whole plant is the most effective approach (see more on this in the Entourage Effect section in Chapter 2).

"In addition to active cannabinoids, cannabis plants also contain a multitude of other therapeutic agents," said Dr. David Meiri, a lead researcher in an Israeli study considered the most in-depth so far on cancer patients and cannabis and involving fifty different strains of cannabis and over two hundred cancer cell lines. "Terpenoids and flavonoids are usually present in small quantities, but can have beneficial therapeutic effects, especially as synergistic compounds to cannabinoids."[270] Varieties high in myrcene, limonene, and linalool are recommended.[271]

115

A 2013 British study demonstrated that a spectrum of cannabinoids was more effective in the treatment of leukemia cells, compared to each individual compound.[272] Dr. Meiri and his team are conducting a number of studies documenting the effects of cannabinoids and other phytochemicals on tumor growth:

> The effects were further investigated in vitro, in various cancer cell lines, and revealed pro-apoptotic (promoting cancer cell death) and anti-proliferative response to cannabinoids, as well as inhibition of invasion and migration. However, the medical use of cannabis remains rather limited due to the large number of active compounds that, together with variability among different cannabis strains and cultivation methods, impairs our ability to predict the specific clinical effect and determine the recommended dose.[273]

While the other active compounds in cannabis such as terpenes (see the section on terpenes) are being further researched, and higher-caliber studies on human subjects are starting to be published, some cancer patients don't have time to wait. Hundreds of stories exist of patients whose cancer was cleared after cannabinoid therapy. It is important to note that all of the anti-cancer effects of cannabinoids come from either test tube or animal studies, with no data yet available from studies in humans to support these individual patient testimonials. See the box for one dramatic case involving a young woman with brain cancer.

In April 2012, successful fashion designer AP, age thirty-nine, went into the hospital with neurological symptoms, and was told she had one of the rarest forms of brain tumor. It was inoperable, and even with radiation and chemo-therapy, her doctors gave her about eighteen months to live. AP was skeptical of conventional treatment, but felt the pressure of being told she would likely die sooner if she didn't submit to six weeks of daily radiation and chemo at the University Hospital. "I was told my brain would start to swell and push against my skull at week three, and that I would need steroids," she wrote. "I would lose my hair permanently where they did radiation. After six weeks of treatment, they told me I needed another round—six months this time. My skin felt like it was crawling, I could not bear it, I finally decided to tell the doctors I refused their treatment."

Over the next few months, she was told the treatment appeared to have failed, but it was difficult to confirm because of swelling. She then discovered stories of people whose brain tumors were healed with cannabis oil. She contacted the author, Leonard Leinow, for guidance and advice, whom she now lovingly calls "The Wizard of Woodacre."

In January 2013, she began taking a high-dose regimen of 200 mg/day (120 mg CBD + 80 mg THC). In June 2013, her oncologists confirmed that the tumor was still growing, but more slowly than expected. They gave her less than six months to live. "I went into fight mode and decided to double my dose of cannabinoids. Then, in November, after my MRI, my oncologist sat us down looking very serious, but she gave us expected news—my tumor was starting to regress . . . my medicine was working! The doctor told me that many of her patients had tried to find their own treatment, but all had failed. She was amazed, and, while she couldn't get involved, she was excited for me."

A year later, the tumor had shrunk to a point that only scar tissue remained. By April 2015, she reduced her dose down to maintenance level, and by January 2016 tests showed that the damage to her brain caused by the radiation had also disappeared. "My oncologist had never seen this kind of amazing result. Every other patient she had with the same diagnosis had died. The cannabis not only shrunk my incurable grade 3-4 anaplastic astrocytoma brain tumor, but also mopped up damage to my brain. It is my opinion that cannabis has 100 percent saved my life. In addition to my cannabis treatment, I eat a very clean alkaline diet and exercise every day of the week. I now help families with advice on cannabis treatment for cancer. This medicine should be legal everywhere. I want to spend the rest of my life campaigning for low-THC, high-CBD plant-based cannabis concentrates as a cure for cancer and many other illnesses, and help those who need healing."

How to Take the Medicine: Dosage and Delivery

It is suggested that patients work with a health-care practitioner experienced in recommending CBD or medicinal cannabis so that dosage and delivery methods can be developed and fine-tuned on an individual basis. At the same time, educated and aware patients can be their own highly informed health consultants (see p.75 for information about the subjective-intuitive approach to using cannabis-based medicines).

For all orally administered medicines, refer to the dosage tables on pp. 61–63 for guidelines on CBD dosage by body weight. Always start with the micro dose to test sensitivity and go up as needed within the dosing range by body weight until symptoms subside.

Dosage for advanced cancer is generally in the **macro dose** range, with a suggested range of 200 mg to 2,000 g of total cannabinoids per day. The most commonly suggested ratio of CBD to THC is 1:1. However, at the macro dose level, patients often have difficulty tolerating medication with the higher amount of THC. At the beginning stages of taking macro doses, most are not able to tolerate more than 20–30 mg THC from an oral application. Over a four-to-six-week period, patients are able to increase their tolerance level and become acclimated to high doses. See p. 65 for various protocols to titrate up THC dosages while minimizing side effects or impairment.

When high doses are required, many patients use concentrated forms of cannabis oil and take it orally, either in capsule form or by adding to food (nut butters seem to work well). The purest, most potent concentrates are made using a CO_2-extraction process. More information about various forms of delivery (e.g., sublingual, edible, inhaled) for cannabinoid-based medication can be found starting on p. 38.

For relief of immediate symptoms such as pain, loss of appetite, or nausea, vaporized or smoked cannabis can be highly effective. The medication lasts one to three hours, whereas most ingested products take thirty to sixty minutes before taking effect and last six to eight hours. The most effective vaporizers use a cartridge filled with the CO_2 concentrate, and these are available in various ratios of CBD to THC.

The Cannabis Health Index (CHI) is an evidence-based scoring system for cannabis (in general, not just CBD) and its effectiveness on various health issues based on currently available research data. Refer to p. 86 for more on CHI scores, and check cannabishealthindex.com for updated information.

Effectiveness: Current Science—Cancer

Bone Cancer:	2.7	
Bladder Cancer:	3.0	
Brain Cancer:	2.0	
Breast :	1.5	
Cervical Cancer:	1.0	
Colon:	1.3	
Gastric:	1.0	
Kaposi's Sarcoma:	0.0	
Kidney Cancer:	2.0	
Leukemia:	1.3	
Liver Cancer:	1.2	
Lung Cancer:	1.2	
Lymphoma:	1.2	
Pancreatic:	1.2	
Prostate:	1.5	
Skin Cancer (Melanoma):	1.0	
Skin Cancer (Non-Melanoma):	3.7	
Thyroid Cancer:	1.5	

FIGURE 35

BLADDER CANCER

A study in 2010 showed that CBD induced the death of human urothelial carcinoma cells and concluded that it had identified a potential therapeutic target for bladder cancer.[274] Another study in 2013 found that cannabis use appeared to reduce the risk of bladder cancer in the evaluation of nearly eighty-five thousand men in California.

BRAIN CANCER

A 2004 study showed that CBD was able to produce significant anti-tumor activity both in vitro and in vivo, thus suggesting a possible application of CBD as an antineoplastic agent.[275] Authors of a 2010 research study wrote:

> "The CB1 and CB2 receptor agonist Δ-^{9} tetrahydrocannabinol (THC) has been shown to be a broad-range inhibitor of cancer in culture and in vivo, and is currently being used in a clinical trial for the treatment of glioblastoma. It has been suggested that other plant-derived cannabinoids, which do not interact efficiently with CB1 and CB1 receptors, can modulate the actions of Δ-^{9} THC.[276]

In several glioblastoma cell lines, THC and cannabidiol acted synergistically to inhibit cell proliferation. The treatment of glioblastoma cells with both compounds led to significant modulations of the cell cycle and induction of reactive oxygen species and apoptosis as well as specific modulations of extracellular signal-regulated kinase and caspase activities. These specific changes were not observed with either compound individually, indicating that the signal transduction pathways affected by the combination treatment were unique. The results suggest that the addition of CBD to THC regimens may improve the overall effectiveness in the treatment of glioblastoma in cancer patients.[277]

In 2013, GW Pharmaceuticals began the first human trials to study the potential benefits of its 1:1 ratio product Sativex in the treatment of glioblastoma multiforme, an aggressive form of brain cancer that accounts for half of all new brain cancer diagnoses in the United States. The organization announced positive top-line results from the exploratory Phase 2 placebo-controlled study in early 2017.[278] A 2014 literature review confirmed that, in numerous experimental studies, cannabinoids exerted anti-tumor activity in vitro and/or produced anti-tumor evidence in vivo in several models of tumor cells and tumors. The anti-tumor activity included anti-proliferative effects (cell cycle arrest), decreased viability and cell death by toxicity, apoptosis, necrosis, autophagy, as well as anti-angiogenic and anti-migratory effects. Anti-tumor evidence included reduction in tumor size, anti-angiogenic, and anti-metastatic effects. Additionally, most of the studies described that the cannabinoids exercised selective anti-tumor action in several distinct tumor models. Thereby, normal cells used as controls were not affected. The various cannabinoids tested in multiple tumor models showed anti-tumor effects both in vitro and in vivo. These findings indicate that cannabinoids are promising compounds for the treatment of gliomas.[279] Cristina Sanchez, cancer researcher at University of Spain, stated in an interview in 2015 that glioblastoma tumors are more responsive to a higher THC content in the CBD:THC ratio.[280]

Breast Cancer

A 2006 study acknowledged the anti-tumor effect of THC and focused on the anti-tumor activities of other plant cannabinoids including CBD for breast and other cancers. Results obtained in a panel of tumor cell lines clearly indicate that, of the five natural compounds tested, CBD is the most potent inhibitor of cancer cell growth.[281]

Preclinical research in 2010 focused on ErbB2-positive types of breast cancers that are typically resistant to treatment. It concluded that there is strong evidence for the use of cannabinoids to treat this type of cancer.[282]

In 2015, a study focused on the anti-tumor role and mechanisms of CBD against highly aggressive breast cancer cell lines including triple-negative (TNBC). It showed for the first time that:

> CBD inhibits breast cancer growth and metastasis through novel mechanisms by inhibiting EGF/EGFR signaling and modulating the tumor microenvironment. These results also indicate that CBD can be used as a novel therapeutic option to inhibit growth and metastasis of highly aggressive breast cancer subtypes including TNBC, which currently have limited therapeutic options and are associated with poor prognosis and low survival rates.[283]

In an interview in 2015, Cristina Sanchez stated her research showed breast cancer was responsive to cannabis therapy, and it was even more responsive when the CBD:THC ratio was much higher in CBD.[284]

At age thirty, SLR was diagnosed with stage 4 metastatic breast cancer and given less than one year to live. After surgery and chemotherapy, the cancer returned. She then refused traditional treatments and chose CBD-rich cannabis therapy. "Cannabis oil killed all of the tumors in my body. My monthly lab and quarterly scan results are proof that the cannabis oil treatment worked," she says. Her doctor, who had previously been skeptical, now credits these "alternative" treatments as the reason for her speedy recovery.[285]

Colon Cancer

A 2011 study showed that CBD could promote the death of prostate and colon cancer cells and that the activity was linked to enzymes that remove phosphates from proteins and modulate the activities of these enzymes. The following year, an animal trial showed that in colorectal carcinoma cell lines, "cannabidiol protected DNA from oxidative damage, increased endocannabinoid levels and reduced cell proliferation in a CB(1)-, TRPV1- and PPARγ-antagonists sensitive manner. It is concluded that cannabidiol exerts chemopreventive effect in vivo and reduces cell proliferation through multiple mechanisms."[286]

DH was diagnosed with colon cancer along with infected lymph nodes and received chemotherapy and radiation treatment. After the surgical removal of the cancer from his large intestine, he was deemed cancer free. One year later, the cancer returned to the lungs and was now being called terminal. "I then started taking about one gram of CBD-rich cannabis oil a day," he reported. "A subsequent PET scan revealed that the cancer in my lung had disappeared. The doctor then wanted to remove my lymph nodes and administer conventional treatment afterwards. I refused the treatment and have remained cancer free since then with a maintenance dose."[287]

Endocrine Cancer

A 2008 research analysis reported that "recent evidence indicates that endocannabinoids influence the intracellular events controlling the proliferation of numerous types of endocrine and related cancer cells, thereby leading to both in vitro and in vivo anti-tumor effects. In particular, they are able to inhibit cell growth, invasion and metastasis of thyroid, breast and prostate tumors."[288]

Kaposi's Sarcoma

A 2012 study found a potential biochemical mechanism for the effects of CBD on tumors caused by Kaposi's sarcoma–associated herpesvirus (KSHV). This type of cancer is prevalent among the elderly in the Mediterranean region, inhabitants of sub-Saharan Africa, and immune-compromised individuals such as organ transplant recipients and AIDS patients. Current treatments for Kaposi's sarcoma can inhibit tumor growth but are not able to eliminate KSHV from the host. When the host's immune system weakens, KSHV begins to replicate again, and active tumor growth ensues. "New therapeutic approaches are needed," the authors wrote, reporting that CBD "exhibits promising anti-tumor effects without inducing psychoactive side effects."[289]

Leukemia

A 2013 initiative led by Dr. Wai Liu and colleagues carried out laboratory investigations using a number of cannabinoids, either alone or in combination with each other, to measure their anti-cancer actions in relation to leukemia. Of six cannabinoids studied, each demonstrated anti-cancer properties as effective as those seen from THC. Importantly, they had an increased effect on cancer cells when combined with each other.

> These agents are able to interfere with the development of cancerous cells, stopping them in their tracks and preventing them from growing. In some cases, by using specific dosage patterns, they can destroy cancer cells on their own.

> Used in combination with existing treatment, we could discover some highly effective strategies for tackling cancer. Significantly, these compounds are inexpensive to produce and making better use of their unique properties could result in much more cost effective anti-cancer drugs in future. [290]

The study examined two forms of cannabidiol (CBD), two forms of cannabigerol (CBG), and two forms of cannabigevarin (CBGV), which represent the most common cannabinoids found in the cannabis plant apart from THC.

Lung Cancer

A 2010 study first provided evidence for the mechanism underlying the anti-invasive action of CBD on human lung cancer cells. German research published in 2012 demonstrated for the first time the chemical process by which CBD induces cancer cell death in human lung cancers.[291]

> SK was diagnosed with stage 4 terminal lung cancer. She was told there was no viable treatment and was given six to nine months to live. She took cannabis oil for seven months. The second scan found no active cancer cells in her body—she was cancer free. The oncologist said this was new territory for her as she had never heard of "full metabolic response" on the standard pharmaceutical treatments.[292]

Prostate Cancer

Research published in 2013 provided comprehensive evidence that plant-derived cannabinoids, especially cannabidiol, are potent inhibitors of prostate carcinoma viability in vitro. The study also showed that the extract was active in vivo, either alone or when administered with drugs commonly used to treat prostate cancer (Taxotere or Casodex), and explored the potential mechanisms behind these antineoplastic effects.[293] The following year, authors of another study on CBD and prostate cancer wrote that the results clearly indicate that CBD is a potent inhibitor of cancer cell growth, with significantly lower potency in non-cancer cells. Treatment with CBD "may effectively inhibit spheroid formation in cancer stem cells. This activity may contribute to its anti-cancer and chemosensitizing effect against prostate cancer."[294]

> Three years ago, after a prostate biopsy, DH was given the diagnosis of aggressive stage 3 adenocarcinoma. Using a 1:1 CBD:THC oil, in three months the primary cancer was gone, with only minor metastatic lesions left. After another three months, the metastasis was completely gone. He continues to take a maintenance dose to prevent reoccurrence.[295]

SKIN CANCER

Skin cancer is the most common form of cancer, with 3.5 million new people diagnosed every year in the United States.[296] A 2013 study showed the anti-cancer activity of anandamide in human cutaneous melanoma cells.[297] CBD may be effective by making anandamide, the endogenous neurochemical most similar to THC, more available to the body.

DT had melanoma-type skin cancer on his nose that was treated with conventional medicine and then came back. His doctor recommended a chemotherapy cream, which he refused. He used the CBD+THC oil for three to four weeks before he saw any results, and then the results were dramatic. Not only was the oil healing his nose, it appeared to have "brought cancer to the surface that they didn't even know was there." This was treated and he remains cancer free.[298]

ON MITIGATING THE SIDE EFFECTS FROM CHEMOTHERAPY

The National Cancer Institute, an organization run by the U.S. Department of Health and Human Services, recognizes cannabis as an effective treatment for providing relief of a number of symptoms associated with cancer and chemotherapy treatments, including pain, nausea and vomiting, anxiety, and loss of appetite.[299] Cannabis has long been demonstrated to effectively reduce the nausea and vomiting that often occur after chemotherapy treatments. Studies have found that CBD is effective at treating the more intractable symptoms of nausea, as well as preventing anticipatory nausea in chemotherapy patients[300,301] (see the separate entry on nausea and vomiting).

In one study, cancer patients with neuropathic pain who had previously and unsuccessfully tried to manage their discomfort with opioids saw, after two weeks, significant reductions in pain levels after being treated with cannabis containing both THC and CBD[302] (see more in the section on pain).

Cannabis can also help prevent weight loss and a loss of appetite in chemotherapy patients. THC has been shown to significantly stimulate appetite in patients who have cachexia related to cancer. In addition, patients undergoing chemotherapy and treated with THC have a larger appetite and report that food "tastes better"[303] (see the separate entry on eating disorders). Usually, a small dose of THC, around 2.5 mg, treats weak appetite with very few side effects.

Research also suggests that cannabis may help reduce the swelling in the hands and feet that can occur alongside chemotherapy. Both THC and CBD have shown to have anti-inflammatory properties.[304]

A survey of 131 cancer patients participating in cannabis treatments for six to eight weeks reported significant improvements in all of the measured symptoms, including nausea, vomiting, mood disorders, fatigue, weight loss, anorexia, constipation, sexual function, sleep disorders, itching, and pain.[305] Patients treated with THC have also been shown to experience a higher quality of sleep and relaxation.[306]

Concussions, Brain and Spinal Cord Injuries, and Related Syndromes

Cannabidiol has been reported to promote neuroprotection in several experimental models of brain injury. A 2003 trial that used a 1:1 ratio of CBD to THC to treat neurogenic symptoms from several causes, including spinal cord injury, found that a number of related symptoms improved, including pain, muscle spasms, and bladder control.[307] And in 2012, a study showed improved locomotor functional recovery and reduced injury extent, suggesting that it could be useful in the treatment of spinal cord lesions.[308] The following year, researchers wrote that "the modulation of the endocannabinoid system has proven to be an effective neuroprotective strategy to prevent and reduce neonatal brain injury in different animal models and species."[309] This conclusion has huge clinical implications for post-stroke and brain-injured patients as well as infants affected by perinatal brain injury.

A couple of prominent former NFL quarterbacks, Jake Plummer and Jim McMahon, have been speaking out about the benefits of CBD for brain trauma. In a 2016 publicity video, Plummer explains, "I've had friends, guys I played alongside, whose mood changed from night to day. I know others who've replaced hellacious amounts of painkillers with CBD . . . and I hope this gets even more guys involved. The bigger the number, the better chance we have to get in front of [NFL commissioner] Roger Goodell and say, 'You need to fund this.' Not just for football players, but for the millions of others it could help."[310]

How to Take the Medicine: Dosage and Delivery

It is suggested that patients work with a health care practitioner experienced in recommending CBD or medicinal cannabis so that dosage and delivery methods can be developed and fine-tuned on an individual basis. At the same time, educated and aware patients can be their own highly informed health consultants (see p. 75 for information about the subjective-intuitive approach to using cannabis-based medicines).

CBD products with a ratio of 20:1 or higher are recommended and administered as drops, capsules, or edibles. When appropriate, products containing various ratios of THC from indica-leaning strains can work on intractable pain, and THCV is also recommended for its anti-inflammatory effect. For all orally administered medicines, refer to the dosage tables on pp. 61–63 for guidelines on CBD dosage by body weight. Always start with the micro dose to test sensitivity, and go up as needed within the dosing range before going to the next, until symptoms subside. The **standard dose** is usually recommended to treat brain and spinal cord injuries.

When high doses are required, many patients use concentrated forms of cannabis oil and take it orally, either in capsule form or by adding to food (nut butters seem to work well). The purest, most potent concentrates are made using a CO2-extraction process.

For relief of pain or other immediate symptoms, vaporizing or smoking work well. The medication effect is immediate and lasts one to three hours, whereas most ingested products take thirty to sixty minutes before taking effect (faster on an empty stomach) and last six to eight hours. Vaporizers that use a cartridge filled with the CO2 concentrate are highly effective, and these are available in various ratios of CBD to THC. Herbal vaporizers that use the whole plant are also an effective delivery method. More information about various forms of delivery (e.g., sublingual, oral, inhaled) for cannabinoid-based medication can be found starting on p. 38.

A 2016 randomized, placebo-controlled experiment studied two different doses of vaporized THC on forty-two patients with neuropathic pain related to spinal cord injury or disease. "The reduction in pain intensity remained significant. . . . The lower dose [of THC] appears to offer the best risk-benefit ratio in patients."[311] See the entry on pain in this chapter for more information on dosing and how cannabinoids work on pain.

Effectiveness: Current Science—Spinal Cord Injury

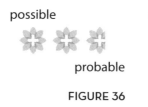

possible   actual

probable

FIGURE 36

The Cannabis Health Index (CHI) is an evidence-based scoring system for cannabis (in general, not just CBD) and its effectiveness on various health issues based on currently available research data. Refer to p. 86 for more on CHI scores, and check cannabishealthindex.com for updated information. Using this rubric, cannabis treatment for spinal cord injury has a rating of likely probable efficacy.

Depression and Mood Disorders

Clinical depression is a serious mood disorder characterized by persistent sadness and loss of interest, sometimes leading to decreased appetite and energy and suicidal thoughts. Commonly used pharmaceuticals for depression often target serotonin, a chemical messenger that is believed to act as a mood stabilizer. The neural network of the endocannabinoid system works similarly to the way that serotonin, dopamine, and other systems do, and, according to some research, cannabinoids have an effect on serotonin levels. Whereas a low dose of THC increases serotonin, high doses cause a decrease that could worsen the condition.[312] In 2009 researchers concluded that there was substantial evidence pointing to endocannabinoid signaling as a target for the pharmacotherapy of depression.[313] Authors of a 2016 study wrote that "CBD could represent a novel fast antidepressant drug, via enhancing both serotonergic and glutamate cortical signaling through a 5-HT1A receptor-dependent mechanism."[314]

CBD might especially be effective for depression related to chronic stress, which has been shown to cause a decrease in endocannabinoid levels.[315,316]

How to Take the Medicine: Dosage and Delivery

It is suggested that patients work with a health care practitioner experienced in recommending CBD or medicinal cannabis so that dosage and delivery methods can be developed and fine-tuned on an individual basis. At the same time, educated and aware patients can be their own highly informed health consultants (see p. 75 for information about the subjective-intuitive approach to using cannabis-based medicines).

CBD products with a ratio of 20:1 or higher are recommended and administered as drops, capsules, or edibles. Specifically, products made with Valentine X or Electra 4 are more energizing, helping relieve depression. When low energy is an issue, sativa or other stimulating strains (see more on these classifications in Chapter 7) can be helpful for improving energy and focus when THC can be tolerated. Varieties that are high in the terpene limonene are recommended for mood elevation.

For all orally administered medicines, refer to the dosage tables on pp. 61–63 for guidelines on CBD dosage by body weight. Always start with the micro dose to test sensitivity and go up as needed within the dosing range before going to the next, until symptoms subside. The **micro to standard dose** is usually recommended to treat depression.

Vaporized or smoked cannabis is recommended for relief of immediate symptoms, or a boost in dosage, and it can also be useful for sleep issues. Sublingual sprays or tinctures taken as liquid drops take effect quickly and last longer than inhaled products. More information about various forms of delivery (e.g., sublingual, oral, inhaled) for cannabinoid-based medication can be found starting on p. 38.

Effectiveness: Current Science—Depression

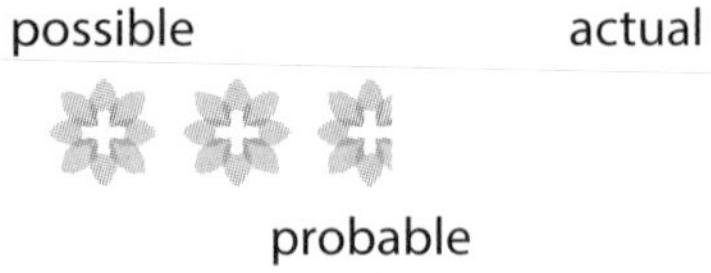

possible   actual

❁ ❁ ❁

probable

FIGURE 37

The Cannabis Health Index (CHI) is an evidence-based scoring system for cannabis (in general, not just CBD) and its effectiveness on various health issues based on currently available research data. Refer to p. 86 for more on CHI scores, and check cannabishealthindex.com for updated information. Using this rubric and based on twenty-one studies, cannabis rated in the possible-to-probable range of efficacy for treatment of depression.

Research in 2005 called for clinical trials to look into the effectiveness of cannabinoids for bipolar disorder (manic depression).[317] In 2010, a study suggested that CBD was not useful for the manic episodes associated with bipolar disorder.[318] However, for depressive episodes, the evidence points to greater potential for effectiveness.[319]

Authors of a 2013 review of animal studies wrote that CBD showed anti-anxiety and antidepressant effects in several models and suggested that the compound worked by interacting with the 5-HT1A neuroreceptor.[320]

"It is important to remember that CBD improves the activity in the endocannabinoid system by increasing the time anandamide works on the CB1 and CB2 receptors," writes Dr. Michael Moskowitz. "Anandamide works on the serotonin, norepinephrine, and dopamine systems. It also works on the GABA-glutamate system and the hypothalamic-pituitary-adrenal axis. Its main role is restoring balance through inhibition when levels are too high and enhancement when they are too low. This is the most likely reason phytocannabinoids in general and CBD specifically are able to regulate depression and anxiety."[321]

Diabetes

Diabetes mellitus refers to a group of metabolic diseases characterized by hyperglycemia caused by defects in insulin secretion, insulin action, or both.

The chronic hyperglycemia of diabetes is associated with long-term damage, dysfunction, and failure of various organs, especially the eyes, kidneys, nerves, heart, brain, and blood vessels. Several pathogenic processes are involved in the development of diabetes. These range from autoimmune destruction of the β-cells of the pancreas with consequent insulin deficiency to metabolic abnormalities and inflammation that result in insulin resistance.

Cannabinoid treatment may be helpful for both type 1 and type 2 diabetes. Researchers in 2011 concluded that "both central and peripheral aspects of endocannabinoid regulation of energy balance can become skewed and contribute to obesity, dyslipidemia, and type 2 diabetes, thus raising the possibility that CB1 antagonists might be used for the treatment of these metabolic disorders. Evidence is emerging that some non psychotropic plant cannabinoids, such as CBD, CBDV and THCV can be employed to retard β-cell damage in type 1 diabetes."[322]

In 2013 one of the largest studies on human patients related to cannabis and metabolic processes found that marijuana use was associated with lower levels of fasting insulin and HOMA-IR, not to mention smaller waist circumference.[323]

POTENTIAL BENEFITS OF CANNABINOIDS FOR PEOPLE WITH DIABETES INCLUDE

- the stabilization of blood sugars
- neuroprotective effects that help thwart inflammation of nerves and reduce the pain of neuropathy by activating receptors in the body and brain
- anti-spasmodic agents that help relieve muscle cramps and the pain of gastrointestinal (GI) disorders
- vasodilator that keeps blood vessels open and improves circulation, contributing to lower blood pressure over time (vital for diabetics)
- anti-inflammatory action that may help quell some of the arterial inflammation common in diabetes[324]

How to Take the Medicine: Dosage and Delivery

It is suggested that patients work with a health care practitioner experienced in recommending CBD or medicinal cannabis so that dosage and delivery methods can be developed and fine-tuned on an individual basis. At the same time, educated and aware patients can be their own highly informed health consultants (see p. 75 for information about the subjective-intuitive approach to using cannabis-based medicines).

CBD products with a ratio of 20:1 or higher are recommended and administered as drops, capsules, or edibles. For all orally administered medicines, refer to the dosage tables on pp. 61–63 for guidelines on CBD dosage by body weight. Always start with the micro dose to test sensitivity and go up as needed within the dosing range before going to the next, until symptoms subside. The **standard dose** is recommended to treat diabetes.

Vaporized or smoked cannabis is recommended for relief of immediate symptoms, such as neuropathic pain or "restless legs syndrome." It is also useful for sleep issues. Sublingual sprays or tinctures taken as liquid drops take effect quickly and last longer than inhaled products. More information about various forms of delivery (e.g., sublingual, oral, inhaled) for cannabinoid-based medication can be found starting on p. 38.

When neuropathic pain is present, topical products can be applied. These can be made using CBD-dominant cannabis or other strains. Topicals affect the cells near application and through several layers of tissue but do not cross the blood-brain barrier and are, therefore, not psychoactive. These may be available as oils, ointments, salves, or other forms, with varying ratios of CBD and THC (a ratio of 1:1 is often recommended as ideal for skin application). The skin has the highest amount and concentration of CB2 receptors in the body.

Effectiveness: Current Science—Diabetes

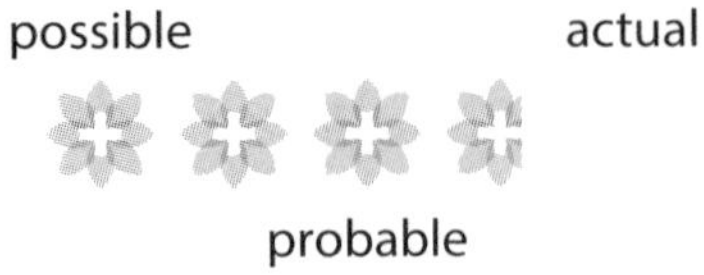

possible   actual

probable

FIGURE 38

The Cannabis Health Index (CHI) is an evidence-based scoring system for cannabis (in general, not just CBD) and its effectiveness on various health issues based on currently available research data. Refer to p. 86 for more on CHI scores, and check cannabishealthindex.com for updated information.

Using this rubric and based on twenty-three studies, cannabis rated in the possible-to-probable range of efficacy for treatment of diabetes.

Research in 2006 and 2008 indicated that CBD treatment could reduce the manifestation of diabetes in animals induced with the disorder. The disease was diagnosed in only 32 percent of the mice in the CBD-treated group, compared to 86 percent and 100 percent in the emulsifier-treated and untreated groups.[325,326]

Authors of a 2010 study concluded that, "collectively, these results, coupled with the excellent safety and tolerability profile of CBD in humans, strongly suggest that it may have great therapeutic potential in the treatment of diabetic complications, and perhaps other cardiovascular disorders, by attenuating oxidative/nitrative stress, inflammation, cell death and fibrosis."[327]

Eating Disorders
(Anorexia, Cachexia, Obesity)

A number of diseases that involve extreme weight gain and loss, including obesity related to binge eating, have similar biological and psychological factors.[328] Emerging evidence has shown a link between defects in the endocannabinoid system and eating disorders, and some research has shown promise in the use of cannabinoids to treat them.

Interestingly, cannabis has been used historically both to increase and suppress appetite. Animal and human studies indicate that CB1 receptor *agonists* relate to appetite enhancement and an increase in the perceived reward value of food, while CB1 *antagonists* have been shown to inhibit food intake. This has led to the clinical development of several pharmaceutical drugs that modulate the endocannabinoid system in the treatment of eating disorders, with mixed success.[329] Current science is limited and suggests that certain cannabinoids tend to increase eating while others reduce food intake.[330] Add to this the fact that cannabinoids can sometimes affect people in opposite ways (see p. 69 for more on the bidirectional effect), which supports the hypothesis that cannabinoids may adapt to different body chemistries to facilitate homeostasis.

Research in 2016 examined the relationship between CBD and what is known as brown fat, the type of fat cell that burns calories in order to generate heat rather than store them. The study data suggested that "CBD plays dual modulatory roles in the form of inducing the brown-like phenotype as well as promoting lipid metabolism. Thus, CBD may be explored as a potentially promising therapeutic agent for the prevention of obesity."[331]

Conversely, anorexia and cachexia involve physical wasting and malnutrition. While anorexia is both biological and psychological in nature, cachexia accompanies cancer, AIDS, pulmonary disease, multiple sclerosis, heart failure, tuberculosis, severe neurological diseases, heavy metal poisoning, and extreme hormonal imbalance. Characteristics of both conditions include loss of weight, muscle atrophy, fatigue, weakness, and loss of appetite. Research has confirmed that cannabinoids help alleviate cachexia symptoms in many sufferers and offers treatment of related conditions as well.[332]

In 2013 two studies showed promising results related to the use of cannabinoids with anorexia patients. THC activates the CB1 receptor, which helps increase appetite. CB1 is also involved with the receptor for ghrelin, a hormone that contributes to an increase in the sensation of hunger. One involved use of a synthetic cannabinoid, dronabinol, which led to small but significant weight gain in anorexia nervosa patients,[333] and another that found cannabinoids helped anorexia-stricken mice recover and return to a healthy weight.[334]

How to Take the Medicine: Dosage and Delivery

It is suggested that patients work with a health care practitioner experienced in recommending CBD or medicinal cannabis so that dosage and delivery methods can be developed and fine-tuned on an individual basis. At the same time, educated and aware patients can be their own highly informed health consultants (see p. 75 for information about the subjective-intuitive approach to using cannabis-based medicines).

For obesity, CBD products with a ratio of 20:1 or higher are recommended and administered as drops or capsules. Varieties high in THCV may retard appetite.[335]

Sativa strains like Sour Diesel are usually the most effective, if THC can be tolerated, to stimulate appetite in anorexia and cachexia patients, but it bears individual experimentation with strains and dose. Usually, a small dose of THC (around 2.5 mg) treats weak appetite with very few side effects. A person without experience with THC should use caution and titrate slowly up to higher doses (read more on how to do this on p. 65). A 1:1 ratio of CBD to THC can be used when patients report too much psychoactivity, as CBD is anti-psychoactive. Another cannabinoid being studied for its use in stimulating appetite is CBG, so varieties high in this compound may be beneficial.

For all orally administered medicines, refer to the dosage tables on pp. 61–63 for guidelines on CBD dosage by body weight. Always start with the micro dose to test sensitivity and go up as needed within the dosing range before going to the next, until symptoms subside. The **micro to standard dose** is usually recommended to treat eating disorders.

For immediate effect on appetite, vaporized or smoked cannabis can be highly effective in quickly increasing or suppressing the desire for food (depending on individual body chemistry and the type of cannabis). The medication lasts one to three hours, whereas most ingested products take thirty to sixty minutes before taking effect and last six to eight hours. The most effective vaporizers use a cartridge filled with the CO2 concentrate, and these are available in various ratios of CBD to THC. Sublingual sprays or tinctures taken as liquid drops take effect quickly and last longer than inhaled products. More information about various forms of delivery (e.g., sublingual, oral, inhaled) for cannabinoid-based medication can be found starting on p. 38.

Effectiveness: Current Science— Anorexia/Cachexia and Obesity

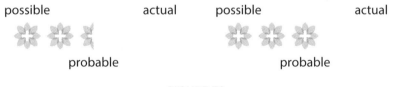

possible   actual   possible   actual

probable   probable

FIGURE 39

The Cannabis Health Index (CHI) is an evidence-based scoring system for cannabis (in general, not just CBD) and its effectiveness on various health issues based on currently available research data. Refer to p. 86 for more on CHI scores, and check cannabishealthindex.com for updated information. Using this rubric and based on thirteen studies, for anorexia and cachexia, cannabis rated in the possible-to-probable rate of efficacy (2.5 points). For obesity, based on six studies, it rates in the range of likely probable efficacy (3 points).

There have also been several studies investigating the possibility that mutations in genes related to the endocannabinoid system may render bearers more susceptible to eating disorders such as anorexia. A study published in 2009 concluded that a single nucleotide change in the gene that encodes for the expression of the CB1 receptor, as well as a second polymorphism in a gene controlling production of the anandamide-degradation molecule FAAH, may contribute to a biological sensitivity to anorexia and bulimia nervosa.[336]

Inflammatory Bowel Syndromes and Diseases (IBS and IBD)

Inflammatory bowel disorders are classified according to the primary symptoms, usually characterized by diarrhea, constipation, or alternating symptoms of both, and worsened by stress (see the entry on anxiety and stress in this chapter). These disorders include ulcerative colitis, a form that can also affect other parts of the body, and Crohn's disease, among other similar syndromes. The epithelium of the GI tract is embedded with the enteric nervous system, a web of neurons that regulate gut function and where both CB1 and CB2 receptors are found in abundance. This is one aspect of the overall relationship between metabolism and energy balance and the endocannabinoid system.

Inflammatory bowel disease affects millions of individuals; nevertheless, pharmacological treatment is disappointingly unsatisfactory. CBD has antioxidant and other pharmacological effects that are potentially beneficial for the inflamed gut.[337]

A number of studies over the past decade have demonstrated the chemical messengers and endocannabinoid receptors involved in modulating and balancing the GI system. Specifically, FAAH is an enzyme crucially involved in the modulation of intestinal physiology through anandamide and other endocannabinoids.[338] CBD specifically has been shown to stimulate the endocannabinoid system by blocking the FAAH enzyme responsible for breaking down anandamide, thereby increasing its availability. A 2016 study was the first to show in the lab that inhibiting FAAH may suppress colitis by reducing activated T cells and inflammatory response in the colon.[339]

"These processes might link stress with abdominal pain," researchers wrote that year. "The endocannabinoid system (ECS) is also involved centrally in the manifestation of stress, and endocannabinoid signaling reduces the activity of hypothalamic-pituitary-adrenal pathways via actions in specific brain regions, notably the prefrontal cortex, amygdala, and hypothalamus. Agents that modulate the ECS are in early stages of development for treatment of gastrointestinal diseases. Increasing our understanding of the ECS will greatly advance our knowledge of interactions between the brain and gut and could lead to new treatments for gastrointestinal disorders."[341]

How to Take the Medicine: Dosage and Delivery

It is suggested that patients work with a health-care practitioner experienced in recommending CBD or medicinal cannabis so that dosage and delivery methods can be developed and fine-tuned on an individual basis. At the same time, educated and aware patients can be their own highly informed health consultants (see p. 75 for information about the subjective-intuitive approach to using cannabis-based medicines).

CBD products with a ratio of 20:1 or higher are recommended and administered as drops in oil, capsules, or edibles. Patients should assess which delivery system is least disruptive and best absorbed by their bodies. Cannabinoids can be very effective in reducing chronic inflammation, treating temporary stress, and protecting the body from the physiological effects of both. Beyond CBD, a promising cannabinoid for gastrointestinal inflammation is CBG. "Purple" and "Afghan" varieties and those high in limonene are popular with patients with inflammatory bowel disorders.[341] Alcohol-based tinctures usually should be avoided for IBS patients. Also, be aware that varieties high in THCV may suppress appetite.[342]

For all orally administered medicines, refer to the dosage tables on pp. 61–63 for guidelines on CBD dosage by body weight. Always start with the micro dose to test sensitivity and go up as needed within the dosing range before going to the next, until symptoms subside. The **micro to standard dose** is usually recommended to treat inflammatory bowel disorders.

For relief of nausea or other immediate symptoms, vaporizing or smoking work well. The medication effect is immediate and lasts one to three hours, whereas most ingested products take thirty to sixty minutes before taking effect (faster on an empty stomach) and last six to eight hours. Vaporizers that use a cartridge filled with the CO_2 concentrate are highly effective, and these are available in various ratios of CBD to THC. Herbal vaporizers that use the whole plant are also an effective delivery method. Sublingual sprays or tinctures taken as liquid drops also take effect quickly and last longer than inhaled products. More information about various forms of delivery (e.g., sublingual, oral, inhaled) for cannabinoid-based medication can be found starting on p. 38.

Effectiveness: Current Science—Bowel and Chron's

possible   actual

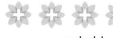

probable

FIGURE 40

The Cannabis Health Index (CHI) is an evidence-based scoring system for cannabis (in general, not just CBD) and its effectiveness on various health issues based on currently available research data. Refer to p. 86 for more on CHI scores, and check cannabishealthindex.com for updated information. Using this rubric and based on nine studies, cannabis rated in the possible range of efficacy for treatment of inflammatory bowel disorders (1.9 points), and in the possible-to-probable range based on studies related specifically to Crohn's disease (3.3 points).

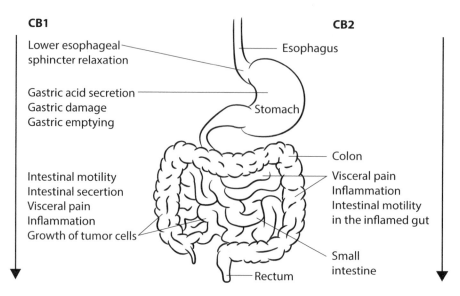

FIGURE 41

Research in 2012 indicated that intrarectal delivery of cannabinoids (via suppository) may represent a useful therapeutic administration route for the treatment of colonic inflammation.[343] The following year, researchers commented that the activity of cannabinoids had been enigmatic for gastroenterologists and pharmacologists, but that new evidence pointed toward CBD as a potential candidate for the development of a new class of anti-IBD drugs.[344,345]

Migraine

A migraine is a headache disorder characterized by recurrent moderate-to-severe headaches that most often affect one half of the head. Migraines tend to be pulsating in nature and last from four to seventy-two hours or longer. Symptoms can be disabling in nature: visual disturbances; nausea; vomiting; dizziness; extreme sensitivity to sound, light, touch, and smell; and tingling or numbness in the extremities or face.[346] Physical activity can exacerbate the pain.[347] Migraines impact approximately one billion people globally and about thirty-eight million men and women in the United States. Migraines are the third-most prevalent illness and the sixth-most disabling illness in the world.[348] In many cases, migraines cause such severe symptoms that patients are unable to focus on work, children, or other responsibilities. The underlying mechanisms are not fully known. Migraines are commonly believed to involve the nerves and blood vessels of the brain but may also be caused by problems in the cervical spine. Depression, anxiety, and sleep disturbances are common for those with chronic migraine.[349]

Interestingly, medication overuse is the most common reason episodic migraine turns chronic. Furthermore, the health care and lost-productivity costs associated with migraine are estimated to be as high as $36 billion annually in the United States. And, although 25 percent of sufferers would benefit from preventive treatment, only 12 percent of all sufferers receive it.[350]

These numbers indicate that improved treatment options for this debilitating condition must be developed. Recent studies show that migraine headaches may be due to endocannabinoid deficiency and abnormal inflammatory response. In fact, patients suffering from migraines have reported feeling as if the brain tissue itself is inflamed and physically bumping against the skull. The use of CBD and THC can augment endocannabinoid deficiencies and mitigate or reduce inflammation.

GN suffered from severe ocular migraines that interrupted his daily life and often came with a great deal of discomfort and pain. In discovering CBD derived from cannabis, he has almost entirely eliminated these migraines without much need for pain meds. Where he was having occurrences almost weekly before, he has only had a few very mild occurrences in the last few years. His strain of choice has been Valentine X, taken in small doses as liquid drops, as a preventative two to three times daily.

In case he does have a migraine, GN has a Sumatriptan prescription to support the CBD therapy. He reports, however, "the drug mostly sits in my medicine cabinet past the expiration date. In addition to this, I find that I am much less interested in any form of alcohol or caffeine, which can be a migraine-triggering substance. With CBD from cannabis available now, my quality of life has improved many times over."

How to Take the Medicine: Dosage and Delivery

It is suggested that patients work with a health care practitioner experienced in recommending CBD or medicinal cannabis so that dosage and delivery methods can be developed and fine-tuned on an individual basis. At the same time, educated and aware patients can be their own highly informed health consultants (see p. 75 for information about the subjective-intuitive approach to using cannabis-based medicines).

Oral CBD products with a ratio of 20:1 or higher, administered as drops, capsules, or edibles, can be very effective in treating pain. Most discussions of treating pain with CBD suggest that finding the right dosage is critical. Refer to the dosage tables on pp. 61–63 for guidelines on CBD dosage by body weight. Always start with the micro dose to test sensitivity and go up as needed within the dosing range by body weight until symptoms subside. The **micro to standard** dose is usually recommended to treat migraines, but patients need to carefully monitor their condition and experiment to find the right formula.

For the most part, using CBD to prevent symptoms from manifesting is much easier than treating migraines after the onset of symptoms as, at that point, the patient often needs to augment CBD with some quantity of THC. A person without experience with THC should use caution and titrate slowly up to higher doses. A 1:1 ratio of CBD to THC can be used when patients report too much psychoactivity, as CBD reduces this. Specific anti-inflammatory strains of cannabis high in CBD, such as Swiss Gold, Sour Tsunami, and Harlequin, can be excellent in reducing symptoms. Sour Diesel, while having a higher THC profile and lower CBD profile, is another strain highly effective in reducing pain, especially after the onset of more severe symptoms. Researchers have found inhalation a more effective delivery than ingestion, as cannabinoids are able to act faster without any delay in getting into the bloodstream.

Dr. Allan Frankel, a physician who treats migraine-suffering patients with CBD, stated, "Every migraine patient I have seen has always suffered with anxiety and tight cervical muscle issues. So, whether it is a true migraine, cluster or other non-vascular headache, my recommendation is almost always modest doses of a high ratio CBD:THC capsule."[351]

Another method of delivery for migraines recommended by Dr. Michael Moskowitz involves applying a few drops of alcohol-based tincture to the inner cheek by the jaw muscle, where sensory and motor branches of the trigeminal nerve are located (the spot where a dentist applies anesthetic to numb the jaw). A sativa strain strong in THC and in an alcohol tincture can be administered with a cotton swab or your finger. This is a very fast-acting and effective method for migraines. Also, a 1:1 ratio of CBD to THC (sativa-leaning strains are recommended) can be very effective in bringing medication directly to the site. Even a high-CBD, low-THC, oil-based tincture can be effective. None of these treatments causes psychotropic effects in the vast majority of patients.

Anxiety that develops after several bouts of migraines is known as an anticipatory symptom and can be treated best with a minimal dose of CBD in the morning. The cervical muscle tension that can precipitate a migraine can similarly be treated with the same CBD regime. Dr. Frankel added, "I have seen this nearly always works."[352]

Other cannabinoids are also shown to relieve pain, including CBC, CBG, THCV, and THCA. Varieties high in beta-caryophyllene, myrcene, and linalool provide additional pain relief and increase the effectiveness of other cannabinoids for analgesia.

For relief of immediate symptoms, as in a flare-up of pain, vaporizing or smoking work well. The medication effect is immediate and lasts one to three hours, whereas most ingested products take thirty to sixty minutes before taking effect (faster on an empty stomach) and last six to eight hours. Vaporizers that use a cartridge filled with the CO2 concentrate are highly effective, and these are available in various ratios of CBD to THC. Herbal vaporizers that use the whole plant are also an effective delivery method. Sublingual sprays or tinctures taken as liquid drops also take effect quickly and last longer than inhaled products. More information about various forms of delivery (e.g., sublingual, oral, inhaled) for cannabinoid-based medication can be found starting on p. 38.

Effectiveness: Current Science—Migraine

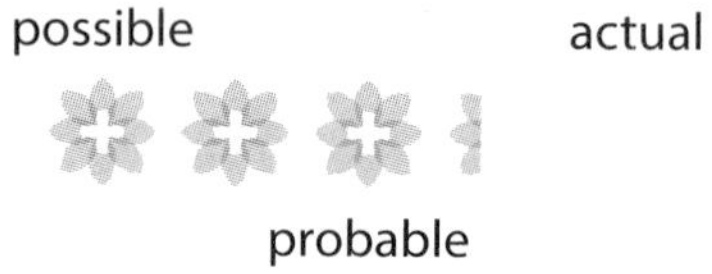

possible   actual

probable

FIGURE 42

The Cannabis Health Index (CHI) is an evidence-based scoring system for cannabis (in general, not just CBD) and its effectiveness on various health issues based on currently available research data. Refer to p. 86 for more on CHI scores, and check cannabishealthindex.com for updated information. Using this rubric and based on six studies, cannabis rated in the possible-to-probable range.

A 2014 study suggested that medical cannabis could reduce migraine frequency. The study found that, on average, migraine-suffering patients who used medical marijuana saw their frequency of migraines drop significantly.[353] While initial findings are encouraging with regards to CBD and migraine treatment, future research may shed more light onto how migraines manifest and what CBD does to decrease symptoms.

Multiple Sclerosis and Spasticity

Spasticity, or painful muscle rigidity and spasms, is one of the primary symptoms of multiple sclerosis (MS), cerebral palsy, ALS, and spinal cord injury (see separate sections on the latter two disorders in this chapter). An autoimmune and inflammatory disorder with unknown causes, MS results in the degeneration of the nerve fibers of the brain and is fairly common in developed countries in the West. Symptoms can range from mild to severely disabling, and for years MS sufferers have claimed significant benefit from cannabis (see separate section on autoimmune disorders), though results can vary from dramatic to subtle. In the past few years, science has gained a foothold in understanding the role of the endocannabinoid system in regulating the neural signaling that controls spasticity and its underlying conditions. Cannabis-based medicines have been approved in a number of states and countries for the treatment of pain and spasticity associated with MS, including a pharmaceutical 1:1 CBD:THC ratio mouth spray called Sativex (see more on Sativex on p. 56). Sativex is plant-based and is not a synthetic cannabinoid.

EK was diagnosed with MS in 1995. About a decade passed and the chronic, overall body pain that typically accompanies MS began to increase and adversely affect her functional capability and mental state (depression from constantly feeling ill). After experiencing the undesirable side effects of various doctor-prescribed opioids, which did not help with her MS pain, her doctor asked if she would consider medicinal marijuana. She was more than willing to try anything that would return her toward normalcy. The doctor put her in contact with a nurse who had been using CBD (which had very limited availability at the time) and THC strains to help with her own health issues, and the information she provided initiated the educated path that EK has developed and that really works for her.

She started with THC-dominant strains, which were all she could find. They significantly reduced daily pain, but she was not thrilled with the psychoactive effects that resulted. Then she found Synergy Wellness and started using CBD-dominant strains. EK says the tinctures made from AC/DC, Valentine X, and other high-CBD strains have worked a near miracle on her pain and, consequently, on her general quality of life. She seldom has really horrible days since having developed a feel for how to use the various strains and ratios. On those days, when the pain level is high, she adjusts her baseline CBD by blending in a little THC (usually about 4:1 ratio). With ratios of 4:1 or higher, the pain is controlled without significant psychoactive effects. This responsible use of cannabis enables her to live a fairly normal life, in spite of this devastating disease.

The benefit of cannabinoid activity for MS is "supported both by the biology of the disease and the biology of the cannabis plant and the endocannabinoid system," according to the authors of a 2012 study. "MS impairs neurotransmission, and this is controlled by cannabinoid receptors and endogenous cannabinoid ligands. [Cannabinoids] can limit spasticity and may also influence the processes that drive the accumulation of progressive disability."[354]

How to Take the Medicine: Dosage and Delivery

It is suggested that patients work with a health care practitioner experienced in recommending CBD or medicinal cannabis so that dosage and delivery methods can be developed and fine-tuned on an individual basis. At the same time, educated and aware patients can be their own highly informed health consultants (see p. 75 for information about the subjective-intuitive approach to using cannabis-based medicines).

Oral CBD products with a ratio of 20:1 or higher, administered as drops, capsules, or edibles, can be very effective in treating pain, especially the inflammatory type. Most discussions of treating symptoms with CBD suggest that finding the right dosage is critical. Other cannabinoids with low psychoactivity are also shown to relieve pain, including CBC, CBG, THCV, and THCA. Chemotypes high in beta-caryophyllene, myrcene, and linalool provide additional pain relief and increase the effectiveness of other cannabinoids for analgesia.

For treatment of spasticity, products with a higher ratio of THC are sometimes recommended to better manage symptoms. In general, for pain, and especially for evening and nighttime, strains that lean toward broad-leaf indica are favored for the sedative effect. A person without experience with THC should use caution and titrate slowly up to higher doses.

For all orally administered medicines such as drops, capsules, or edibles, refer to the dosage tables on pp. 61–63 for guidelines on CBD dosage by body weight. Always start with the micro dose to test sensitivity and go up as needed within the dosing range before going to the next, until symptoms subside. The **standard to macro dose** is usually recommended to treat multiple sclerosis.

For immediate delivery, vaporizing or smoking work well. The medication effect is immediate and lasts one to three hours, whereas most ingested products take thirty to sixty minutes before taking effect (faster on an empty stomach) and last six to eight hours. Vaporizers that use a cartridge filled with the CO2 concentrate are highly effective, and these are available in various ratios of CBD to THC. Herbal vaporizers that use the whole plant are also an effective delivery method. Sublingual sprays or tinctures taken as liquid drops also take effect quickly and last longer than inhaled products. More information about various forms of delivery (e.g., sublingual, oral, inhaled) for cannabinoid-based medication can be found starting on p. 38.

Effectiveness: Current Science—MS

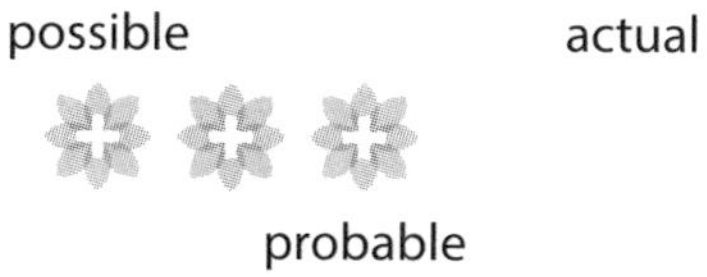

possible   actual

✻ ✻ ✻

probable

FIGURE 43

The Cannabis Health Index (CHI) is an evidence-based scoring system for cannabis (in general, not just CBD) and its effectiveness on various health issues based on currently available research data. Refer to p. 86 for more on CHI scores, and check cannabishealthindex.com for updated information. Based on thirty-seven studies from 1981 to present and according to this rubric, cannabis has a rating of likely probable efficacy for treatment of MS.

A 1997 study in the United Kingdom found that 30 percent of the MS sufferers surveyed reported relief from symptoms such as spasticity, chronic pain, and memory loss.

GW Pharmaceuticals has been developing a product with a 1:1 balanced ratio of THC to CBD called Sativex, available as an oromucosal spray. Several clinical trials have shown it to be effective,[355,356] and it has been approved for use for treatment of MS symptoms in numerous countries, including Canada, the United Kingdom, Australia, and at least twenty more.[357]

Nausea and Vomiting

The anti-emetic (effective against nausea and vomiting) properties of cannabis are probably one of the most recognized and studied medicinal application of the plant, and a clear body of evidence supports its efficacy. The research demonstrates that manipulation of the endocannabinoid system regulates nausea and vomiting in humans and other animals, whether the condition is related to toxins, hormones, or motion.[358] Cannabis has been used to treat nausea and vomiting across cultures for millennia, and in the mid-1970s scientific research began to focus on the treatment of these symptoms among chemotherapy patients. The first studies used high-THC cannabis successfully and resulted in the development of a synthetic THC pharmaceutical called Marinol, still prescribed today for nausea and appetite stimulation related to cancer and AIDS. However, evidence shows that Marinol and other synthetic versions of cannabinoids are not as effective as plant-based products for many diseases. For nausea and vomiting in particular, inhaled products have proven to have a higher success rate since they bypass the GI system and have immediate effect, but oral cannabinoids can also work for chronic issues.

By 2002, researchers began to turn toward cannabinoids without psychoactive side effects, namely CBD, for their therapeutic value in the treatment of nausea.[359] Unlike THC, CBD has a low affinity for the CB1 and CB2 receptors[360] but appears to work indirectly on the 5-HT receptor, in the serotonin family of neurotransmitters.[361]

How to Take the Medicine: Dosage and Delivery

It is suggested that patients work with a health care practitioner experienced in recommending CBD or medicinal cannabis so that dosage and delivery methods can be developed and fine-tuned on an individual basis. At the same time, educated and aware patients can be their own highly informed health consultants (see p. 75 for information about the subjective-intuitive approach to using cannabis-based medicines).

For relief of immediate symptoms, vaporizing or smoking works well, and many nausea patients prefer this delivery system as it doesn't require ingestion (and potentially not being able to keep the medicine down long enough to take effect). Often, the very thought of having to ingest anything, including medicine, will cause the nausea to worsen. The medication effect is immediate and lasts one to three hours, whereas most ingested products take thirty to sixty minutes before taking effect (faster on an empty stomach) and last six to eight hours. Vaporizers that use a cartridge filled with the CO_2 concentrate are highly effective, and these are available in various ratios of CBD to THC. Herbal vaporizers that use the whole plant are also an effective delivery method. Sublingual sprays or tinctures taken as liquid drops also take effect quickly and last longer than inhaled products. More information about various forms of delivery (e.g., sublingual, oral, inhaled) for cannabinoid-based medication can be found starting on p. 38.

When more chronic nausea is an issue, CBD products with a ratio of 20:1 or higher are recommended and administered as drops, capsules, or edibles. For all orally administered medicines, refer to the dosage tables on pp. 61–63 for guidelines on CBD dosage by body weight. Always start with the micro dose to test sensitivity and go up as needed within the dosing range before going to the next, until symptoms subside. The **micro to standard dose** is usually recommended to treat nausea and vomiting. For chemotherapy-induced nausea, a higher dose may be required (see more in the section on cancer). Most varieties of cannabis work effectively for nausea, and some treatment plans include starting with 5 mg of THC and scaling up to 15 mg before chemotherapy begins.

Effectiveness: Current Science—Nausea

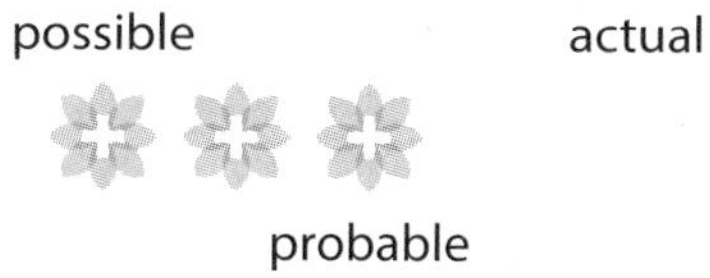

possible   actual

probable

FIGURE 44

The Cannabis Health Index (CHI) is an evidence-based scoring system for cannabis (in general, not just CBD) and its effectiveness on various health issues based on currently available research data. Refer to p. 86 for more on CHI scores, and check cannabishealthindex.com for updated information. For treatment of nausea and vomiting, according to this rubric, cannabis rates as likely probable efficacy (3 points).

Over forty studies have been conducted on the use of cannabinoids to effectively treat nausea and vomiting, and it is considered one of the best-supported therapeutic uses of cannabis according to American and British medical association reviews. One study pooled available data of over one thousand chemotherapy patients and found that oral synthetic THC provided relief of nausea in 76–88 percent of users and smoked cannabis provided relief in 70–100 percent.[362]

Commonly prescribed drugs for chemo-related nausea are 5-HT antagonists, which suppress vomiting but do not minimize nausea, and are not effective for delayed nausea and vomiting. Cannabinoids are effective for these symptoms according to a 2011 study.[363]

Neurodegenerative Diseases (Huntington's and Parkinson's)

While Parkinson's and Huntington's diseases have different origins and are typically found in different populations, both affect the part of the brain that controls movement (see also the entries for ALS and Alzheimer's). Parkinson's usually affects people over fifty and can cause tremors, slowed movement, rigidity, and impaired balance and coordination. Huntington's appears in a younger population and always has genetic origins, affecting movement, cognition, and mood. Evidence suggests that cannabinoids can be very effective as treatment for this class of disorder as they are able to suppress the excitotoxicity, glial activation (a source of centralized pain), and oxidative injury that cause neural degeneration. They work on multiple levels as neuroprotectants that potentially slow progression of these diseases, while also treating a number of the symptoms.[364]

Researchers in 2008 and again in 2014 concluded that CBD has a demonstrated ability to recover memory deficits induced by brain iron accumulation, which is involved in the pathogenesis of a number of neurological diseases.[365] It can also improve the function of mitochondria in cells and activate the clearance of debris, further encouraging neuron health.[366] In addition, CBD may help patients experiencing neurodegenerative-related psychosis.[367]

THC has also been shown to help in the treatment of neurodegenerative diseases by protecting against damage caused by free radicals and activating the formation of new mitochondria.[368] For improving symptoms, products with various ratios of CBD to THC have been shown to produce significant improvements in motor impairments, bradykinesia, tremors, pain, and sleep.[369,370,371] A 2014 study on Parkinson's patients found a measurable improvement in well-being and quality of life scores in general after one week of treatment with CBD.[372]

Although a study in 1991 involving CBD and Huntington's yielded disappointing results,[373] twenty years later GW Pharmaceuticals, mentioning limitations of previous research, began preclinical trials using Sativex, its 1:1 CBD:THC oral spray that has been approved in numerous countries outside the United States for spasticity associated with multiple sclerosis.[374] Preliminary results didn't show statistically significant improvement in motor or cognitive deficits, but the drug was well tolerated and studies using higher doses are underway.[375] In 2015, a study showed that CBG has promise as a neuroprotectant with numerous beneficial actions on brain health.[376]

How to Take the Medicine: Dosage and Delivery

It is suggested that patients work with a health care practitioner experienced in recommending CBD or medicinal cannabis so that dosage and delivery methods can be developed and fine-tuned on an individual basis. At the same time, educated and aware patients can be their own highly informed health consultants (see p. 75 for information about the subjective-intuitive approach to using cannabis-based medicines).

For all orally administered medicines, refer to the dosage tables on pp. 61–63 for guidelines on CBD dosage by body weight. Always start with the micro dose to test sensitivity and go up as needed within the dosing range by body weight until symptoms subside. Patients should be cautious about titrating slowly up to a target **standard to macro dosing range** to ensure minimal psychoactive effects. Varieties that are high in myrcene have a more relaxing effect, and strains high in THCV are indicated for their potential neuroprotective properties.

That being said, products made with broad-leaf, indica-dominant varieties that are higher in THC can be helpful for sleep issues (see more in the entry for sleep disorders in this chapter) or produce a calming and sedating effect. A maximum range of 5–10 mg of THC per dose is suggested. Avoid products containing sativa-dominant strains as they can promote hyperactivity and dissociation. Vaporized or smoked cannabis is recommended for relief of immediate symptoms, or a boost in dosage, and it can also be useful for sleep issues. Sublingual sprays or tinctures taken as liquid drops take effect quickly and last longer than inhaled products. For safety reasons, smoked or vaporized products are not recommended for patients with advanced cognitive symptoms.

When high doses are required, many patients use concentrated forms of cannabis oil and take it orally, either in capsule form or by adding to food (nut butters seem to work well). The purest, most potent concentrates are made using a CO2-extraction process. More information about various forms of delivery (e.g., sublingual, edible, transdermal) for cannabinoid-based medication can be found starting on p. 38.

LS is a former police captain who had suffered from Parkinson's for decades and exhausted every conventional method of treatment, every drug, and even brain surgery. Refusing to give up, he discovered medical cannabis. His experimentation included the use of high-CBD products such as sublingual drops, which greatly benefitted him. In 2011 filmmakers began documenting his experience, which has been released as a multipart series. LS has become a campaigner, raising awareness about the disease, and has been healthy enough to continue completing educational and fundraising long-distance bike rides.[377]

Effectiveness: Current Science—Huntington's/Parkinson's

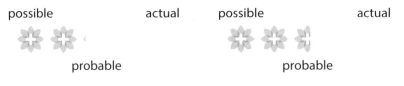

FIGURE 45

The Cannabis Health Index (CHI) is an evidence-based scoring system for cannabis (in general, not just CBD) and its effectiveness on various health issues based on currently available research data. Refer to p. 86 for more on CHI scores, and check cannabishealthindex.com for updated information. For treatment of Huntington's disease, based on thirty-two studies, cannabis scored in the possible-to-probable range of efficacy (2.1 points). For Parkinson's the score was in the same range and was based on twenty-eight studies (2.6 points).

Results of a 2007 study indicated that cannabinoids provide neuroprotection against the progressive degeneration of nigrostriatal dopaminergic neurons occurring in Parkinson's. In 2009 data suggested that CBD might be effective, safe, and well-tolerated for the treatment of the psychosis in neuro-degenerative disorders,[378] and in 2011 a study on THCV concluded it had "a promising pharmacological profile for delaying disease progression and also for ameliorating parkinsonian symptoms."[379]

CB2 receptor up-regulation has been found in many neurodegenerative disorders including Huntington's and Parkinson's, which supports the ben-eficial effects found for CB2 receptor agonists in both disorders. Evidence reported so far supports those cannabinoids' antioxidant properties and/or capability to activate CB2 receptors as promising therapeutic agents in treat-ing both disorders, thus deserving a prompt clinical evaluation.[380,381]

Pain

"For the relief of certain kinds of pain, I believe, there is no more useful medicine than Cannabis within our reach," wrote Sir John Russell Reynolds, neurologist, epilepsy research pioneer, and physician to Queen Victoria back in 1859.[382] In fact, cannabis was used for pain relief in all of the major ancient civilizations from Asia through the Middle East and into Europe and the Americas. The scientific inquiry into cannabis over the past several decades has confirmed that it is an effective and safe analgesic for many kinds of pain.

Of all the reasons that people use CBD today, pain is the most common. The same can be said of cannabis in general. In the United States, over sev-enty million people suffer from chronic pain, which is defined as experienc-ing over one hundred days per year of pain. Physicians differentiate between neuropathic (usually chronic) and nociceptive pains (usually time-limited), and cannabis works on most neuropathic and many nociceptive types of pain. A number of studies have demonstrated that the endocannabinoid system is both centrally and peripherally involved in the processing of pain signals.[383] Most discussions of treating pain with CBD suggest that finding the right dosage is critical.

Cannabinoids can be used along with opioid medications, and a number of studies have demonstrated that they can reduce the amount of opioids needed, lessen the buildup of tolerance, and reduce the severity of with-drawal.[384] At least ten randomized, controlled trials on over one thousand patients have demonstrated efficacy of cannabinoids for neuropathic pain of various origins.

BV has bone-on-bone arthritis and was in need of a full knee replacement. He was in a lot of pain and having trouble with mobility. In addition, he has Hashimoto's disease. He started taking CBD oil for both. In just a few weeks, he was feeling so much better, free of the nerve and deep muscle pains that he usually had from the Hashimoto's. It was when he skipped a daily dose that he realized how much the oil was really helping.[385]

How to Take the Medicine: Dosage and Delivery

It is suggested that patients work with a health care practitioner experienced in recommending CBD or medicinal cannabis so that dosage and delivery methods can be developed and fine-tuned on an individual basis. At the same time, educated and aware patients can be their own highly informed health consultants (see p. 75 for information about the subjective-intuitive approach to using cannabis-based medicines).

Oral CBD products with a ratio of 20:1 or higher and administered as drops, capsules, or edibles can be very effective in treating pain, especially the inflammatory type. Most discussions of treating pain with CBD suggest that finding the right dosage is critical. Refer to the dosage tables on pp. 61–63 for guidelines on CBD dosage by body weight. Always start with the micro dose to test sensitivity and go up as needed within the dosing range by body weight until symptoms subside. The **micro to standard** dose is usually recommended to treat pain, but patients need to carefully monitor their condition and experiment to find the right formula; 10–40 mg of CBD or CBD+THC together is usually enough.

If CBD-dominant products alone are not enough to treat a particular case, products with a higher ratio of THC are sometimes recommended to better manage pain. For day use, more stimulating, sativa varieties with higher concentrations of myrcene could be added to the formula (see more on these classifications in Chapter 7). In general, for pain, and especially for evening and nighttime, indica strains are favored for their relaxing, sedative effect. A person without experience with THC should use caution and titrate slowly up to higher doses (read more on strategies for increasing THC doses with minimal side effects on p. 65). Research as well as patient feedback have indicated that, in general, a ratio of 4:1 CBD:THC is the most effective for both neuropathic and inflammatory pain. Each individual is different, however—for some, a 1:1 ratio of CBD:THC can be more effective, and others prefer a high-THC strain when it can be tolerated. Each patient's tolerance and sensitivity will differ, and through titration the correct strain and ratio combination can be found.

Other cannabinoids are also shown to relieve pain, including CBC, CBG, THCV, and THCA. Chemotypes high in beta-caryophyllene, myrcene, and linalool provide additional pain relief and increase the effectiveness of other cannabinoids for analgesia.

For relief of immediate symptoms, as in a flare-up of pain, vaporizing or smoking work well. The medication effect is immediate and lasts one to three hours, whereas most ingested products take thirty to sixty minutes before taking effect (faster on an empty stomach) and last six to eight hours. Vaporizers that use a cartridge filled with the CO2 concentrate are highly effective, and these are available in various ratios of CBD to THC. Herbal vaporizers that use the whole plant are also an effective delivery method. Sublingual sprays or tinctures taken as liquid drops also take effect quickly and last longer than inhaled products. More information about various forms of delivery (e.g., sublingual, oral, inhaled) for cannabinoid-based medication can be found starting on p. 38.

When pain is localized, topical products can be applied. These can be made using CBD-dominant cannabis as well as THC strains. Topicals affect the cells near application and through several layers of tissue but do not cross the blood-brain barrier and are, therefore, not psychoactive. These may be available as oils, ointments, salves, or other forms, and with varying ratios of CBD and THC (a ratio of 1:1 is often recommended as ideal for skin application). The skin has the highest amount and concentration of CB2 receptors in the body.

Effectiveness: Current Science—Pain

possible   actual

probable

FIGURE 46

The Cannabis Health Index (CHI) is an evidence-based scoring system for cannabis (in general, not just CBD) and its effectiveness on various health issues based on currently available research data. Refer to p. 86 for more on CHI scores, and check cannabishealthindex.com for updated information and more about studies related to specific types of pain. Considering all of the studies together, which number over forty (for various types of pain), cannabis is shown to have a rating of likely probable efficacy. It is one of the best-substantiated medical uses of cannabinoids.

Sativex, a cannabis plant–derived oromucosal spray containing equal proportions of THC and CBD, has been approved in a number of countries for use to treat specific types of pain. Numerous randomized clinical trials have demonstrated the safety and efficacy of Sativex for treatment of central and peripheral neuropathic pain, rheumatoid arthritis, and cancer pain.[386]

Cannabinoids affect the transmission of pain signals from the affected region to the brain (ascending) and from the brain to the affected region (descending). A 2011 study showed that CBD and CBC stimulated descending pain-blocking pathways in the nervous system and caused analgesia by interacting with several target proteins involved in nociceptive control. Authors concluded that the cannabinoids "might represent useful therapeutic agents with multiple mechanisms of action."[387] The following year, researchers reported that CBD significantly suppressed chronic inflammatory and neuropathic pain without causing apparent analgesic tolerance in animals.[388] And then in 2013, researchers concluded that chronic pain patients prescribed hydrocodone were *less likely* to take the painkiller if they used cannabis.[389]

Post-Traumatic Stress Disorder (PTSD)

Post-traumatic stress disorder (PTSD) is a debilitating condition affecting the body, mind, and spirit, related to the failure of what scientists call the brain's "extinction process," which diminishes the impact of traumatic memories. It results from direct or witnessed exposure to an extreme traumatic event and is characterized by symptoms such as anxiety, nightmares, flashbacks, and depression, and is sometimes accompanied by alcohol or substance abuse. Veterans with PTSD appear to be at particular risk of developing high-THC cannabis dependence, and many studies have focused on this despite the many reports that cannabis provided relief from symptoms. Recent research confirms that CBD has the potential to treat symptoms of PTSD safely and effectively without psychoactivity and underscores a link between the endocannabinoid system and the processing of traumatic memories in the brain.

Evidence has shown a reduction in circulating endocannabinoid levels in individuals with PTSD, including a 2013 study of individuals following exposure to the World Trade Center attacks. "These data support the hypothesis that deficient eCB [endocannabinoid] signaling may be a component of the glucocorticoid dysregulation associated with PTSD," the authors concluded.[390]

Even the U.S. Department of Veterans Affairs acknowledges on its website that the link between PTSD and the endocannabinoid system has been clearly demonstrated and that cannabis may help with symptoms in the short term, but warns about the long-term risks of addiction to high-THC cannabis. It mentions that CBD has been proven to be effective at treating anxiety related to other causes, but that research on its use for treating PTSD is not yet adequate.

MP struggled with PTSD linked to a string of experiences including sexual abuse, service in the Israeli army, and being personally affected by terrorist violence. She found relief through the use of both THC and high-CBD products and reported that using a variety of strains is critical for her. "For nightmares, taking CBD at night reduces anxiety before bed. Early awakening is a problem for people with PTSD—you wake up at night and can't get back to sleep . . . a little bit of indica at that point will help make you tired."[391]

How to Take the Medicine: Dosage and Delivery

It is suggested that patients work with a health care practitioner experienced in recommending CBD or medicinal cannabis so that dosage and delivery methods can be developed and fine-tuned on an individual basis. At the same time, educated and aware patients can be their own highly informed health consultants (see p. 75 for information about the subjective-intuitive approach to using cannabis-based medicines).

For all orally administered medicines, refer to the dosage tables on pp. 61–63 for guidelines on CBD dosage by body weight. Always start with the micro dose to test sensitivity and go up as needed within the dosing range by body weight until symptoms subside. A **micro to standard dose** is generally recommended to treat PTSD. Varieties that are high in myrcene and linalool, a terpene shared with lavender, have a more relaxing effect and also help with sleep.

Products made with indica-dominant varieties that are higher in THC can also be helpful for sleep issues (see more in the entry for sleep disorders in this chapter) or produce a calming and sedating effect. A maximum range of 5–10 mg of THC per dose is suggested. Avoid products containing sativa strains as they can promote hyperactivity and dissociation. Products with a higher CBD content with a ratio above 20:1 should be tried first to prevent too much psychoactivity. If this does not work, THC can be introduced into the protocol slowly, working toward a 1:1 ratio.

While CBD-dominant products help some people sleep, in others it promotes wakefulness (see p. 69 for more on the bidirectional effect). Orally administered THC, especially products from heavier broad-leaf indica "Kush" strains and purple cannabis varieties, are very effective for sleep disorders. These tend to be high in myrcene and linalool, a terpene shared with lavender, known to be effective for relaxation. A 1:1 ratio of CBD to THC can be used when patients report too much psychoactivity, as CBD reduces this.

For immediate delivery, vaporizing or smoking work well. This can be helpful for wakefulness in the middle of a rest period but only lasts one to three hours. The medication effect is immediate, whereas most ingested products take thirty to sixty minutes before taking effect (faster on an empty stomach) and last six to eight hours. Vaporizers that use a cartridge filled with the CO2 concentrate are highly effective, and these are available in various ratios of CBD to THC. Herbal vaporizers that use the whole plant are also an effective delivery method. Sublingual sprays or tinctures taken as liquid drops also take effect quickly and last longer than inhaled products.

When high doses are required, many patients use concentrated forms of cannabis oil and take it orally, either in capsule form or by adding to food (nut butters seem to work well). The purest, most potent concentrates are made using a CO2-extraction process. More information about various forms of delivery (e.g., sublingual, edible, transdermal) for cannabinoid-based medication can be found starting on p. 38.

Effectiveness: Current Science—PTSD

possible   actual

probable

FIGURE 47

The Cannabis Health Index (CHI) is an evidence-based scoring system for cannabis (in general, not just CBD) and its effectiveness on various health issues based on currently available research data. Refer to p. 86 for more on CHI scores, and check cannabishealthindex.com for updated information. For treatment of PTSD, based on sixteen studies, cannabis rated in the possible-to-probable range of efficacy (2.8 points).

A 2016 animal study reconfirmed the antipsychotic properties of CBD in relation to schizophrenia and identified the mechanism for its function in the brain, closely related to that of other pharmaceutical drugs prescribed for PTSD-related psychosis. "CBD can produce effects similar to antipsychotic medications by triggering molecular signaling pathways associated with the effects of classic antipsychotic medications."[392] A study a few years earlier on human patients in Germany showed that CBD was as effective as regularly prescribed antipsychotics and had fewer side effects.[393]

Schizophrenia

The relationship between the endocannabinoid system and schizophrenia has been the subject of scientific research for several decades. Early studies showed that schizophrenics had elevated levels of anandamide (an endogenous neurotransmitter that works on the same receptor as THC), which caused speculation that this could be part of the cause of the illness. By 2012, a study demonstrated that, as CBD relieved patients' symptoms, anandamide levels rose in concert. One of the main authors of the study, D. Piomelli, hypothesized that the high levels seen in people with schizophrenia aren't the cause of the problem, but the result of the brain's attempts to solve it are. "It looks like anandamide is a signaling molecule that has evolved to help us cope with stress," Piomelli wrote. "In the brain, everything it does seems to be related to ways of relieving stress. It can relieve anxiety and reduce the stress response. It is involved in stress-induced analgesia [when you stop feeling pain while fighting or fleeing]. These are all mechanisms to help us prevent [negative outcomes related to stress]."[394]

Evidence suggests that inhibition of anandamide deactivation may contribute to the antipsychotic effects of cannabidiol, potentially representing a completely new mechanism in the treatment of schizophrenia.[395]

In 2016, a study on the mechanisms by which CBD produces antipsychotic effects identified a neurological basis for its efficacy, reporting that it "triggered molecular signaling pathways associated with the effects of classic antipsychotic medications."[396]

Two weeks ago, I saw a twenty-eight-year-old male with schizophrenia. He had been using hemp-based CBD and had taken as much as 150 mg daily. In spite of this high daily dosage, his symptoms, which included hallucinations, paranoia, anxiety, and more, were not relieved and he was getting desperate. I suggested he stop taking the hemp-based products and instead take whole-plant cannabis-derived CBD at a 20:1 ratio. He slowly ramped up to 30 mg daily and is now around 80 percent better. We *may* need to increase his dose, but I will have him stay at this comfortable dose for a couple more weeks. I imagine that he, like many of my other schizophrenic patients, will do well even if we need to increase to 60 mg of CBD daily.

Serious illnesses such as schizophrenia require the best medicines, and, in my experience, I do not find hemp-based medicines fit that requirement.

ALLAN FRANKEL, MD

How to Take the Medicine: Dosage and Delivery

It is suggested that patients work with a health care practitioner experienced in recommending CBD or medicinal cannabis so that dosage and delivery methods can be developed and fine-tuned on an individual basis. At the same time, educated and aware patients can be their own highly informed health consultants (see p. 75 for information about the subjective-intuitive approach to using cannabis-based medicines).

For all orally administered medicines, refer to the dosage tables on pp. 61–63 for guidelines on CBD dosage by body weight. Always start with the micro dose to test sensitivity and go up as needed within the dosing range by body weight until symptoms subside. To ensure minimal psychoactive effects, patients with schizophrenia should be cautious about titrating slowly up to a target range between a **standard to macro dose.** It is highly recommended to use products that have a 20:1 ratio of CBD:THC or higher for this condition. Often, *minimal doses of THC can make the condition worse.* AC/DC has proven to be very effective for schizophrenia. Varieties that are high in myrcene have a more relaxing effect.

Effectiveness: Current Science—Schizophrenia

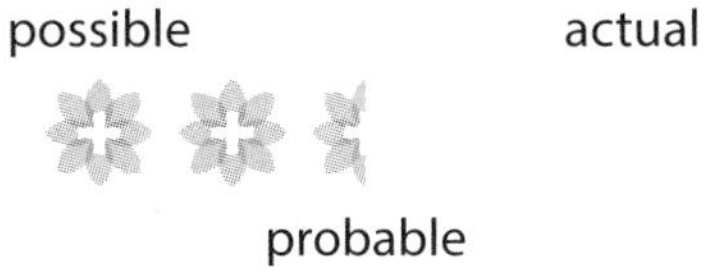

possible   actual

probable

FIGURE 48

The Cannabis Health Index (CHI) is an evidence-based scoring system for cannabis (in general, not just CBD) and its effectiveness on various health issues based on currently available research data. Refer to p. 86 for more on CHI scores, and check cannabishealthindex.com for updated information. For treatment of schizophrenia, based on eight studies, cannabis has a rating of likely probable efficacy, according to this rubric (2.5 points).

A 2011 study found that using cannabis with high CBD content was associated with significantly lower degrees of psychotic symptoms, providing further support for the antipsychotic potential of cannabidiol.[397] The following year, a review of thirty years of research data on CBD and psychosis concluded that the results "support the idea that CBD may be a future therapeutic option in psychosis, in general and in schizophrenia, in particular."[398]

In a 2015 mid-stage trial involving eighty-eight patients, an experimental cannabis-based pharmaceutical for treating schizophrenia, developed by UK-based GW Pharmaceuticals, was found to be superior to a placebo.[399]

Seizure Disorders

Out of all of the many medicinal uses of CBD, using it for seizure control has shown some of the most spectacular and well-publicized results. It is dramatic and potentially life threatening when a person, especially an infant or child, has a grand mal epileptic seizure. After administration of the proper dose of medical-grade, plant-based CBD medicine, for many patients seizures are greatly reduced and in some cases stop altogether. Studies vary on the efficacy rate (see more information later in this section), but many experience a reduction in frequency, intensity, and duration of seizures.

Most children who have epilepsy or one of the many similar disorders have tried or are using many different pharmaceutical drugs in combination to control their seizures. The drugs used may cause dependency. Sedation and cognitive impairment are common side effects. Often, they are taking

---

Dr. Sanjay Gupta researched and created a documentary series *Weed* on CNN. In the first installment of that series in 2013, he showcased a three-year-old girl with epilepsy named Charlotte Figi. He filmed her having seizures before using CBD and after. The results were like night and day. Before, her seizures could not be controlled, and the drugs put her into a stupor. After administration of CBD-based plant medicine, she became a different person, fully alive, playing, laughing, and able to be a normal toddler. A popular CBD strain, "Charlotte's Web," was named after her, and thousands of parents of children with similar issues flocked to Colorado, where it was being grown.

ZJ was fortunate enough to live near the farm that was growing this strain in the summer of 2012. At nine years old, he had suffered since infancy from seizures, which had become a potentially fatal type called tonics in the past year. After trying seventeen different pharmaceuticals to treat the condition unsuccessfully, the family looked toward cherishing the time they had together. Following the very first night ZJ was given the Charlotte's Web extract, he went for forty-eight hours without an episode, which was unheard of. His mother raised the dose over subsequent months, and the fall of 2012 marked his last major seizure. "It has literally put his condition into remission," she said in an interview. "He used to have very severe autistic tendencies. Now he is like a normal boy. He has friends he plays with and rides a bike."[400]

several different types of drugs at the same time. In many cases, the patient has "intractable epilepsy" (also called refractory or uncontrolled epilepsy), which means all pharmaceutical drugs simply do not work.

How to Take the Medicine: Dosage and Delivery

It is suggested that patients work with a health care practitioner experienced in recommending CBD or medicinal cannabis so that dosage and delivery methods can be developed and fine-tuned on an individual basis. At the same time, educated and aware patients can be their own highly informed health consultants (see p. 75 for information about the subjective-intuitive approach to using cannabis-based medicines).

Bonnie Goldstein, MD, suggests 0.5 mg/lb/day of CBD as a starting dose for pediatric epilepsy, increasing by 0.5 mg/lb/day every two weeks, depending on response. It is preferable to divide this daily dose into three separate doses of 0.16 mg/lb, taken every seven to eight hours, preferably between meals. Consistently monitor the results. Most of her patients who respond positively end up taking between 2 and 8 mg/lb/day. Following this recommendation, a 50-pound child would take 25 mg of CBD per day to begin, or 8.3 mg three times daily.

Refer to the dosage tables on pp. 61–63 for guidelines on CBD dosage by body weight. Always start with a micro dose to test sensitivity and go up as needed within the dosing range by body weight until seizures subside.

For children, CBD-only oil infusions, glycerin tinctures, sublingual products, or pure CO2-extracted concentrates are recommended (no alcohol tinctures). The oil can be given straight or mixed with yogurt or other food. Concentrates can also be mixed with food such as nut butters, made into capsules, or made into suppositories for infants. If seizures are not reduced or eliminated, blends that add a small amount of THC or THCA are sometimes effective. See p. 65 for more on introducing THC while minimizing side effects or impairment.

Adults can take any of the above, as well as alcohol-based tinctures, capsules, and other edibles. For more immediate symptoms, vaporizing or smoking work well. The medication effect is immediate and lasts one to three hours, whereas most ingested products take thirty to sixty minutes before taking effect (faster on an empty stomach) and last six to eight hours. Vaporizers that use a cartridge filled with the CO2 concentrate are highly effective,

and these are available in various ratios of CBD to THC. Herbal vaporizers that use the whole plant are also an effective delivery method. Sublingual sprays or tinctures taken as liquid drops also take effect quickly and
last longer than inhaled products. More information about various forms of
delivery (e.g., sublingual, oral, inhaled) for cannabinoid-based medication
can be found starting on p. 38.

Changing strains or changing the ratios of CBD to THC can sometimes
be effective if a patient is not responding or builds a tolerance to a certain
strain. AC/DC and Valentine X have proven to be effective strains to control
seizures (Saint Valentine is the patron saint of epilepsy, and this strain was
named after him). Charlotte's Web and Remedy are also effective strains.

Effectiveness: Current Science—Seizure

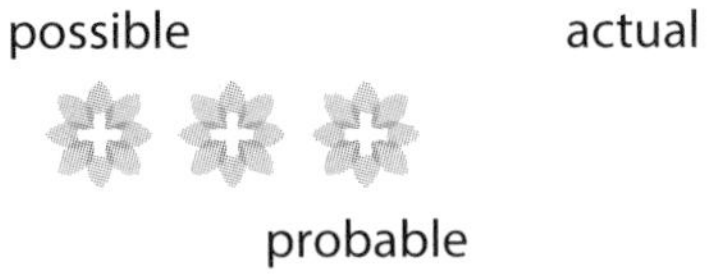

possible   actual

probable

FIGURE 49

The Cannabis Health Index (CHI) is an evidence-based scoring system for cannabis (in general, not just CBD) and its effectiveness on various health issues
based on currently available research data. Refer to p. 86 for more on CHI
scores, and check cannabishealthindex.com for updated information. Using
this rubric, seizure disorders scored in the likely probable range of efficacy for
treatment based on approximately twenty-eight studies available at press time.

Though cannabis has been used to treat epilepsy dating back to the
Middle Ages, according to Arabic medical texts,[401] scientific research has
only recently broken through toward an understanding of the relationship
between cannabinoids and seizure disorders. Clinical trials are still few in
number. It has been shown that cannabinoids can be both proconvulsant
and anticonvulsant,[402] that dosage is key, and that it is important to know
the chemical makeup of the strain being used. CBD shows the most promising results among the cannabinoids studied for seizure control, but some
types of seizures appear to respond better to higher ratios of THC. Research
indicates that the effects of CB1 receptor signaling on seizures are related to

the way in which specific cannabinoids interact with the receptor, as either agonist or antagonist.[403]

In a 2015 open-label study of 162 pediatric epilepsy patients at centers across the United States, researchers administered CBD at a rate of 4–10 mg/lb per day and up-titrated until intolerance or to a maximum dose of 50 mg/lb/day. The approach reduced seizures at a rate similar to existing drugs, a median of 36.5 percent. In addition, 4 percent of patients became completely free of motor seizures.

In a study presented in 2016 of 201 children with epilepsy using high-CBD oils, with doses recommended by Dr. Bonni Goldstein, 68 percent of epileptic patients had greater than 50 percent improvement and 15 percent are seizure free. Over 40 percent of those studied were able to reduce or totally eliminate pharmaceutical drugs.[404] Positive side effects included improved energy, mood, and sleep; improved appetite and focus; and reduced ER visits and hospitalizations. Negative side effects included drowsiness and diarrhea.

A 2016 retrospective study of seventy-four pediatric patients in Israeli clinics found that 89 percent reported a reduction in seizure load with CBD therapy. Five patients reported aggravated seizures.[405]

GW Pharmaceuticals has conducted several randomized, double-blind, placebo-controlled clinical trials of its investigational medicine Epidiolex (CBD as oral drops derived from whole-plant cannabis) for the treatment of seizures with positive results and is in the process of approval by the FDA in the next few years.[406]

Skin Conditions
(Including Acne, Dermatitis, Psoriasis)

Just as the endocannabinoid network facilitates homeostasis in various systems of the body, these same receptors are found in cutaneous cells. They maintain the immune competence of the skin as well as the proper and well-balanced proliferation, differentiation, and survival of skin cells. The disruption of this delicate balance might facilitate the development of multiple pathological conditions and diseases of the skin (e.g., acne, seborrhea, allergic dermatitis, itch and pain, psoriasis, hair growth disorders, systemic sclerosis, and cancer).[407]

Cannabinoids are well-known for their role in regulating inflammation, and it appears that this role may be key to their ability to treat eczema and psoriasis. A 2006 study reported that highly concentrated cannabinoid-based creams were effective for itching.[408] When applied topically, compounds in cannabis bind to cell receptors in the skin's immune cells and treat allergic reactions on the skin—because cannabinoids are immunosuppressant, they dampen the overactive immune response causing the inflammatory rash.[409] The skin has the highest amount and concentration of CB2 receptors in the body.

Psoriasis is an inflammatory disease also characterized in part by epidermal keratinocyte hyper proliferation. Cannabinoids are anti-inflammatory and have inhibitory effects on a number of tumorigenic cell lines, some of which are mediated via cannabinoid receptors. Researchers in a 2007 study concluded, "Our results show that cannabinoids inhibit keratinocyte proliferation, and therefore support a potential role for cannabinoids in the treatment of psoriasis."[410]

In an informal study involving a patient with acute psoriasis at the Gwynedd Cannabis Club in Wales, a woman who had previously tried conventional pharmaceutical therapy (involving a chemotherapy drug called Methotrexate) applied three treatments of topical cannabis oil per day for nine days. Within that nine-day period, she experienced a complete healing of her skin with no negative side effects. In fact, she was able to go swimming with her family for the first time in years following the cannabis therapy.[411]

CBD appears to treat acne by inducing sebocyte apoptosis, and a number of other terpenes present in cannabis may offer complementary activity. Limonene has been shown to inhibit *Propionibacterium acnes* (at a potency higher than that of triclosan). Pinene also inhibits *P. acnes,* and linalool suppresses inflammation in response to acne. Authors of a 2014 study concluded that "findings suggest that due to the combined lipostatic, antiproliferative, and anti-inflammatory effects, CBD has potential as a promising therapeutic agent for the treatment of acne vulgaris."[412]

How to Take the Medicine: Dosage and Delivery

It is suggested that patients work with a health care practitioner experienced in recommending CBD or medicinal cannabis so that dosage and delivery methods can be developed and fine-tuned on an individual basis. At the same time, educated and aware patients can be their own highly informed health consultants (see p. 75 for information about the subjective-intuitive approach to using cannabis-based medicines).

Topical products can be made using CBD-dominant cannabis or other strains. Topical products containing THC affect the cells and layers of tissue near application but do not cross the blood-brain barrier and are, therefore, not psychoactive. They may be available as oils, ointments, sprays, and other forms. Select carefully, and look for ingredients most appropriate for the particular skin issue. Products can work well with varying ratios of CBD and THC (a ratio of 1:1 is often recommended as ideal for skin application). Studies show that products containing any of the major cannabinoids can be effective for skin disorders and that a higher concentration of cannabinoids can be used safely when a stronger dose of topical medication is required. For serious conditions, like skin cancer, pure cannabis oil in a 1:1 ratio of CBD to THC is recommended to be applied topically. The skin has the highest amount and concentration of CB2 receptors in the body.

For immediate treatment of itching associated with skin issues, vaporized and smoked cannabis is effective, as are cannabinoids taken orally. Be aware it has been suggested that extremely high doses of THC can aggravate acne. For all orally administered medicines, refer to the dosage tables on pp. 61–63 for guidelines on CBD dosage by body weight. Always start with the micro dose to test sensitivity and go up as needed within the dosing range by body weight until symptoms subside. More information about various forms of delivery (e.g., sublingual, edible, transdermal) for cannabinoid-based medication can be found starting on p. 38. Popular strains for skin conditions include Harlequin, Cannatonic, and Purple indica varieties.

Effectiveness: Current Science—Skin Disorders

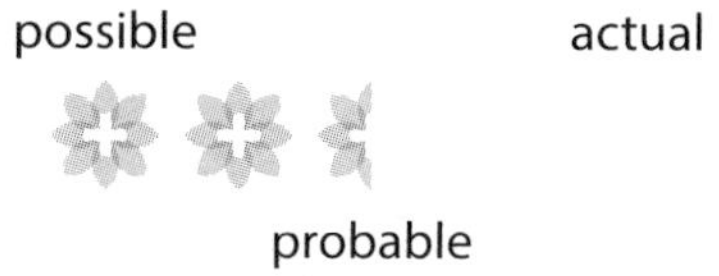

possible   actual

❀ ❀ ❅

probable

FIGURE 50

The Cannabis Health Index (CHI) is an evidence-based scoring system for cannabis (in general, not just CBD) and its effectiveness on various health issues based on currently available research data. Refer to p. 86 for more on CHI scores, and check cannabishealthindex.com for updated information. Using this rubric, the use of cannabis-based products for treating skin disorders rated in the possible-to-probable range of efficacy based on the four studies available at press time (2.5 points).

A study published in 2007 showed that the major cannabinoids all demonstrated some level of effectiveness in inhibiting keratinocyte production in the epidermis, which is involved in psoriasis. Authors wrote that "cannabinoid receptors have been found in even the smallest nerve fibers controlling hair follicles; keratinocytes have also been shown to bind and metabolize anandamide, the most prolific endocannabinoid."[413]

Research in 2013 showed that the phytocannabinoids CBD and CBG are transcriptional repressors that can control cell proliferation and differentiation. "This indicates that they (especially cannabidiol) have the potential to be lead compounds for the development of novel therapeutics for skin diseases."[414]

MM had endured five bouts of squamous cell carcinoma on his neck and face. He did traditional treatments of chemotherapy, radiation, and surgery, and, while the treatments would temporarily destroy it, the condition kept coming back. When the doctor diagnosed him with another recurrence of the same cancer, he decided to use a pure form of cannabis oil as a topical application. In ten days, the condition started to heal, and in three months the cancer totally disappeared.[415]

Sleep Disorders (Insomnia, Sleep Apnea)

Cannabis and sleep have a complex relationship that is only beginning to be understood by science. In general, for most people, indica strains are more relaxing and effective for sleep disorders, whereas sativa strains are more stimulating and tend to keep people awake (see more on these classifications in Chapter 7).

Several studies conducted between 2004 and 2008 demonstrated the variable effect of different cannabinoids on sleep. In one, 15 mg of THC appeared to have sedative properties, while 15 mg of CBD appeared to have alerting properties.[416] Another tested the effects of CBD on animal models in both lights-on and lights-off environments and found that this non-psychoactive cannabis compound increased alertness with the lights on and had no discernable effects on lights-off sleep. The study's authors concluded that CBD might actually hold therapeutic promise for those with somnolence, or excessive daytime sleepiness from a not-so-good night's rest. Another study found CBD to be wake-inducing for most subjects, though some reported better sleep a few hours after taking it.[417]

"Many of my patients report either better energy or sleepiness on the same high-CBD/low-THC plants," Dr. Michael Moskowitz reported. "Most, however, feel more energy on high-CBD cannabis." [418]

In general, indica varieties of THC appear to work best as a sleep aid for most people. However, a significant number of people find THC, even indica strains, will make the mind more active. For these people, CBD tends to work well, providing the relaxation and calm for the mental as well as the physical body. For these people, CBD taken at nighttime as part of a bedtime regime produces a restful sleep, not the alertness produced in the daytime. This bidirectional effect of CBD is the result of balancing the endocannabinoid system.

In relation to sleep apnea, a 2002 animal study observed the ability of THC to restore respiratory stability by modulating serotonin signaling and reducing spontaneous sleep-disordered breathing.[419] In 2013 a trial using the pharmaceutical drug dronabinol, a synthetic THC mimic, noted improvements in fifteen out of seventeen study participants following twenty-one days of treatment.[420]

LS had suffered from sleep apnea for a while when CBD was recommended to him. The first night he took a few drops of the tincture, he had uninterrupted sleep for the first time in weeks. He began incorporating changes to his diet, exercise, and schedule, and also started seeing an acupuncturist regularly. Especially when stress is a factor, he adds the CBD drops and has significantly fewer to no episodes of sleep apnea. "I use it sparingly as I do not wish to rely on it," he wrote. "But I respect it as gift and medicine."

How to Take the Medicine: Dosage and Delivery

It is suggested that patients work with a health care practitioner experienced in recommending CBD or medicinal cannabis so that dosage and delivery methods can be developed and fine-tuned on an individual basis. At the same time, educated and aware patients can be their own highly informed health consultants (see p. 75 for information about the subjective-intuitive approach to using cannabis-based medicines).

As mentioned previously, while CBD-dominant products help some people sleep, in others it promotes wakefulness (see p. 69 for more on the bidirectional effect). Orally administered THC, especially products from heavier "Kush" strains and Purple cannabis varieties, are very effective for sleep disorders. These tend to be high in myrcene and linalool, a terpene shared with lavender and known to be effective for relaxation. Cannabis combinations with ratios of 1:1, 4:1, or 24:1 CBD:THC can be used when patients want to reduce psychoactivity.

For all orally administered medicines, such as drops, capsules, or edibles, refer to the dosage tables on pp. 61–63 for guidelines on CBD dosage by body weight. Oral consumption is recommended as it usually lasts the whole night. Always start with the micro dose to test sensitivity and go up as needed within the dosing range before going to the next, until symptoms subside. The **micro to standard dose** is usually recommended to treat insomnia and sleep apnea. When relaxing indica strains are used with higher THC levels, a dose of 5–10 mg is usually sufficient. Other people find they need larger doses, such as 15–40 mg. CBD taken as a tincture or edible will aid in a restful six to seven hours of sleep. This type of disorder varies widely from one patient to the next. Often, one needs to perform some experimental research and try strains of different CBD:THC ratios to figure out the best protocol.

For immediate medicinal effects, vaporizing or smoking work well. This can be helpful for either initial sleep onset or for wakefulness in the middle of a rest period but only lasts one to three hours. The medication effect is immediate, whereas most ingested products take thirty to sixty minutes before taking effect (faster on an empty stomach) and last six to eight hours. Vaporizers that use a cartridge filled with the CO_2 concentrate are convenient and highly effective, and these are available in various ratios of CBD to THC. Herbal vaporizers that use the whole plant are also an effective delivery method. Sublingual sprays or tinctures taken as liquid drops also take effect quickly and last longer than inhaled products. More information about various forms of delivery (e.g., sublingual, oral, inhaled) for cannabinoid-based medication can be found on p. 38.

Effectiveness: Current Science—Sleep Disorders

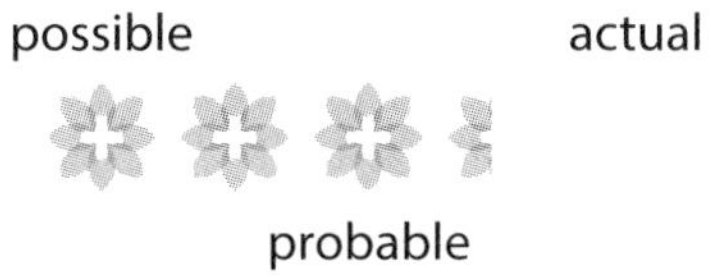

possible   actual

✿ ✿ ✿ ⦂

probable

FIGURE 51

The Cannabis Health Index (CHI) is an evidence-based scoring system for cannabis (in general, not just CBD) and its effectiveness on various health issues based on currently available research data. Refer to p. 86 for more on CHI scores, and check cannabishealthindex.com for updated information. Using this rubric, the use of cannabis-based products for treating insomnia has a rating of likely probable efficacy based on the four studies available at press time (3.4 points).

A 2007 study with the pharmaceutical 1:1 CBD:THC spray showed good results in helping patients with chronic pain sleep better.[421]

REM sleep behavior disorder (RBD) is characterized by the loss of complete muscle relaxation during REM sleep, associated with nightmares and physical activity during dreaming. Four patients in a case series treated with CBD in 2014 had prompt and substantial reduction in the frequency of RBD-related events without side effects.[422]

NOTE *For updates to this chapter, visit www.CBD-book.com/Updates.*

5

Women's Health Issues

Cannabinoids are helpful in treating a number of conditions that commonly affect women, such as osteoporosis, symptoms related to menopause, thyroid issues, fibromyalgia (see the sections on pain and sleep disorders in Chapter 4), and breast cancer (see Cancer section in Chapter 4). Scientific inquiry into the endocannabinoid system has specific implications for women's health. Endocannabinoids are found in the cells of the uterus and reproductive system as well as breast milk.

The endocannabinoid system is directly related to the endocrine system, particularly to the relationship between the hypothalamus, the pituitary, and other hormonal regulators, such as the adrenals (called the hypothalamus-pituitary-adrenal axis, or HPA axis).

The pituitary gland controls key functions within the reproductive system, including the release of the follicle-stimulating hormone (FSH) responsible for prompting ovulation. In the years leading up to menopause, as the body is attempting to regulate its hormones in a new way, the release of this hormone may be sporadic while it gradually decreases (once a woman reaches menopause, the pituitary stops producing FSH altogether).[423]

This chapter starts with a brief anthropological review of the use of cannabis to treat female health issues throughout history. It contains a detailed section on using cannabinoid-based products for menstrual disorders with information on dosage and forms of the medicine. It also includes a discussion of the controversial topic of their use in relation to fertility and pregnancy.

Historical Review

While many of the traditional medicines used to treat women's health conditions were kept secret through the millennia, and some have been lost over time,[424] records of the use of cannabis in relation to labor, birth, and the treatment of menstrual disorders date back to seven centuries before Christ in ancient Mesopotamia.[425] During the Middle Ages in Europe, several references are noted of the topical use of cannabis in fat or oil to ease breast soreness and for nursing mothers to prevent mastitis.[426] Historically, it appears people believed it promoted uterine muscle tone, therefore reducing excess blood flow during menstruation and after childbirth. It was often used as a tincture or infused oil, but there are also records of it being used as a vaginal or rectal suppository. It was said to work synergistically with ergot, a compound commonly used as an abortifacient and to prevent excess blood loss after birth (a derivative, Methergine, is still used for this purpose in hospital settings).

There are many references to the use of cannabis for uterine hemorrhage in more modern Western medicine, starting from the mid-nineteenth century. It was also recorded during this era as an agent to facilitate the birth process. Most texts credit it with shortening labor by strengthening uterine contractions while also controlling pain and anxiety. It was generally understood to have few side effects for women or babies.[427] Another traditional medical use of cannabis with numerous references across cultures is treatment of disorders involving the bladder and urinary tract.[428]

An 1889 medical text by Boston-area doctor J. W. Farlow describes using cannabis suppositories to ease menopausal symptoms: "the irritability, the pain in the neck of the bladder, flashes of heat and cold, according to my experience, can frequently be much mitigated."[429]

Cannabis and the Monthly Cycle:
Menstrual Symptoms and Fertility

Cannabis has long been used for treating premenstrual syndrome (PMS), endometriosis, and menstrual cramps (it was most notably used by Queen Victoria in England who was prescribed cannabis tincture by her doctor Sir

John Russell Reynolds for dysmenorrhea; she used it monthly for years). Still, science has yet to focus much research on the use of cannabinoids for these common ailments that affect millions of women. Commonly used tinctures for menstrual cramps, patented by U.S. pharmaceutical companies, included cannabis in their formulas.

Hormonal fluctuations during the premenstrual phase can cause a wide range of symptoms, including pain, irritability, mood swings, fatigue, and bloating. Levels of hormones such as progesterone significantly increase during this phase, while other hormones such as estrogen decrease.

The endometrium, or interior lining of the uterus, is also governed by hormonal changes. When the cells that make up this lining proliferate outside the uterus, painful growths and adhesions occur in a condition known as endometriosis.

Estrogen levels are linked to endocannabinoid levels, and both peak at ovulation and drop off after menopause. FAAH, the enzyme that breaks down the endocannabinoid anandamide and controls its levels, is regulated by estrogen. In fact, activation of estrogen receptors and cannabinoid receptors on the same cells often works synergistically to produce greater effects.

Women are often prescribed supplementary progesterone as a treatment for PMS and premenstrual dysphoric disorder (PMDD) as well as a combination of hormones as replacement therapy during menopause, but research shows it is important to have one's individual hormonal levels checked to best assess if supplementation is needed. Indeed, although it is generally thought that abnormal premenstrual symptoms are linked to low progesterone levels at a time when they should be high, some forms appear in fact to be linked to excessive progesterone levels and reduced estrogen levels.[430]

Evidence suggests that cannabis use lowers progesterone during the luteal (post-ovulatory) phase[431] and possibly alters levels of other important hormones such as prolactin and cortisol.[432] A 1986 study showed that THC affected the luteinizing hormone connected to ovulation. Its impact on fertility is not fully understood, but it is possible that a woman's cycle may be affected enough to alter the chances of ovulation and implantation, so it is advisable for women trying to get pregnant to avoid THC if they are new to cannabis. However, it has been shown that the bodies of regular users adapt, and fertility returns to normal levels. The effect of THC on fertility is relatively short-lived, and hormones return to baseline within one or two cycles of abstinence.

CBD has not been adequately studied for an understanding to be reached regarding its effect on fertility, though some stories and research suggest that, when properly timed, it could have beneficial effects for women suffering from infertility, especially related to endometriosis.[433,434] High levels of anandamide are helpful for promoting ovulation (CBD allows this endocannabinoid to be more available in the system), but for an embryo to implant, anandamide levels must be low.[435,436] One hypothesis suggests that cannabinoids such as CBD could decrease the likelihood for pregnancy in women with naturally high anandamide levels, and alternatively could increase the likelihood in women whose anandamide levels are low.[437,438]

Menopause

Reduction in endocannabinoid signaling may be responsible for some of the negative symptoms associated with menopause, and many women report relief from the use of cannabis products. A 2007 review found that cannabinoids relieved menopause-related insomnia.[439] Estrogen recruits the endocannabinoid system to regulate emotional response and relieves anxiety and depression through its actions on the brain. Lowered levels of estrogen during and after menopause means less activation of the endocannabinoid system and poor ability to respond to stress and elevate mood accordingly.[440] Another symptom that can be addressed is hot flashes—body temperature is generally lowered by cannabis. Finally, issues related to sex, including changes in libido, lubrication levels, and sensitivity, can accompany menopause. Research on the potential use of cannabinoids for these sexual health concerns is badly needed, but anecdotal evidence points to the fact that they may work well for some women. Lubricants infused with THC have appeared on the market, and stimulating sativa strains are often recommended for improving sex and increasing drive.

Endocannabinoid levels that are too low may spur early menopause. Underweight women, or women with anorexia who tend to enter menopause early, also have low endocannabinoid levels. As an endocannabinoid deficiency can be balanced by boosting these levels with phytocannabinoids it is hypothesized that this could help delay menopause in such cases. The endocannabinoid system regulates the bone loss seen after menopause. CB2 receptors are found on bone cells, called osteoblasts. A common mutation in the gene that codes CB2 in humans, resulting in fewer CB2 receptors, is associated with osteoporosis after menopause.[441] Anandamide is the endocannabinoid-signaling agent responsible for forming bone at the CB1 receptor in bone, while 2-AG contributes to breaking it down at the CB2 receptor, thus keeping a balance and allowing bone to remodel throughout life.[442]

How to Take the Medicine: Dosage and Delivery

It is suggested that patients work with a health care practitioner experienced in recommending CBD or medicinal cannabis so that dosage and delivery methods can be developed and fine-tuned on an individual basis. At the same time, educated and aware patients are often their own most informed health consultants (see p. 75 for information about the subjective-intuitive approach to using cannabis-based medicines).

CBD products with a ratio of 20:1 or higher are recommended for endometriosis, premenstrual and menopause-related syndromes, and for relief from menstrual cramps. Medicines can be administered as drops, capsules, or edibles. For all orally administered medicines, refer to the dosage tables on pp. 61–63 for guidelines on CBD dosage by body weight. Always start with the micro dose to test sensitivity and go up as needed within the dosing range before going to the next range, until symptoms subside. The **micro to standard dose** is usually recommended to treat menstrual disorders.

If CBD-dominant products alone are not enough to treat a particular case, products with a higher ratio of THC are sometimes recommended to better manage pain or other symptoms. For day use, more stimulating, narrow-leaf sativa varieties with higher concentrations of myrcene could be added to the formula (see more on these classifications in Chapter 7). In general, for pain, and especially for evening and nighttime, broad-leaf indica strains are favored for their relaxing, sedative effect. A person without experience with THC should use caution and titrate slowly up to higher doses. A 1:1 ratio of CBD to THC can be used when patients report too much psychoactivity, as CBD reduces that effect.

Women are more responsive to the pain-relieving effects of cannabis and THC when their estrogen levels are at their highest. Because menopausal and postmenopausal women have low levels of estrogen, they will be less responsive to THC and require higher doses than premenopausal women to achieve the same amount of pain relief. Premenopausal women develop tolerance to

THC quickly and may be more vulnerable to negative side effects of cannabis such as paranoia, anxiety, or dependence. Postmenopausal women may be able to stay on a stable dosage of THC or cannabis for the long term and may be less likely to feel anxious or paranoid from cannabis.[443]

Other cannabinoids are also shown to relieve pain, including CBC, CBG, THCV, and THCA. Chemotypes high in beta-caryophyllene, myrcene, and linalool provide additional pain relief and increase the effectiveness of other cannabinoids for analgesia.

For fast relief of pain, insomnia, or other immediate symptoms, vaporizing or smoking work well. The medication effect is immediate and lasts one to three hours, whereas most ingested products take thirty to sixty minutes before taking effect (faster on an empty stomach) and last six to eight hours. Vaporizers that use a cartridge filled with the CO2 concentrate are highly effective, and these are available in various ratios of CBD to THC. Herbal vaporizers that use the whole plant are also an effective delivery method. Sublingual sprays or tinctures taken as liquid drops also take effect quickly and last longer than inhaled products. Recently, cannabis-based vaginal suppositories and topical products in which the medicine is absorbed into the muscle tissue of the pelvic floor and surrounding area have become available. More information about various forms of delivery (e.g., sublingual, oral, inhaled) for cannabinoid-based medication can be found starting on p. 38.

Effectiveness: Current Science—Menstrual Disorders

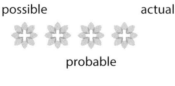

possible · actual · probable

FIGURE 52

The Cannabis Health Index (CHI) is an evidence-based scoring system for cannabis (in general, not just CBD) and its effectiveness on various health issues based on currently available research data. Refer to p. 86 for more on CHI scores, and check cannabishealthindex.com for updated information. Using this rubric, for menstrual pain, hormone-related nausea, and endometriosis, cannabis scored in the probable-to-demonstrable range of treatment efficacy. The effect of the endocannabinoid system on reproduction is complex, and more research is badly needed on cannabinoids and women's health.

Cannabis and Maternity

The jury is still out on the effect of plant-based cannabinoids on pregnancy and the developing child, though it is clear that the endocannabinoid system is intimately involved in regulating the chemical messengers central to fertility and breastfeeding. Studies on the potential risks of prenatal exposure are limited and sometimes contradictory.

A landmark 2017 research review[444] of current studies on medical cannabis for many health concerns concluded that smoking high-THC cannabis has been linked to slightly lower infant birth weights (as has tobacco use), but that its relationship to other pregnancy and childhood outcomes is unclear. A 2002 survey of 12,060 British women did not demonstrate significant differences in growth among newborns exposed to cannabis in utero versus those with no exposure when controlling for co-founding factors such as the mother's age, pre-pregnancy weight, and the self-reported use of tobacco, alcohol, caffeine, and other illicit drugs.[445]

Many challenges to research in this area are related to the difficulties of controlling alcohol and other substances and the legal sanctions that women could face in certain states for admitting to cannabis use while pregnant. As a result, much of the published data assessing the extent of maternal cannabis use and its health implications remain limited to historical texts, studies from non-Western cultures where the use of cannabis has greater social acceptability, and retrospective survey data.[446]

CBD on its own has not been adequately researched in relation to pregnancy, and neither have most cannabinoids. Almost all research has focused on THC, and not all of these properly control the use of alcohol or other substances. Among those that do control other substances, most report cannabis's apparent impact on birth weight and other adverse perinatal outcomes as minimal. However, adverse reproductive outcomes have been reported in rodents given large doses of synthetic THC.

While some studies have shown no effect from cannabis use during pregnancy and long-term fetal and child development,[447] and one study even reported a positive effect on infant health, mood, and milestones,[448] a 2002 study review reported measurable differences related to attention/impulsivity and complex problem solving in children over three years old whose mothers were heavy users.[449] One 2014 laboratory study reported that the neurological development of fetuses exposed prenatally to high doses of THC is altered in the area connected to this type of brain activity.[45]

While the impact of cannabis on pregnancy and fetal development is still only marginally understood by science and remains a source of controversy, women report anecdotally that very small doses are effective in relieving nausea, anxiety, and depression during pregnancy. The historical use of cannabis for pregnancy-associated concerns is also referenced in African, Indian, and Southeast Asian cultures.[451] It was also a common part of a Western midwife's pharmacopeia in some periods in history. In addition, it has shown effective for reducing pain and anxiety during labor in some women. If the thought of women using cannabis-based products during labor sounds "out there," it should be noted that narcotics commonly used for these same purposes in many hospitals include Fentanyl or other similar opioids, including morphine. And the majority of women in the United States receive epidural medication such as bupivacaine and other synthetic derivatives of cocaine.[452] All of these have rare but potentially dangerous side effects.

A systematic review of available evidence completed in 2016 concluded that maternal cannabis use (with unknown THC or CBD levels) was not associated with adverse neonatal outcomes such as low birth weight or preterm delivery. The authors concluded that the risk previously associated with it appeared to be associated with use of tobacco, alcohol, or other drugs at the same time.[453] The longer-term effects of heavy prenatal exposure are more nebulous. Some studies have shown lower test scores for school-aged children who were exposed prenatally to high-THC smoked cannabis but were limited to groups with low socioeconomic status and numerous compounding factors.[454]

However, pregnant women and health care practitioners must be mindful of possible risks and are advised to err on the side of caution with all cannabis and especially avoid synthetic cannabinoids and high-potency THC products.

EATING FOR TWO:
HYPEREMESIS GRAVIDARUM (HG)

In 2002, Dr. Wei-Ni Lin Curry published a first-person account documenting her own use of therapeutic cannabis to alleviate symptoms of hyperemesis gravidarum (HG), a potentially life-threatening condition for both mother and baby characterized by severe nausea and vomiting, malnutrition, and weight loss during pregnancy. (While general nausea and vomiting, colloquially known as "morning sickness," is experienced by an estimated 70 to 80 percent of all expectant mothers, approximately 1 to 2 percent suffers from the persistent vomiting and wasting associated with HG.)

"Within two weeks of my daughter's conception, I became desperately nauseated and vomited throughout the day and night," Curry wrote. "I vomited bile of every shade, and soon began retching up blood. . . . I felt so helpless and distraught that I went to the abortion clinic twice, but both times I left without going through with the procedure. . . . Finally, I decided to try medical cannabis. . . . Just one to two little puffs at night, and if I needed it in the morning, resulted in an entire day of wellness. I went from not eating, not drinking, not functioning, and continually vomiting and bleeding from two orifices to being completely cured. . . . Not only did the cannabis save my [life] during the duration of my hyperemesis, it saved the life of the child within my womb."

Canadian survey data published in 2006 reported that cannabis is therapeutic in the treatment of both morning sickness and HG. Of the eighty-four women who responded to the anonymous questionnaire, thirty-six said that they had used cannabis intermittently during their pregnancy to treat symptoms of vomiting, nausea, and appetite loss. Of these, 92 percent said that cannabis (inhaled or ingested) was "extremely effective" or "effective" in combating their symptoms.

NOTE *For updates to this chapter, visit www.CBD-book.com/Updates.*

PART III

Veterinary CBD

By Gary Richter, MS,
Doctor of Veterinary Medicine

6

CBD for Animals

As more and more people discover the benefits of medical cannabis, many pet owners are wondering if there are similar benefits for their furry family members. As it turns out, the use of cannabis in animals is nothing new. Cannabis has been used in veterinary medicine for nearly as long as humans have used it to treat common health issues. Thousands of years ago, the ancient Greeks used cannabis to treat horses for colic, inflammation, and even to heal battle wounds.[455]

The first published research related to cannabis and companion animals appeared in 1899 in the *British Medical Journal*. Written by English physician and pharmacologist Walter E. Dixon, the article included Dixon's observations on the response of dogs and cats to high-THC cannabis.[456] Since that time, most medical cannabis research has focused on humans, although, more recently, benefits for animals are being explored.

In the last couple of years, veterinarians have re-discovered the benefits of cannabis to treat medical conditions in pets, and we have seen successes in treating many of the same diseases from which humans suffer. Pets suffering from pain, inflammation, arthritis, cancer, seizures, and digestive issues have all found relief through the use of medical cannabis. Dosing considerations, however, must be taken very seriously. Due to their small size and physiological differences, pets cannot be dosed like "small humans."

Annie was a two-year-old black Labrador retriever brought to my office by her owners in search of an effective treatment. Annie had been diagnosed with epilepsy. She was having multiple seizures per day despite being on two different anti-seizure medications.

Epilepsy is occasionally seen in dogs. The seizures normally begin when the dog is young (two or three years old) and can range in severity from very mild to quite severe. Annie's seizures were relatively mild, but she was having multiple episodes per day. A full workup by a neurologist, including an MRI, yielded no abnormal findings.

After examining Annie and consulting with her owners, we decided to try CBD-rich cannabis oil. We discussed the exact product and dosing that would be the safest and most effective for her.

Within two weeks, Annie's seizures were reduced by 75 percent. Her quality of life was significantly improved and her owners were thrilled. With a little fine-tuning of her dosing, we were able to further improve her seizure frequency. Although she still has the occasional seizure, Annie's life (and that of her owners) has been greatly changed for the better.

Animals and the Endocannabinoid System

From an evolutionary perspective, the endocannabinoid system is quite old. All higher forms of animals have an endocannabinoid system, and it is even found in many primitive forms of life such as slugs. Just as in humans, the complex web of neurotransmitters in the endocannabinoid system is involved in physiological processes such as appetite, pain sensation, mood, and memory (see Chapter 2 on the endocannabinoid system for more details on how it works). While the overall function of the endocannabinoid system is similar in all animals, there are differences between species.

Dogs are particularly unique with regard to the endocannabinoid system because they have a greater concentration of endocannabinoid receptors in their brainstem and cerebellum than any other species does. These structures within the brain control heart rate, breathing, and muscle coordination. The dramatic response seen when dogs ingest excessive levels of cannabis containing THC is due to the high concentration of cannabinoid receptors as well as their relatively smaller size.

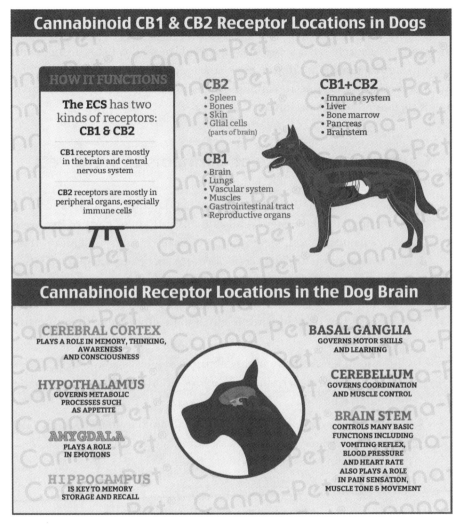

FIGURE 53: COURTESY OF CANNA-PET.COM

When dogs ingest excessive levels of cannabis containing THC, they lose muscle coordination, have difficulty with balance, and may lose bowel and bladder control. They will stand in a "sawhorse" stance and sway back and forth. This response is known as static ataxia and is unique to dogs. Depending on the size of the dog and the dose ingested, signs of toxicity can last from hours to days and may result in the dog being unable to eat or drink.

Conversely, cats react to overdoses of THC much the same as humans, although their small size frequently means the effects are severe and prolonged. While rarely fatal, some pets may require medical care to maintain their hydration during the time they are incapacitated. The few fatalities that have occurred in pets due to cannabis ingestion usually involve other toxic foods such as chocolate or coffee.

Cautions on the Use of Cannabis to Treat Pets

- Dogs have a higher number of endocannabinoid receptors in their cerebellum and brainstem than humans do. These parts of the brain control coordination, heart rate, respiratory rate, and more. This makes dogs particularly susceptible to toxicity from too much THC.

- Dogs intoxicated with THC may show signs of static ataxia. These dogs will seem rigid and have difficulty standing. This condition is unique to the dog and, while not fatal, often requires supportive medical therapy.

- Cannabis in any form is a highly pharmacologically active drug. Always consult with your veterinarian before administering any cannabis product to your pet.

- Because of the extreme sensitivity of small animals to THC, high-CBD products with little or no THC are frequently favored due to their greater margin of safety.

Delivery Methods

Oral Administration

Cannabis oil, which is usually diluted in a carrier such as olive oil or coconut oil, is one of the simplest ways to administer the medicine to pets. It can be added to food or given directly by mouth. Preparations of a highly concentrated extract (CO_2 or alcohol extraction are the cleanest methods) are diluted in the carrier to make appropriate dosing possible. Without dilution, the concentrated extracts (especially those containing THC) are difficult to dose with accuracy in small animals. Using undiluted concentrates greatly increases the chance of accidental overdose.

In addition to oils, cannabis-infused treats are available for pets. Most of these are CBD treats made from hemp and are sold over the counter nationwide. Hemp-based CBD treats have little to no THC, are very safe, and are often effective for mild to moderate aches and pains. Most practitioners agree, however, that, when higher doses are needed, hemp-based CBD treats and supplements are not as potent as those made from marijuana.

Topical Use

Cannabis oils, salves, or sprays can be used on pets with skin allergies or even for arthritis and back pain. The cannabinoid receptors in the skin and hair follicles provide both surface (skin) and deeper (muscle and joint) relief. Many of these animals otherwise require steroids or other medications that may have harmful side effects. The effects of topicals in some patients are nothing short of amazing. Topicals are a great option for pets, although sometimes fur may need to be shaved and it is important to prevent the pet from licking off the medicine.

Smoking and Vaping

Under no circumstances should any attempt be made to dose a pet with cannabis by blowing smoke or vapor into its face. Pets have highly sensitive respiratory systems that are not equipped for this type of delivery. In addition, it is currently impossible to accurately dose medicine for pets this way. There may come a time when accurate dosing is available through a metered dose inhaler, such as is used with pets and people to administer asthma medication. Until then, stick to oral and/or topical administration only.

Choosing a Cannabis Product for Your Pet

With the advent of CBD products and effective low-dose THC therapy, cannabis products are becoming more common for treating animals safely and effectively. "The results are almost immediate," says Darlene Arden, a certified animal behavior consultant. "Elderly dogs are running around like puppies, and their last months or years are far more comfortable. Those with cancer are no longer in any sort of pain. It increases the appetite. In other words it improves the quality of life. Not surprisingly, few veterinarians are prescribing medical marijuana yet, but I think we'll see a trend that way once some testing is done."

"Marijuana should be dispensed under medical care," Arden continued. "I think the benefits far outweigh any negative connotations, if it's used judiciously, people are educated about how to use and store it, and it is carefully dosed to the size of the dog."[457]

There may have been a day when CBD was "riding the coattails" of THC when it came to how people viewed cannabis as medicine, but no more. CBD has become a major player in its own right. THC and CBD are both highly active compounds that overlap in their pharmacological use. However, while both can be effectively used for pain, inflammation, and treatment of cancer, CBD has particular affinities for treating conditions such as gastrointestinal disease and seizures. The primary goal when using cannabis as medicine in pets (and people) is determining which compounds can be used most safely and effectively.

Like all botanical medicines, cannabis is made up of many active compounds. It is theorized that there is a synergistic effect between these chemicals that ultimately is greater than the sum of its parts. This phenomenon, known as the "entourage effect" (see p. 25), is one of many reasons utilizing a whole plant as medicine is often better than attempting to isolate a single compound for pharmaceutical use. In the future, the full spectrum of cannabinoids, terpenes, and flavonoids within cannabis will be utilized to achieve the greatest medical effect. For now, however, product selection is most commonly based on the ratio of CBD to THC.

The relative ratio of CBD to THC is as important to successful treatment as is the actual amount of each compound present in a medication. THC and CBD each mimic a different neurotransmitter in the endocannabinoid system and thus have different effects on the body. The individual amounts of THC and CBD in a formula create a medicine that affects the body relative to the specific ratio used. For example, a formula that is well suited to fight cancer often will have a higher THC content, whereas one designed for seizures will have a higher CBD content. Since formulas can be created with specific ratios, it is possible to create medicines to help a wide variety of conditions.

When choosing a cannabis product for use in pets, it is imperative to know both the concentration of the medicine and the ratio of CBD to THC. The table below is a guide to product selection for specific diseases or conditions and the most appropriate CBD-to-THC ratio.

Recommended CBD: THC Product Ratios for Specific Diseases or Conditions in Pets/Animals

CBD:THC	DISEASE OR CONDITION
High CBD, low THC (between 4:1 to 30:1)	Epilepsy/seizures Pain, inflammation Cancer Stroke or head injury Anxiety, restlessness (as an aid for pets who are not sleeping well)
Equal CBD and THC (1:1)	Inflammatory bowel disease Pain, inflammation Cancer, especially involving tumors Spinal cord injuries
Low CBD, high THC (between 1:4 to 1:20)	Severe pain such as advanced arthritis or cancer pain Appetite stimulation Cancer, especially involving tumors

For many conditions and in smaller pets, it is beneficial to begin with a lower-THC, higher-CBD medicine. This allows for a greater margin of safety and, if needed, acclimation to THC, which helps limit the chances of toxicity. Depending on the pet's response to the initial product, changes to higher-THC doses can be made under veterinary supervision.

We had a thirteen-year-old golden retriever who developed a growth on his lip. It was removed and diagnosed as an oral melanoma. His vet told us that in all cases it would return, and at this stage of the cancer, these tumors would have metastasized to various other parts of the mouth, jawbone, and internal organs. Life expectancy was given as three weeks to three months with no treatment. The veterinary options were to cut back to the bone on the jaw line, along with standard cancer treatments of chemo and radiation, without any indication of extending life expectancy. When we asked about survival rates and any alternatives, we were told: "under the law of the land its the only thing we can offer!"

After researching alternatives, we settled on a mixture of medical hemp CBD and medical cannabis oil, mixed as 1:1, complemented with 1/4 teaspoon of baking soda in his food (to alkalize the body) on a daily basis, plus we changed his food to The Honest Kitchen. After six weeks, we returned to the vet and had a full examination, x-rays, and other "cancer" determining tests. The vet later returned with a look of seeing a ghost. "There's nothing there, absolutely nothing, its completely gone, not even the growth on the lip has reappeared." Now six months later, our golden continues to be fit and healthy, and we continue with a maintenance regimen of a lower dosage of the CBD and medical cannabis oil, mixed as 1:1.

RAY WRIGHT, PET OWNER[458]

Accuracy in Labeling

Like any drug, the most important consideration with cannabis is to know exactly how much active ingredients are in the medication. With conventional pharmaceuticals, this is easy because standardized labeling allows us to know exactly what is contained within every liquid, pill, and capsule on the market.

Because our friends at the FDA have stated that cannabis has no legitimate medical use, they do not regulate or oversee product manufacturing or labeling. The upside of this is the presence of a lot of "boutique" companies making artisan products much like fine wine. A lot of love goes into these products. The downside, however, is inconsistency and/or inaccuracy in labeling. A cannabis preparation needs to be labeled with both the amount of CBD and THC in a given quantity, such as milligrams per milliliter (mg/ml), *and* the ratio of CBD to THC. We must have both pieces of information for safe and successful medical use.

Many cannabis products do not contain enough information on their labels to be safe to give to pets. Additionally, in this "let the buyer beware" environment, some product labels contain inaccurate information that may lead to the medicine being ineffective or even potentially dangerous.

CBD from Cannabis versus Hemp

Although never fatal, concerns for THC-related toxicity in pets is a real thing. It may arise from a dosing miscalculation or through using a mislabeled medicine. Either way, the result is a stressful (and potentially expensive) situation for both pets and their owners. By comparison, the relatively wide margin of safety of high-CBD products coupled with their efficacy makes a compelling case for the use of CBD in pets.

Medical cannabis containing CBD comes from either marijuana or hemp. They are both essentially the same plant, although, legally, hemp contains less than 0.3 percent THC. So, does it matter where the CBD comes from?

The answer is both yes and no. Many people who use CBD as medicine report that marijuana products are more effective than hemp. The reason is most likely due to the entourage effect, in which a full spectrum of cannabinoids used in therapy seems to have a synergetic effect and work better. Recall that marijuana contains much more than just THC and CBD. A variety of other cannabinoids, terpenes, and flavonoids make up the whole plant. It is very likely that complex interaction between these phytochemicals leads to their medical efficacy. While hemp contains some of these compounds, higher levels are found in medical-grade cannabis.

The CBD in hemp is the same CBD found in cannabis. That said, the specifics of the plant of origin and the methods of manufacture are critical to efficacy and safety. Historically, CBD from hemp comes from "industrial" sources where focus on plant genetics is on fiber production rather than cannabinoid, terpene, and flavonoid content. These products are also sometimes manufactured with non-organic solvents that potentially leave harmful residues behind. Today, however, there are hemp producers growing plants specifically for CBD and using safe methods such as CO_2 extraction to produce higher-quality medicine.

Regarding the use of CBD made from hemp, veterinarian Matthew J. Cote said, "What we've seen is that some of these dogs respond very rapidly. One woman from Fort Bragg was ready to put down her dog due to how sick and in pain he was, but the day before he was scheduled to go under, she administered our [CBD] treats and just like that the dog was up, walking around and acting normally again."[459]

Guidelines for Product Selection

- CBD products made from hemp can be safe and effective, provided they come from high-quality plants and are manufactured safely, but this can be a challenge (see p. 203 for more on hemp vs. medical cannabis–grade products). It's a good idea to research companies and manufacturing methods thoroughly before purchasing.

- Complete and accurate labeling of medical cannabis is critical for safety and success with medicine containing THC. Product labels should contain both the concentration of CBD and THC (usually expressed in milligrams) as well as the ratio of CBD to THC.

- Always begin at a low dose and slowly work up as needed (see dosing information in the next section). This process will limit the chances of adverse reactions.

- Think of cannabis as a prescription-strength medication. Use it with appropriate caution and always consult your veterinarian at every step of the way.

Safe and Effective Dosing

We know cannabis is a complex combination of various forms of THC, CBD, terpenes, and flavonoids. It is, however, impractical to calculate the concentration of all of the compounds present in a given plant as a means of determining dosage. Since THC and CBD are the most biologically active cannabinoids, medical cannabis dosing is based on these two components.

When determining the dosing of cannabis for pets, the primary necessity is accurate labeling. Without this information, carefully calculated doses mean nothing. Assuming the product being used is labeled accurately, the other consideration to take into account is the biphasic dosing curve.

Biphasic Dosing Curve

Cannabis displays a phenomenon called a biphasic dosing curve; in short, it refers to the optimal dose for a given condition and individual. Dosing below *or* above this optimum can result in a decreased effect of the medication. There is effectively a "sweet spot" with cannabis where it works optimally.

Given that there is no way to know exactly what the ideal dose is for any individual, the best strategy is to begin with a low dose and slowly increase on a weekly basis until the optimal response is found. Decreased efficacy from exceeding the optimal dose is different from overdosing in the sense of toxicity.

Dose Calculations

When purchasing a product specifically designed for pets, determining a dose should be easy: simply follow the directions on the label. But, even with CBD, and as stated previously, it is still advisable to start at the low end of the dosing range provided and slowly increase over time. This will prevent excessive sedation, which can occur even with CBD products.

Cannabis products produced for human consumption may have dosing information on them, but, once again, dogs and cats are not "small humans." Dosing them as such may result in a trip to the emergency room.

The following dosage guidelines for dogs and cats have been derived from a combination of research data and veterinary experience. Recommendations vary by individual and condition, so always consult an experienced veterinarian prior to giving cannabis to your pet.

THC*

- Dose: 0.1–0.25 mg/kg/day

- Calculated dose should be divided for twice-daily dosing

- Start low and slowly increase to develop tolerance and adjust for the biphasic dosing curve

---

*Although the amount of CBD in a given medicine is important, THC is the compound in cannabis that has the potential for toxicity. Thus, THC is always the limiting factor for any product containing THC. In order to prevent toxicity and a trip to the emergency room, accurate dosing is critical. Consult your veterinarian to assist you with the dosing calculations.

CBD

- Dose: 0.1–0.5 mg/kg/day
- Calculated dose should be divided for twice-daily dosing
- Doses up to 5 mg/kg/day have been reported for difficult seizure cases
- Start low and slowly increase to adjust for the biphasic dosing curve

The Future of Medical Cannabis for Pets

By anyone's estimation, the future of medical cannabis is bright. More and more states are legalizing cannabis, and it is inevitable that the FDA will ultimately be forced to reschedule marijuana and admit it has medical benefits. No one knows what is going to happen when Big Pharma tries to monopolize the industry, but, regardless, medical cannabis is here to stay.

Hesitation on the part of veterinarians to discuss the benefits of CBD (and THC) for pets is mostly founded in a lack of familiarity of how it works and the legal landscape. All of this is changing, however. Veterinarians are becoming more educated on the topic and are increasingly enthusiastic about how we can improve quality and quantity of life with this incredible medicine.

Until rescheduling and the entry of the pharmaceutical industry into the world of medical cannabis happen, the movement will continue to be a grass-roots effort. Both veterinarians and pet owners are part of this process. The more cannabis is discussed and results shared with other pet owners and medical professionals, the greater the response will be within the veterinary community.

NOTE *For updates to this chapter, visit www.CBD-book.com/Updates.*

PART IV

Varieties of Cannabis

Understanding Genetics to Match Strain to Condition

Cannabis farmers identify the varieties of the plant by its genetics, often called a *strain*. New strains are continually being bred, and there are now over one thousand varieties. For the patient looking for the best medicine for his or her condition, though it can be confusing, identifying strains is important. Often, the name of the strain is the only information the patient has when purchasing finished medicine, seeds, or clones, and selection of the strain should be based on understanding the varying medicinal effects of the different strains. The important facts to know are:

- the potency of the CBD and THC

- the ratio of CBD:THC

- the genetics, usually described in terms of sativa, indica, and hybrid (see more in the next section)

- the terpene content (when possible)

Once a patient finds a strain that works for his or her condition, he or she can experiment with other strains having similar ratios and genetic traits. Unfortunately, not all plants with the same strain name are identical. Mother Nature has a way of creating variety and adding different cultivators to the mix. Even within one farm, there will be variations from plant to plant, even variations from the top of the plant to the bottom. Much of the variation comes from the nutrients used, growing techniques, weather conditions, and location. Two samples with the same strain name can vary quite widely in characteristics. Whenever possible, it is important to know any other relevant strain-specific information that can help patients identify which strain will be best for their condition. Ideally, information would come from laboratory test results.

Each strain has been developed using various techniques of crossbreeding, selective breeding, feminization, and other genetic processes. The strains are often crossbred with themselves to make them more stable. When the female plant is pollinated with a male, it produces seeds, and, like human offspring, the brothers and sisters often have a lot of variety in personality, physical characteristics, and so on. The plants that grow from these seeds also have a wide variety of features, including their CBD:THC ratio, potency, terpene content, as well as their medicinal efficacy.

Once a specific plant is found with the ideal characteristics, that plant can be "cloned." Cloning is a propagation process that involves taking new sprouts from a mother plant still in its vegetative growth cycle. Female plants are used since the oil from the female flowers has the vast majority of the medicinal material. The baby clones are then processed to develop their own roots and eventually become large productive plants. Cannabis plants are all annual plants, and this process is repeated each year. The advantage of cloning plants is that the offspring has almost the exact characteristics of the mother. Therefore, specific medicinal qualities will be reproduced clone after clone, crop after crop. In nature, cannabis plants that grow to maturity and make seeds that fall to the ground and propagate in this way year after year are known as "land race strains."

Most of the very high–CBD strains that have been developed are only available as clones, known as "clone only." If you want to grow your own medicine, beware of sources of clone-only strains that are sold as seeds, as not all seed companies are reputable. Granted, seeds are more convenient to ship and source, and plants from seeds do offer some benefits to the grower over cloned plants, including more robust plants with a nicely developed tap root. However, seeds can have a very wide variety of medicinal properties and other characteristics. Not only will half of them be male or female, the CBD:THC ratio will be all over the map, varying from 1:1 to 25:1 within the same strain. If you're interested in growing plants with specific traits, like a very high 20:1 CBD:THC ratio, then its best to look for plants generated from clones.

Cannabis Subspecies:
Sativa, Indica, and Ruderalis

Reporting contributed by Heather Dunbar

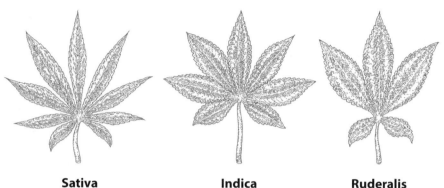

| Sativa | Indica | Ruderalis |

FIGURE 54: [Eschved] © 123RF.com

Cannabis Family/Pharmacology

- Family: Cannabaceae

- Genus: Cannabis

- Species: Sativa, Indica, Ruderalis

Cannabis is the botanical genus of the plant, and although cannabis is biologically classified as one single species (*Cannabis sativa L.*) there are at least three distinct plant subspecies that have been identified and debated for many years: *Cannabis sativa, Cannabis indica,* and *Cannabis ruderalis*. There are also many hybrids, of which there are many crosses, between mostly sativa and indica varieties. Cannabis used for fiber and food, typically referred to as hemp, is grown for the use of seeds and fiber, and it has only traces of the psychoactive cannabinoid THC, generally less than 0.5 percent. Hemp varieties of cannabis appear to be the genetic origin of CBD strains and are often very high in CBD content.

The biologist Carl Linnaeus first identified a single species he named *C. sativa* in 1753. He listed several varieties, assuming they all belonged to a single species. In 1785, a plant biologist named Jean-Baptiste Lamarck delineated a second species he called *C. indica.* He noted that *C. sativa* grows taller, is more fibrous, and has narrow leaflets, whereas *C. indica* grows shorter, has wider leaflets, and is more psychoactive. More recently in 2005, Karl Hillig, from Indiana University, investigated the diversity of genetics among cannabis varieties of the world and made an interesting discovery. He revealed that all drug/psychoactive strains shared a relatively narrow range of genes and that the fiber/hemp strains shared another, smaller set of genes.[460]

Hillig is supportive of the original two-species concept of *C. sativa* and *C. indica,* with *C. indica* being more diverse genetically due to its larger worldwide cultivation. He decided that all fibrous strains should be classified as *C. sativa,* and all drug varieties classified as *C. indica.* He further grouped *C. indica* into four subspecies: *indica, afghanica, chinensis,* and *kafiristanica.* He ultimately divided indica varieties into broad-leaf drug (BLD) and narrow-leaf drug (NLD) varieties.[461] Most hybrids found today are a combination of these two.

In a most recent publication, *Cannabis: Evolution and Ethnobotany,* authors Clarke and Merlin also divide modern cannabis into four categories, with the genus *Cannabis* and species *sativa* and *indica* belonging to all four categories. These are classified as: broad-leaf hemp (BLH), broad-leaf drug (BLD), narrow-leaf hemp (NLH), and narrow-leaf drug (NLD). According to their work, Clarke and Merlin concluded these four species are a combination of *C. sativa* and *C. indica.*[462]

Presently, almost all modern medical cannabis varieties are hybrids between members of two *C. indica* subspecies: *indica,* representing the traditional and geographically widespread NLD land race marijuana varieties, and *afghanica,* representing the geographically limited BLD hashish land race varieties of Afghanistan. The combination of land race strains from such geographically isolated and genetically diverse populations allowed for the blossoming of the great variety of modern-day hybrid medical as well as recreational cannabis.

Cannabis strain differences are in part a result of geographic origin, the outcome of plant evolution, and breeder interaction with different strains within subspecies. Modern-day genetic "breeders" of cannabis have developed thousands of different strains that are crossbreeds called *hybrids.* Hybrid strains produce varieties that carry some characteristic of each parent. Therefore, knowing the parent lineage will give clues to the medicinal properties.

The characteristics of these plants and their effects are more similar than different, but different ratios of cannabinoids and terpene content can produce noticeably different effects. Cannabis cannot be oversimplified into sedative and stimulant these days. Michael Backes, in his book *Cannabis Pharmacy*, states, "eventually, the distinction between indica and sativa effects will be based on a variety's terpene, rather than its cannabinoid, content."[463]

Certainly, the medicinal effects are a much better way to classify strains than the traditional "sativa versus indica" categorization. Most strains available today are the result of much breeding and crossbreeding, rendering most strains as hybrids with a various blend of both qualities.

Cannabis sativa

Cannabis sativa originated close to the equator and thrives in warmer climates, such as Colombia, Mexico, Thailand, and Southeast Asia. The plant is characterized by narrow leaves and lanky branches that are farther apart compared to the indica and ruderalis strains. These plants tend to be taller and skinnier and produce fewer flowers than indica and ruderalis strains do.

Sativa strains are generally felt more cerebrally, produce stimulating effects, and are preferred for daytime use. Sativa strains can be traced back to hemp varieties and have the enzyme that is responsible for converting CBG into CBD. From an energetic or yogic perspective, sativa strains have been said to activate the upper chakras.

BENEFITS:

- Stimulates/energizes
- Increases sense of well-being
- Increases focus
- Stimulates creativity
- Elevates mood
- Reduces depression
- Relieves headaches
- Relieves nausea
- Increases appetite

POTENTIAL NEGATIVE SIDE EFFECTS:

- Increases anxiety
- Increases paranoia
- Increases heartbeat
- Causes hyperactivity
- Decreases focus

Cannabis indica

Indica strains originate in the Hindu Kush region of the Middle East—India, Turkey, Morocco, Afghanistan, Pakistan, and Nepal—and tend to grow better in cool temperatures and higher altitudes. The plant has broad leaves and tends to be shorter and bushier, with denser flower buds, than sativa strains. It has more relaxing and calming qualities than sativa strains do, and on an energetic level it moves the energy down to the lower chakras.

BENEFITS:

- Relieves body pain
- Relaxes muscles
- Promotes sleep
- Relieves spasms
- Reduces seizures
- Relieves headaches
- Reduces anxiety or stress
- Increases appetite

POTENTIAL NEGATIVE SIDE EFFECTS:

- Causes feeling of tiredness
- Causes sluggish/heavy feeling
- Causes overeating
- Decreases motivation

Cannabis ruderalis

Cannabis ruderalis is the least known subspecies. It is characterized by varied leaf sizes, somewhere in the middle of the sativa and indica varieties. These plants tend to be shorter and smaller than the other varieties and are sometimes referred to as "wild" cannabis.

This less common species was identified in 1924 in southern Siberia and grows wild in other areas of Russia. The origin of the name *ruderalis* comes from the Latin word *rudera* or *ruderal*. A ruderal plant species grows on distressed land, on waste ground, and along roadsides and other disturbed areas. This species gives the term weed or ditch weed a deeper meaning. Unlike sativa and indica strains, ruderalis strains do not depend on light cycles to flower and have an automatic flowering cycle given a number of days.[464] Although it has almost no THC, some breeders are choosing ruderalis strains for their higher levels of CBN (cannabinol), which are proving to have many medicinal benefits, including sleep support.[465]

The Genetics of CBD Strains versus THC Strains

Plants that produce high levels of THC express a gene code for THCA, which converts CBG into THCA, which in turn becomes THC when heated, a process called decarboxylation. These plants are both indica and sativa strains, as well as hybrid varieties.

Some plants express genes that are coded for CBDA, which converts CBG into CBDA, which is the precursor of CBD and converts through decarboxylation. These plants are generally hybrid varieties with a tendency toward sativa dominance with varying amounts of both indica and sativa qualities in CBD strains.

Industrial Hemp versus Medical Cannabis–Derived CBD

The key difference between hemp plants and cannabis plants is resin content. Industrial hemp varieties are typically a low-resin agricultural crop, grown from pedigree seed, with about one hundred tall, skinny plants per square meter. They are machine harvested and manufactured into a multitude of products, including rope, cloth, and plastics. It is believed that the word "canvas," the cloth used for the sails of ships, is a variation of the word "cannabis." Modern medicinal or recreational cannabis plants are a high-resin horticultural crop, typically grown from asexually reproduced female clones, one or two plants per square meter, and hand harvested, dried, trimmed, and cured.

Whether extracted from hemp or cannabis, CBD is the same molecule. Industrial hemp usually contains about 3.5 percent CBD plus a very small amount of THC—less than 0.1 percent. To extract CBD, a large amount of hemp is required to make a small amount of CBD-rich product. The challenge, therefore, becomes the extraction method for production. The cheapest way to extract the CBD is to use solvents, such as butane and hexane. However, with this method, toxic residues can remain in the oil. Tests in 2014 conducted by Project CBD found significant levels of dangerous solvent residues such as hexane (a neurotoxin according to the Environmental Protection Agency) in random samples of CBD products derived from industrial hemp. Also, the hemp plant itself is a bio-accumulator, meaning that it tends to absorb toxins from the soil. It does this so effectively that it was used in the post-Chernobyl nuclear disaster cleanup. Thus, if the hemp is to be consumed by human beings, the soil must be monitored closely, and organic approaches are highly recommended. Many CBD products are made from industrial hemp grown in China, and some of them can contain significant levels of heavy metals and pesticides. Toxic chemicals tend to accumulate and increase potency when extraction and concentration are performed. Extraction is the usual process of concentrating the molecules of interest, and the toxic chemicals cannot be separated with this method. It is highly recommended to know the source and growing techniques of any CBD products one consumes.

Much of the cannabis used in today's medical cannabis industry does have higher levels of THC than hemp has, but some strains are also much higher in CBD, up to 20 percent. Because of this, CBD can be extracted from the whole plant using a simple oil infusion method or a tincturing method with high-proof alcohol.

For many reasons, CBD-rich cannabis is a better source of CBD than industrial hemp. Many manufacturers of CBD oil use Chinese-grown hemp and market their products online. They are restricted by the FDA from calling it a dietary supplement, and in 2016 the FDA singled out eight CBD oil producers for making substandard products as well as making unsubstantiated medical claims about treating pain, spasms, cancer, and other ailments.[466] The FDA and DEA have never approved CBD as a supplement for any kind of medical use.

At time of press, according to U.S. state medical cannabis laws, a CBD-infused oil product (from hemp or cannabis) can be used legally for therapeutic purposes if it is consumed by a certified medical patient, following local guidelines, in a state that has legalized medical or recreational cannabis or, in some cases, CBD-only products (read more on legal trends in Chapter 10).

NOTE *For updates to this chapter, visit www.CBD-book.com/Updates.*

Alphabetized List of High-CBD Strains

Reporting contributed by Amalthea Birkholz

Here's a brief partial list and review of some popular CBD strains in Northern California. This is not a complete list of strains by any means, as many other strains have been developed in different locations. The tables and charts below are the results of sample lab tests run by the authors, not averages of the strains. Each plant is unique and can be a little different.

AC/DC (aka ACDC, Oracle, C-6)

AC/DC has improved the lives of countless people. It is a direct phenotype of Cannatonic, meaning that it comes from a Cannatonic seed, one of the original "gold standards" of CBD purity from Resin Seeds in Spain. AC/DC has a 22:1 CBD:THC ratio (between 20:1 and 25:1) and is a clone-only strain.

Often, AC/DC has been recommended as a first strain for new patients to try for a large variety of medical conditions. Popularity has grown partly because it is so effective, and, to a large extent, because it has no psychoactive side effect due to its low THC. Although the plant is relatively small, fragile, and low yielding, it consistently produces some of the very best high-grade medicine that gets results.

AC/DC unfolds a well-rounded cannabinoid and terpene profile. This is important as we know these compounds work synergistically, making the sum greater than the parts. CBD, once an underrated cannabinoid, is a great supporting actor that, even in small quantities, quietly performs internal balance and health. Studies indicate that AC/DC acts as an antidepressant, encourages brain growth, is an anti-inflammatory, fights pain, and is also an antibacterial and anti-fungal. It is well known for helping children and adults with epileptic seizure disorders, anxiety, multiple sclerosis, Crohn's disease, and neurological pain issues. It is often used for cancer medicine and can be blended with other strains to obtain various ratios between 1:1 and 8:1 of CBD:THC. Often, a 4:1 blend is recommended for pain and inflammation. While some people find it beneficial for sleep, others find it makes them more alert in the day time.

AC/DC was propagated by Dr. William Courtney in 2011, who acquired a number of Cannatonic seeds from Resin Seeds in Spain. These seeds were feminized, and most of the seeds had a relative ratio between 1:1 and 2:1 of CBD:THC. However, one of the plants produced a very high ratio of 22:1. Because he was very interested in using raw cannabis plant material and fresh juice as a dietary source for CBDA and THCA, Courtney saved this strain by making clones and gave it the name AC/DC, which stands for "Alternative Cannabinoid/Dietary Cannabis."

While classified as a 50/50 hybrid (50 percent sativa, 50 percent indica), AC/DC is fairly neutral. It has its own characteristics and does not present with either sativa or indica traits. A clone-only strain, it is available at only a few California dispensaries. Growing AC/DC is considered medium difficulty with a nine-to-ten-week flower cycle (the time interval from when buds begin to form until harvest). From a farming point of view, the yields are small and it is a fussy plant, barely able to support its ripened flowers, which always need a trellis. It grows wider than tall with lots of lateral branches. AC/DC grows well both indoors or in full sun. Its aroma is sweet, lemony, and earthy, with a sweet, spicy, citrus taste.

Type: 50% sativa, 50% indica

Potency: 15–19% CBD, .6–.8% THC

Ratio: Between 20:1 and 26:1 CBD:THC

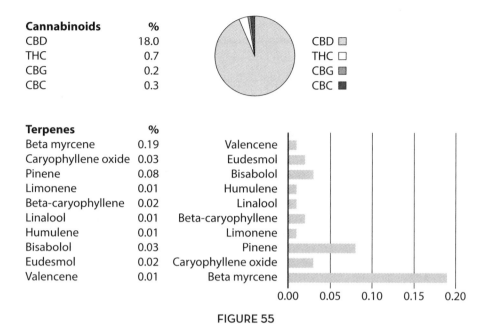

Cannabinoids	%
CBD	18.0
THC	0.7
CBG	0.2
CBC	0.3

Terpenes	%
Beta myrcene	0.19
Caryophyllene oxide	0.03
Pinene	0.08
Limonene	0.01
Beta-caryophyllene	0.02
Linalool	0.01
Humulene	0.01
Bisabolol	0.03
Eudesmol	0.02
Valencene	0.01

FIGURE 55

Cannatonic (aka Canna Tonic)

Cannatonic was one of the very first CBD-rich strains, sparking the start of the CBD revolution. Cannatonic has become the grandmother strain that parented many of the subsequent strains showcased here. A complex and valuable strain that is responsible for much of the CBD awareness and CBD success stories, it was created by Resin Seeds of Spain in 2008. A cross between a female MK Ultra and a famous G13 Haze male, Cannatonic is a unique hybrid strain bred specifically for its low THC content (rarely above 6 percent) and its high CBD content (usually between 7 percent and 15 percent). Usually, flowers have a ratio between 1:1 and 2:1 of CBD:THC. Since it is grown from seeds, the offspring have a wide variety of CBD and THC content, and on a few occasions the ratio has been extremely high, in the 20:1+ range. These exceptional plants have been set aside and cloned, producing other strains such as AC/DC and C-6. Cannatonic's genes live on in some of the most popular strains now arriving on the CBD arena, as it is being crossbred to produce offspring strains such as Canna Tsu, Remedy, and Valentine X.

Cannatonic is one of the premier medicinal strains, good for pain, muscle spasms, insomnia, cancer, relaxation, anxiety, migraines, and a wide variety of psychological disorders. It has been known to help with nausea, stress, and mood disorders and helps focus the mind. CBG and myrcene, which are dominant in Cannatonic, may be responsible for making this strain such a great pain regulator, both chronic and acute. It is also good for fibromyalgia and inflammation.

Cannatonic has an earthy odor with a mild, sweet, and slightly lemon flavor. Its taste is citrus, spice, smooth, and creamy. It soothes and accelerates the healing of many illnesses. While classified as sativa/indica hybrid 50/50, the medicinal effect is more like 40/60 indica dominant. It has a medium difficulty to grow, and it flowers in nine weeks. The potency ranges from 6–17 percent CBD. Seed packs will be 75 percent CBD-rich, and half of them most likely will be 1:1 ratio.

Type: 40% sativa, 60% indica

Potency: 6–17% CBD, .45–7% THC

Ratio: Between 1:1 and 22:1 CBD:THC

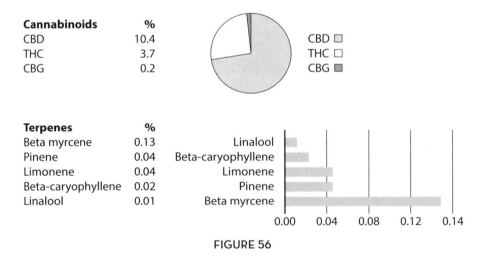

Cannabinoids	%
CBD	10.4
THC	3.7
CBG	0.2

Terpenes	%
Beta myrcene	0.13
Pinene	0.04
Limonene	0.04
Beta-caryophyllene	0.02
Linalool	0.01

FIGURE 56

Canna Tsu (aka Canna Sue)

Canna Tsu is the result of crossbreeding Cannatonic and Sour Tsunami parents. It was developed in 2010 by Lawrence Ringo of SoHum Seeds (Southern Humboldt Seed Company). It is prized by many returning patients because of its medicinal effectiveness. Cannatonic's popular and complex compounds, unveiled in an indica dominance that is tempered by Sour Tsunami's sativa-dominant soothing qualities, results in uplifting clarity for patients. Overall, it offers some of the best of the CBD-hybrid options and manifests with indica-like properties. It has many medicinal applications that include treatment of conditions that need higher CBD ratios, such as pain, stress, Crohn's disease, ALS, inflammation, anxiety, and cancer. It can be used in an extract form for skin conditions, and added to beauty products and anti-aging creams. Its high beta myrcene content means it helps with sleep problems and has a relaxing effect.

This strain produces very beautiful, large colas (flower buds), is bush like, and has a fairly high yield. It is easy to grow and has a strong resistance to mold and mildew. Its flowering time is sixty-three to seventy days, and its flowers have a sweet, spicy, citrus aroma. Seeds are available from SoHum Seeds and Bay Area dispensaries. Because it is not stabilized, Canna Tsu seeds produce a wide variety of ratios of CBD:THC.

Type: 35% sativa, 65% indica

Potency: 9–14% CBD, .45–7% THC

Ratio: Between 2:1 and 22:1 CBD:THC

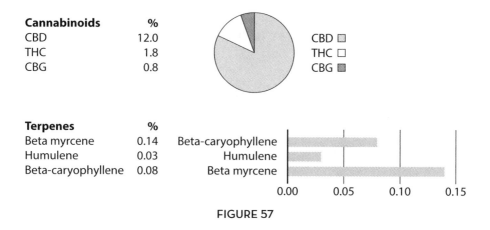

Cannabinoids	%
CBD	12.0
THC	1.8
CBG	0.8

Terpenes	%
Beta myrcene	0.14
Humulene	0.03
Beta-caryophyllene	0.08

FIGURE 57

CBD Therapy (aka Therapy A)

This strain was developed by CBD Crew, an international project by Howard Marks (aka Mr. Nice), Jaime of Resin Seeds (Spain), and Scott Blakey (aka

Shantibaba). Being very experienced breeders of the best cannabis for many years, they decided to work together to produce a line of CBD-rich cannabis strains that are specifically effective for medical marijuana patients. Of their seven CBD-rich strains, CBD Therapy had the highest CBD:THC ratio, averaging 24:1, available as seeds that have been feminized by CBD Crew.

CBD Therapy was derived from high recreational–THC cannabis strains and has taken some four years to stabilize. Because it comes from seeds, there is a lot of variation in the CBD:THC ratio. Most seeds develop into plants with a ratio of between 30:1 and 20:1, while some were closer to 5:1, even a few at 2:1. No seeds produced plants with a higher THC content than the 2:1 ratio.

CBD Therapy is effective for treatment of Dravet syndrome, multiple sclerosis, Crohn's disease, fibromyalgia, inflammation issues, anxiety, depression, or epilepsy. CBD Therapy can be mixed with other strains to create custom medicine for many types of illnesses and conditions. Even though it is a 50/50 indica/sativa hybrid mix, its high beta myrcene content gives it more of an indica effect medicinally and is, therefore, good for treating insomnia and for promoting relaxation and stress reduction. CBD Therapy's flavor and aroma range from fruity and sweet, to dank and earthy.

Type: 50% sativa, 50% indica

Potency: 14–18% CBD, .6–.8% THC

Ratio: Between 20:1 and 30:1 CBD:THC

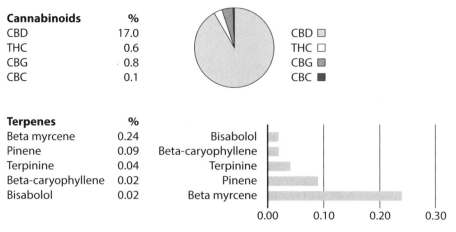

Cannabinoids	%
CBD	17.0
THC	0.6
CBG	0.8
CBC	0.1

Terpenes	%
Beta myrcene	0.24
Pinene	0.09
Terpinine	0.04
Beta-caryophyllene	0.02
Bisabolol	0.02

FIGURE 58

Charlotte's Web

Charlotte's Web was developed by the Stanley Brothers (Joel, Jesse, Jon, Jordan, Jared, and Josh) in 2011 in Colorado. Although somewhat secretive about its origin, it is believed to be a cross between Cannatonic and industrial hemp, and one interview mentioned using "ditch weed" found locally. It is a very high–CBD strain containing a ratio of 25:1 CBD:THC, and the potency runs between 15 percent and 17 percent CBD in the dried flowers. Because the strain does not get one high, it was originally called Hippie's Disappointment.

In 2012, the Stanley Brothers were introduced to the Figi family whose five-year-old daughter, Charlotte, had Dravet syndrome, an intractable form of epilepsy, causing more than three hundred grand mal seizures per week. The Figis had tried all the standard pharmacological options offered, and they all failed to work. They had also tried other CBD strains that were available at the time and some worked, but only a little bit. After trying the Hippie's Disappointment strain, Charlotte experienced a dramatic reduction in epileptic activity: three to four seizures per month. The Stanleys renamed the strain "Charlotte's Web."

In 2013, Dr. Sanjay Gupta featured Charlotte in a CNN documentary called *Weed* and again in 2014 in *Weed 2*. Charlotte and this strain have also been the subject of many documentaries and interviews, including spots on *60 Minutes, Dateline,* and *The Doctors*.[467] The publicity from this exposure has been one of the greatest single events responsible for increased awareness of CBD and its medical properties by a widespread general population of non-cannabis users. It has become the focus of a nationwide effort to legalize marijuana strains high in CBD. Charlotte's story brought public attention to a cause that, in more than a dozen states, has helped secure medical marijuana laws, often called the "Charlotte's Web law," in states that allow CBD only.

Charlotte's Web is a sativa-dominant hybrid. It is highly effective at treating pediatric seizure disorders, as well as helping with pain, muscle spasms, and headaches. The overall effect is entirely in the body, with no intoxication, even in children and first-time users. This strain has a strong pine smell, with floral tones and an earthy taste.

Availability is somewhat limited. The Stanley Brothers have not made the genetics available to other growers, keeping the information within their own organizations, CW Botanicals and the Realm of Caring. In addition, these products are only available within the state of Colorado. However, Charlotte's Web is almost identical to AC/DC in every respect, which is much more readily available.

Type: 60% sativa, 40% indica

Potency: 15–17% CBD, .5–.8% THC

Ratio: Between 22:1 and 26:1 CBD:THC

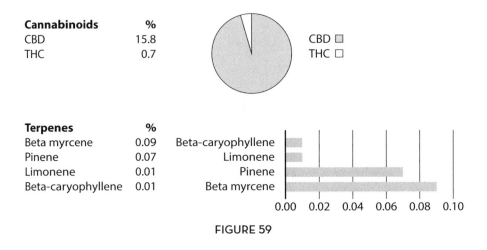

Cannabinoids	%
CBD	15.8
THC	0.7

CBD ☐
THC ☐

Terpenes	%
Beta myrcene	0.09
Pinene	0.07
Limonene	0.01
Beta-caryophyllene	0.01

FIGURE 59

Electra 4

Electra 4 is a cross of AC/DC and Otto, bringing together prominent re-emergent high-CBD strains from California and Colorado. Otto was one of the first CBD strains identified in 2008. Electra 4, like AC/DC, is a clone-only CBD phenotype that offers a ratio between 10:1 and 25:1 of CBD:THC. It was created in Northern California in 2011 by breeder Tim Underwood. It expresses a rich and varied terpene profile.

One of Electra 4's dominant terpenes is beta-caryophyllene, which supports and helps regulate the body's natural response to inflammation caused by irritation or injury. It also provides soothing support to the digestive tract when ingested. Beta-caryophyllene targets CB2 receptors that may combat many inflammatory disorders, ranging from arthritis, bladder cystitis, multiple sclerosis, and HIV-associated dementia, all without the THC high.

Electra 4 was an attempt to meld the bushy shape of AC/DC with the tall, gangly tree-like structure of Otto. Electra 4 grows quite tall like its father, with long heavy branches covered with large flower buds and small sativa-influenced leaves. It resembles industrial hemp more than cannabis, often taking a full twelve weeks to finish growing, and can grow twenty feet tall outdoors. It produces a heavy yield of aromatic flowers with a sparse leaf structure. It resists mold and to some extent mites and budworm, characteristics like its parent, Otto. Its aroma is fruit, pepper, and pine.

Type: 70% sativa, 30% indica

Potency: 12–15% CBD; .6–1.5% THC

Ratio: Between 10:1 and 27:1 CBD:THC

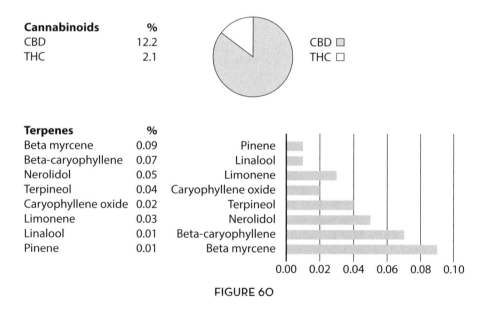

Cannabinoids	%
CBD	12.2
THC	2.1

Terpenes	%
Beta myrcene	0.09
Beta-caryophyllene	0.07
Nerolidol	0.05
Terpineol	0.04
Caryophyllene oxide	0.02
Limonene	0.03
Linalool	0.01
Pinene	0.01

FIGURE 60

Harlequin

Known for soothing a wide variety of ailments ranging from pain and chemotherapy side effects to PTSD, Harlequin is a substantial addition to any medical treatment program. It grows in a dark green Christmas tree shape quite vigorously. Large flower buds (colas) are so dense they can take up to three weeks to dry. The smell and taste are pine and sweet with an almost syrupy heaviness that creates pleasant medicine. It was first noticed in 2007/2008 by Wade Laughter, a pioneer in the re-emergence of CBD. Laughter procured some seeds from a Swiss cannabis farm from a strain called Snowcap, named for its profuse white trichomes. He crossbred it with Colombian Gold, Nepali (indica), and Thai (sativa). Because of his attentive gardening, he managed to save this remarkable plant and later named it Harlequin.

Test results verified a 2:1 CBD:THC ratio, rich in medicinal qualities. It's very high in beta myrcene and beta-caryophyllene, providing both anti-inflammatory and relaxing tendencies. Laughter collaborated with Project CBD and Harborside dispensary to help stock clones and dried flowers. It became popular in local dispensaries and quickly spread throughout California, providing an introduction to CBD for many. It is fairly easy to cultivate, has large trichome-laden colas, has an eight-to-nine-week flower cycle, and is available as a clone-only strain from California dispensaries.

Type: 75% sativa, 25% indica

Potency: 14–18% CBD; 7–9% THC

Ratio: Between 1:1 and 3:1 CBD:THC

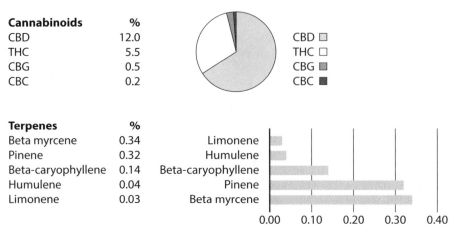

Cannabinoids	%
CBD	12.0
THC	5.5
CBG	0.5
CBC	0.2

Terpenes	%
Beta myrcene	0.34
Pinene	0.32
Beta-caryophyllene	0.14
Humulene	0.04
Limonene	0.03

FIGURE 61

Laughter offered some Harlequin to a friend with a reconstructed shoulder and found that, "although it didn't get him high, it was the only thing he'd found that took away the pain."

Another patient, a veteran in Arizona, found it so effective for his PTSD that he made an agreement with a local sheriff to allow him to grow Harlequin if he offered it free of charge to any veteran in need who could show legal documentation.

Harle Tsu (aka Harle Sue)

Harle Tsu is a 60 percent indica-dominant hybrid. It grows like a strong and dependable queen, exuding confidence that patients can lean on. This plant offers a solid variety of well-known cannabinoids and terpenes producing an almost complete entourage effect in one plant.

Harle Tsu (aka Harle Sue) was developed by Lawrence Ringo of SoHum Seeds in 2012. It is a cross between Harlequin and Sour Tsunami. It is a uniform, light emerald green plant with flowers that elongate in a luxuriant stretch, developing large, dense buds. It is a vigorous, heavy producer of reliable, high-CBD medicine. It develops a notable fruity, woody, and pine fragrance during flowering that reveals an abundant terpene content. If grown and harvested properly, this fragrance remains when cured.

Harle Tsu has been known to help with ALS, anxiety, chemotherapy-related nausea, bipolar disorder, cancer, Crohn's disease, depression, epilepsy, inflammation, multiple sclerosis, Parkinson's disease, PTSD, pain, stress, head trauma, ticks and head shakes (not related to epilepsy), restless legs syndrome, and rheumatoid arthritis.

Harle Tsu is available as seeds from SoHum Seeds in Humboldt County. The seeds often have a ratio of 20:1 CBD:THC. It is fairly easy to cultivate with a high yield that grows tall. Its flowering time is eight weeks. Its aroma is distinct apple and citrus, rooted in earth and wood scents.

Type: 40% sativa, 60% indica

Potency: 12–17% CBD, .6–.8% THC

Ratio: Between 18:1 and 24:1 CBD:THC

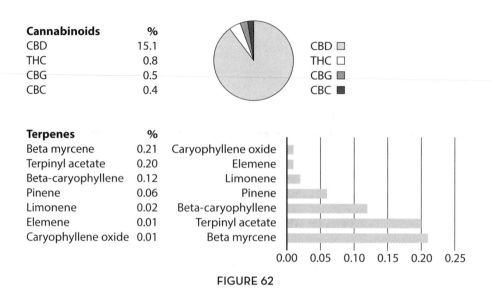

Cannabinoids	%
CBD	15.1
THC	0.8
CBG	0.5
CBC	0.4

Terpenes	%
Beta myrcene	0.21
Terpinyl acetate	0.20
Beta-caryophyllene	0.12
Pinene	0.06
Limonene	0.02
Elemene	0.01
Caryophyllene oxide	0.01

FIGURE 62

Omrita

Omrita RX is a sativa-dominant hybrid from the San Francisco Bay Area. With an average CBD level ranging from 9.5 to 12 percent and THC level of 7 to 8 percent, this strain produces extremely potent medicine. Omrita RX is famous among the medical cannabis community for its treatment of a wide range of medical conditions, including chronic pain due to illness or injury, inflammation, muscle spasms, anxiety disorders, and nausea.

The effect associated with Omrita RX is described as an uplifting sense of cerebral clarity and focus with a mild, warming body glow. With a ratio of 1.5:1 CBD:THC, this strain does have a mild cerebral psychoactive effect. Omrita RX has a fresh earthy aroma with hints of skunk and a fresh earthy taste that is slightly peppery. The Omrita RX buds are long and dense, with leafy dark olive green flowers, rich amber hairs, a layer of fine crystal trichomes, and sticky, sweet, syrupy resin.

Miguel A. acquired ten seeds of a strain called Rx from the Vancouver Island Seed Company (VISC) in late 2009. In its catalog, VISC described Rx as its "favorite medicinal variety"—a double-indica cross of Romulan Joe with a strain called "Fucking Incredible." The ten original Rx seeds Miguel planted produced two female plants that were robust, colorful, and covered with resin. These plants were cloned and propagated. Miguel renamed the strain to emphasize its medical value, adding the Sanskrit word Omrita, which means nectar. He acknowledges that the strain "was the result of someone else's work and any recognition should be directed back to the original breeders at VISC for their incredible creation."

Over the past year, cuttings grown out from his original two Rx females have consistently tested at 9–12 percent CBD and 5–7 percent THC. This strain has a large amount of beta-caryophyllene, known for its anti-inflammatory effects.

Type: 65% sativa, 35% indica

Potency: 9.5–12% CBD, 7–8% THC

Ratio: Between 1.5:1 and 2:1 CBD:THC

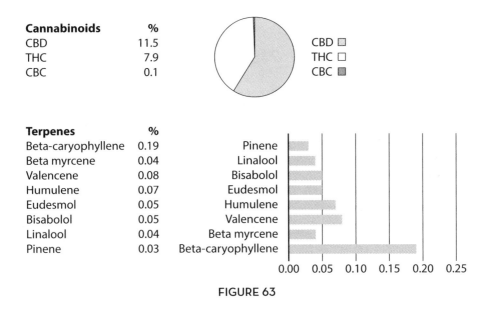

Cannabinoids	%
CBD	11.5
THC	7.9
CBC	0.1

Terpenes	%
Beta-caryophyllene	0.19
Beta myrcene	0.04
Valencene	0.08
Humulene	0.07
Eudesmol	0.05
Bisabolol	0.05
Linalool	0.04
Pinene	0.03

FIGURE 63

Remedy

Remedy brings back to life the Moroccan and Afghan genetics that once naturally produced plants rich in both CBD and THC. These land race plants were commonly used by villagers to maintain health and balance in harsh environments. It is useful for epileptic disorders, like Dravet and Lennox-Gastaut syndromes, as well as anxiety, insomnia, inflammation, nerve disorders, and many other medical issues including cancer.

Similar to Harle Tsu, this strain has an abundance of the favorite cannabinoids and terpenes, like a well-stocked medicine kit offering an "in house" entourage effect. However, Remedy tilts toward the indica side. Remedy grows in a deep blue-green round bush with a lavender flush on its hefty buds. The tips of the flower buds are often magenta. One unique characteristic is its very short flower cycle at just seven weeks. Most other CBD strains take nine to eleven weeks to flower. This rapid growth period allows a grower to yield several crops using light deprivation techniques.

Remedy is an indica hybrid that is 75 percent indica and 25 percent sativa. It was developed by Dark Heart Nursery and is a combination of Cannatonic and Afghan Skunk. It is available as a clone-only plant from Northern California dispensaries. It was bred and released in 2014 and has an easy-to-medium difficulty to grow, with a seven-week flower cycle. It has a lemon, woody, and earthy aroma and a taste with sweet floral notes.

Type: 25% sativa, 75% indica

Potency: 14–19% CBD; .6–.8% THC

Ratio: Between 22:1 and 25:1 CBD:THC

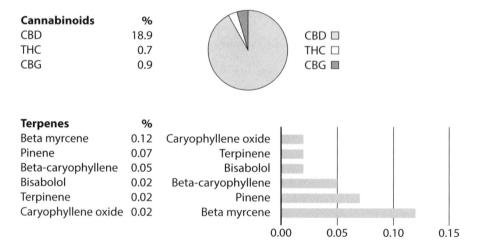

Cannabinoids	%
CBD	18.9
THC	0.7
CBG	0.9

CBD □
THC □
CBG ■

Terpenes	%
Beta myrcene	0.12
Pinene	0.07
Beta-caryophyllene	0.05
Bisabolol	0.02
Terpinene	0.02
Caryophyllene oxide	0.02

FIGURE 64

Ringo's Gift

The result of crossbreeding Sour Tsunami, Harlequin, and AC/DC, this magnificent plant is truly a "gift"—the final strain that Lawrence Ringo of SoHum Seeds created before he departed in 2014. Ringo's Gift is rapidly gaining a reputation for helping a wide variety of conditions, ranging from fibromyalgia, inflammatory diseases, some forms of epilepsy, cancer, and stress as well as many other diseases. It is an abundant powerhouse of medicine, preserving the best aspects of AC/DC while taking its fragile growing traits to a sturdy new evolution. Harlequin and Sour Tsunami bring vigor and abundance to this holy trinity of CBD strains.

Most CBD strains tend to produce low yields, which frustrates most growers. Ringo wanted to produce a strain that combined very high medicinal qualities (20:1+) with vibrant growth and high yield. In 2014, he chose his very best Harle Tsu male to crossbreed with the finest AC/DC female in his garden. After being covered in pollen from the process, he hugged the AC/DC to get all the pollen off him and onto the plant. He knew it would be something special, and in 2015 it won first and second place in San Bernardino for best CBD extract.

> Too many people are not aware of what exactly is in a particular plant. Potencies of cannabinoids and terpenes can vary with seeds, even clones, depending on how they are grown, type of supplemental lighting, and nutrients. Ratios appear to remain the same with clones, both with cannabinoids and terpenes. We still need to do more testing with that, but so far it has shown to be pretty accurate.
>
> SoHum Seeds

Ringo's Gift is available from SoHum Seeds in Humboldt, is easy to cultivate, and has a high yield. Its aroma is floral, citrus, and sweet with a hint of pine. Because it comes from seeds, it has a wide range of CBD:THC ratios.

Type: 60% sativa, 40% indica

Potency: 13–20% CBD; .5–.8% THC

Ratio: Between 15:1 and 25:1 CBD:THC

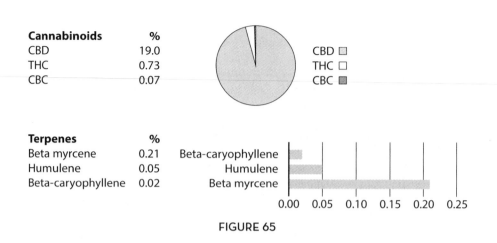

Cannabinoids	%
CBD	19.0
THC	0.73
CBC	0.07

CBD ☐
THC ☐
CBC ■

Terpenes	%
Beta myrcene	0.21
Humulene	0.05
Beta-caryophyllene	0.02

FIGURE 65

Sour Tsunami II (aka Sour-Tsu, Sour-Sue)

Sour Tsunami II is a sativa-dominant strain that provides an uplifting feeling due to its Diesel lineage. CBD content of Sour Tsunami I was first discovered to be 11 percent—a remarkable number in 2011. It now reaches up to 16–19 percent, depending on growing conditions, source seed/clone, and the experience of the growers. Lawrence Ringo spent several years creating the strain to help manage a back injury he'd had since he was thirteen. Vowing to avoid pharmaceutical painkillers and surgery, he wanted to find a cannabis strain that would be healing but not overly sedating. He learned to grow cannabis at age fifteen from some bikers who wanted to reward him for returning a lost ring. At nineteen, he learned organic horticulture in college. This drive and skill set eventually produced a remarkable, stabilized high-CBD strain that he later crossed with a number of other remarkable strains that have greatly increased the effectiveness and availability of CBD to researchers, patients, and doctors.

Being a musician, Ringo saved the seeds of any plant that gave him a creative feeling. In addition to the Diesel strains he had, one day a friend came by with something called Ferrari. Ringo describes his moment of discovery in an article published in the autumn 2011 edition of *O'Shaughnessy's*.

> I'll never forget that creamy taste. I smoked it and my brain just took off. I'm a musician so I grabbed my guitar and was going nuts for hours. . . . It took me about a year to get that clone. It was protected by the rednecks— the good old boys who used to be loggers and now they're pot growers.

They have this little clique going, the good old boys network. At first they weren't going to give it to us but eventually we got it. [468]

Ringo's perseverance and ability to woo bikers and rednecks gave us this mood-uplifting strain. People with ADHD, daytime users, and those looking for a creative or mood lift will be interested in Sour Tsunami II. It's also good for migraine headaches, loss of appetite, anti-inflammatory issues, and cancer.

Sour Tsunami II is a cross of New York Diesel, Sour Diesel, and Ferrari. With continued breeding, it has improved greatly. Sour Tsunami II has up to 24:1 CBD:THC. It grows as a medium-tall, dark green bush with touches of purple on its leaves and dense buds. Later, Ringo crossbred Sour Tsunami II and created several more amazing strains, including Canna Tsu, Harle Tsu, and Ringo's Gift.

Sour Tsunami II is a sativa-dominant hybrid, with 60 percent sativa and 40 percent indica, and is available as seeds from SoHum Seeds and other California dispensaries. Its cultivation is easy-to-medium difficulty, and it flowers in nine weeks. Its aroma is sweet and musky with a taste that is sweet with earth tones.

Type: 60% sativa, 40% indica

Potency: 11–16% CBD; .9–6.0% THC

Ratio: Between 8:1 and 24:1 CBD:THC

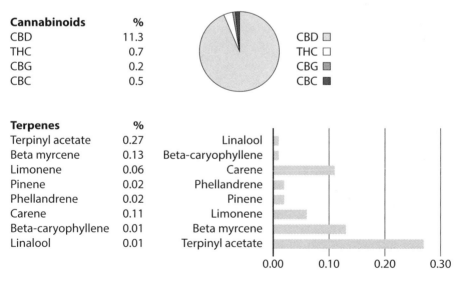

Cannabinoids	%
CBD	11.3
THC	0.7
CBG	0.2
CBC	0.5

Terpenes	%
Terpinyl acetate	0.27
Beta myrcene	0.13
Limonene	0.06
Pinene	0.02
Phellandrene	0.02
Carene	0.11
Beta-caryophyllene	0.01
Linalool	0.01

FIGURE 66

Suzy-Q

Suzy-Q is a high-CBD, low-THC strain from Project CBD in Santa Rosa, California. Finished flowers of this strain have tested as high as 59:1 (CBD:THC) with a potency of 15 percent CBD and 0.25 percent THC. Suzy-Q's unique cannabinoid profile is perfect for treating a wide variety of medicinal ailments, including chronic pain, bacterial diseases, diabetes, nausea, seizures, arthritis, inflammation, cancer, psoriasis, PTSD, muscle spasms, anxiety, bone loss, migraines, and Alzheimer's disease.

The taste is piney, crisp, and slightly reminiscent of the popular strain Trainwreck. The finished flowers are moderately dense with deep shades of green and dark orange hairs. It has a nutty sweet taste and scent. Suzy-Q is excellent for treating chronic pain, anxiety, cancer, and inflammation. This strain is ideal for making concentrates and oil-based medicine and is good for anyone who wants pain relief without the psychoactive effect that THC provides.

Type: 25% sativa, 75% indica

Potency: 15–20% CBD; .4–.8% THC

Ratio: Between 18:1 and 30:1 CBD:THC

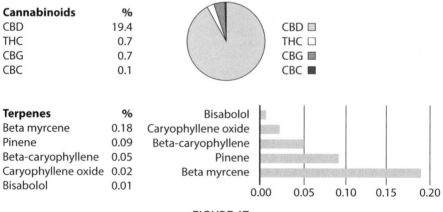

Cannabinoids	%
CBD	19.4
THC	0.7
CBG	0.7
CBC	0.1

Terpenes	%
Beta myrcene	0.18
Pinene	0.09
Beta-caryophyllene	0.05
Caryophyllene oxide	0.02
Bisabolol	0.01

FIGURE 67

> VJS had foot surgery, and the recovery was quite painful. Since she did not like oxycodone, she used Suzy-Q, with amazing results—pain relief, with no high, just a relaxed calm sense of well-being.
>
> SoHum Seeds

Valentine X

Named for Saint Valentine, the patron saint of epilepsy, Valentine X is sought after for its exceptional healing powers and its very high CBD:THC ratio of 25:1. It is a variant of the remarkable AC/DC that is cherished for its healing properties. Many find Valentine X a great help for seizure disorders, inflammation, depression, anxiety, nerve disorders, pain, asthma, and for treating cancer as well as cancer treatment side effects. It's also good for migraine and tension headaches, muscle spasms, and tremors. In addition to its medicinal effects, this strain is known to spark healing and creative thinking. Although it's a 50/50 sativa/indica hybrid, because of its low myrcene content, its effects tend to be more uplifting, providing energy and making it especially good in the daytime.

Valentine X takes effect almost immediately after ingestion, with the result of strong euphoria and a feeling of bliss and tranquility. Any pain felt in both the mind and body as well as any tension or negative effects tend to dissolve due to its high CBD level. The Valentine X flowers have lumpy, dense, and fluffy popcorn-shaped dark olive green flowers with blue undertones and leaves, sparse amber hairs, and a thick frosty coating of blue-tinted crystal trichomes. This flower has an aroma of earthy honey pine that releases a sweetness as the flowers are broken apart and heated. The taste is of sweet honey with an earthy pine aftertaste that has a savory, spicy wood effect that stays on the tongue long after.

Type: 50% sativa, 50% indica

Potency: 14–19% CBD; .6–.8% THC

Ratio: Between 22:1 and 26:1 CBD:THC

CBD

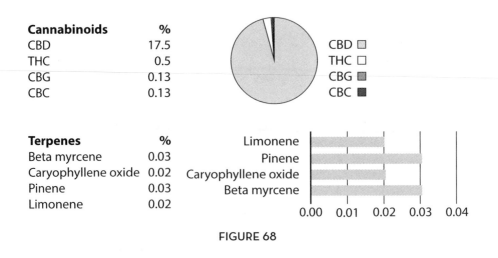

Cannabinoids	%
CBD	17.5
THC	0.5
CBG	0.13
CBC	0.13

Terpenes	%
Beta myrcene	0.03
Caryophyllene oxide	0.02
Pinene	0.03
Limonene	0.02

FIGURE 68

NOTE *For updates to this chapter, visit www.CBD-book.com/Updates.*

PART V

The Future Frontier of Cannabis-Based Medicine

Reporting contributed by Lion Goodman

The tide of cultural opinion regarding cannabis is clearly undergoing a major shift, as more is understood about its wide-ranging health benefits. With the re-emergence of CBD-dominant strains and the increased availability of quality medicine, it seems this long-stigmatized plant is making its way toward a prominent place in the Western pharmacopeia once more.

The future of cannabis medicine is bright, and simultaneously fraught with uncertainty. Our crystal ball is a bit cloudy (like everyone's). In Part V, we touch on three major trends in cannabis medicine with tremendous potential: 1) reducing harm caused by the opioid epidemic, 2) political trends, including legislation, and 3) medical research and the customization of medication.

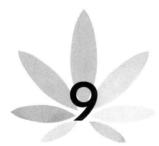

Cannabis as a Tool to Fight the Opioid Epidemic

Overdose deaths in the United States involving opioids (prescription pain-killers and heroin) have quadrupled since 1999. Estimates of the medical costs involved are over $72 billion each year in the United States alone. Dr. Donald Abrams, chief of the Hematology-Oncology Division at San Francisco General Hospital, is among many medical professionals pointing out that anything that weakens this epidemic, which kills eighty Americans every day, is worthy of consideration.

"If we could use cannabis, which is less addictive and harmful than opioids, to increase the effectiveness of pain treatment, I think it can make a difference in this epidemic of opioid abuse." Abrams has investigated the effect of cannabis on pain for over a decade. "We are hampered by the fact that it is still difficult to get funding for studies on cannabis as a therapeutic," he adds.[469]

Dr. Dustin Sulak is a licensed osteopathic physician in Maine who treats a wide variety of his patients' symptoms with medical marijuana. "Cannabis enhances the pain relief of opioids, and if they work together, [the effect] is more powerful," he says.[470] Sulak practices with fifteen other providers in Maine and Massachusetts who treat around twenty thousand people. About 70 percent of their patients use medical marijuana for chronic pain. Others use it for conditions such as nausea from chemotherapy drugs or cancer. Sulak recently surveyed over one thousand patients at the practice, and half said they used cannabis in combination with opioids to treat their pain. The majority of those people said they either stopped opioids completely or reduced their dosage of opioids over time. "You don't see this anywhere else," says Sulak. "Instead you see people coming back and asking for more and more opioids."[471]

CBD and other cannabis-based medicines have the potential to be a major tool in the battle against the current epidemic of pharmaceutical drug abuse and overdose in the United States. They have been used successfully as a substitute for opioid-based pharmaceuticals for pain relief, allowing people to lower their dosages and preventing addiction. Cannabis and narcotic pain-killers are known as co-agonists, which means that each of them magnifies the effect of the other. This allows people to take lower doses with comparable effectiveness. One recent research study of 300 people using high doses of opioids to control pain found they could reduce their opioid intake by 60 percent within a three week period of taking CBD and still manage their pain at the same level. After two months, many of them were able to get off the opioid medicine altogether.

CBD has also been used successfully to ease symptoms from opiate withdrawal during the addiction recovery process. It also decreases the physical craving for the opiates. It has been said in the past that cannabis is a gateway drug. In reality, it is a gateway in the other direction, a gateway out of addiction. It is a drug that is used to facilitate the healing of people addicted to hard drugs. As reported in 2015, the sales of pharmaceutical opioid drugs have dropped by 5 percent in states that have legalized cannabis.

In 2014, University of Pennsylvania researchers published a study examining the rates of opiate-related overdoses in the United States between 1999 and 2010. Results revealed that, on average, states that legalized the use of cannabis for medicinal purposes had nearly a 25 percent lower opioid overdose mortality rate after the laws were implemented. According to Marcus A. Bachhuber, one of the authors of the study, "people already taking opioids for pain may supplement with medical marijuana and be able to lower their painkiller dose, thus lowering their risk of overdose."[472]

The relationship between the passing of a medical marijuana bill and the decrease in opioid overdose deaths has strengthened over time. During the first year after a state's law was implemented, deaths decreased by nearly 20 percent and continued to steadily drop. Five years after implementation, the rate was 33.7 percent lower.

In the June 2016 issue of *The Journal of Pain,* researchers Boehnke, Litinas, and Clauw showed that medical cannabis use was associated with a 64 percent decrease in opioid use in patients with chronic pain. In addition, there was a decrease in the number and side effects of medications and an average of 45 percent improvement in quality of life measures—benefits greater than other classes of medications and with fewer side effects.[473]

Ashley and W. David Bradford, researchers at the University of Georgia, found that, in seventeen states with medical marijuana laws in place by 2013, prescriptions for painkillers fell sharply compared to states that did not have medical marijuana laws. The drops were significant. In medical marijuana states, the average doctor prescribed 1,826 fewer doses of painkillers per year. In addition, average doctors prescribed 265 fewer doses of antidepressants each year, 486 fewer doses of seizure medication, 541 fewer anti-nausea doses, and 562 fewer doses of anti-anxiety medication.[474]

These numbers are likely causing concern among pharmaceutical companies. Big Pharma has been at the forefront of opposition to marijuana reform. It has funded research by anti-pot academics[475] and funneled millions of dollars to groups that oppose marijuana legalization (such as the Community Anti-Drug Coalitions of America).[476,477] Pharmaceutical companies have also lobbied federal agencies directly to prevent the liberalization of marijuana laws.

The biggest players in the anti-marijuana legalization movement are pharmaceutical companies, alcohol and beer companies, private prison corporations, and police unions, all of whom help fund lobby groups that challenge marijuana law reform. Corrections Corporation of America, one of the largest for-profit prison companies in the United States, has spent nearly $1 million a year on lobbying efforts. The company even stated in a report that "changes with respect to drugs and controlled substances . . . could affect the number of persons arrested, convicted, and sentenced, thereby potentially reducing demand for correctional facilities to house them."[478]

According to a report in *The Nation* magazine, among the largest donors to organizations fighting marijuana liberalization are Purdue Pharma, makers of the painkiller OxyContin; Abbott Laboratories, which produces the opioid Vicodin; and Janssen Pharmaceutical, a J&J subsidiary that manufactures the painkiller Nucynta.[479]

"There is big money in marijuana prohibition," notes the Center for Responsive Politics, a non-profit research group based in Washington, DC, that investigated this link to anti-legalization lobbying efforts.[480] The organizations that received money from these companies lobby Congress to maintain marijuana's classification as a Schedule 1 drug, in spite of the fact that more than twenty-two thousand people die every year in the United States from overdoses of pharmaceutical drugs, according to the Centers for Disease Control and Prevention.[481] Three out of every four pharmaceutical overdose deaths involve prescription painkillers—more than heroin and cocaine combined.

It appears that drug companies want to downplay the medical benefits of marijuana in order to maintain or increase the sale of their drugs; alcohol manufacturers do not want competition for their customers from legal cannabis; and private prisons need to fill their beds with convicted drug offenders. Marijuana advocates have some large and well-funded enemies to contend with. The future of legalized cannabis now rests with the efforts of individual citizens to push for changes in state law.

NOTE *For updates to this chapter, visit www.CBD-book.com/Updates.*

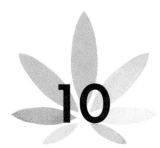

Political and Legal Trends

As this book goes to press, the Trump administration has control of the U.S. White House and the federal government. Because his, as well as the legislative branch's position on cannabis is unclear, we are in a time of real uncertainty about the legal future of medical cannabis. On the one hand, the majority of states have approved marijuana legalization initiatives in one form or another. In 2016, voters in Arkansas, Florida, and North Dakota approved medical marijuana for their citizens, and voters in Montana voted to roll back restrictions on existing medical cannabis laws. These moves bring cannabis access to 20 percent of the population—one in five Americans. The total number of states that have approved marijuana initiatives or decriminalized possession is up to forty. After the 2016 election cycle, 24.5 million more Americans gained access to medical cannabis.

Prior to these ballots, recreational marijuana was only legal in four states (Colorado, Oregon, Washington, and Alaska) and the District of Columbia. Post election, California, Massachusetts, Nevada, and Maine joined the adult-use states. Arizona's adult-use initiative was narrowly defeated. A recent Gallup poll found nationwide support of 60 percent for legalization, the highest level in forty-seven years.

When alcohol prohibition ended in 1933, the government allowed states to pass their own legislation and rules for manufacture, distribution, sale, and consumption of alcoholic beverages. The Feds maintained control (and thus taxation) over interstate commerce, licensing, labeling requirements, importation, and other functions through the Bureau of Alcohol, Tobacco, Firearms and Explosives.

Cannabis has been going in the same direction. In 2014, the Cole Memo II offered an eight-part protocol guideline that curtailed federal enforcement of marijuana laws in states writing their own laws and regulations.[482] However, as long as marijuana is a Schedule 1 drug, it remains illegal at the federal level to operate a cannabis business, even if the state allows it. This is the conundrum that every cannabis business owner, and every consumer, faces. The federal Controlled Substances Act still defines production and sale of marijuana as serious felonies. Banks are not allowed to do business with any companies working in the cannabis or hemp industries for fear of losing their FDIC coverage, and insurance companies are not allowed to reimburse claims for cannabis use as medicine.

Executive branch directives do not bind successive administrations in any way, so Attorney General Sessions could immediately reverse policies on the marijuana industry. Sessions would have broad power under federal law to seize the assets of companies in the industry. Even threats from his office could cause companies to cease public operations, and many probably would go back underground.

In the case of medical cannabis, there are precedents that make it somewhat safer ground. The prior Congress prevented the Department of Justice from spending money to prosecute cannabis-legal state laws or citizens. The current Congress is unlikely to change this—at least, that is our hope.

Because cannabis remains a Schedule 1 drug (including both THC and CBD and "all cannabinoids and molecules" in the plant, as the FDA recently clarified), any interstate commerce continues to be problematic. Companies that supply much-needed medical cannabis to sick patients are forced to stay within clearly defined state boundaries. If they want to expand their services to another state, the entire business must be adjusted to that state's regulation landscape. This makes it difficult for any company to build a national brand identity, and it prevents patients in non-legal states from getting the medicine that could help or cure them.

In early 2016, an international commission published a report in *The Lancet* calling for decriminalization of all drugs, finding that prohibition did not effectively prevent drug use, addiction, or organized crime.[483] At the same time, the United Nations held a special session to discuss global drug policy, the first in almost twenty years.[484] Internationally, some countries have made cannabis legal in some form. Although the International Opium Convention made cannabis (called hashish at the time) illegal in most countries in 1912, since then, many countries have decriminalized the possession of marijuana. As of 2016, countries with the least restrictive cannabis laws include Australia, Bangladesh, Cambodia, Canada, Chile, Colombia, Costa Rica, the Czech Republic, Germany, India, Jamaica, Mexico, the Netherlands, Portugal, Spain, Uruguay, and some U.S. jurisdictions.

On the other side, countries with the most restrictive laws include China, Egypt, France, Indonesia, Japan, Malaysia, Nigeria, Norway, the Philippines, Poland, Saudi Arabia, Singapore, South Korea, Thailand, Turkey, Ukraine, the United Arab Emirates, and Vietnam.[485]

It is challenging to stay on top of the constantly shifting sand that is cannabis legislation. Until the FDA changes the status of cannabis from Schedule 1 to a lesser schedule, or legalizes it completely, business owners, patients, doctors, and citizens will have to follow their own state's regulations and stay informed.

NOTE *For updates to this chapter, visit www.CBD-book.com/Updates.*

What's Next—The Leading Edge of Cannabis-Based Medical Developments

In the past decade since the discovery of the endocannabinoid system, medical research on cannabis has blossomed into an entire scientific discipline, still young and developing. As described in Chapter 10, despite the growing number of states that have made cannabis or CBD legal, the U.S. federal government holds strict control over all research with Schedule 1 drugs. This has limited federally sponsored science and strangled legal access to cannabis as research material—for years there was only one authorized grower of cannabis for scientific research in the entire country, the University of Mississippi. Expressing interest in cannabis experimentation used to be deemed a career killer, so there were few scientists "foolish" enough to even apply for a research grant. In addition, only certain strains were available, and CBD-rich strains were not on the list.

Because of public experimentation on a large scale, and clear medical results from individuals using this substance, a few pioneering individual scientists broke with tradition and began exploring the plant's many potential uses and researching the biological and physiological mechanisms that influenced changes in the brain, nervous system, and body. Today, there are hundreds of scientists at work doing careful scientific research to discover the benefits of specific strains, doses, methods of ingestion, and their impact on specific diseases and conditions.

It has been in laboratories outside the United States, more open-minded in their treatment of cannabis research, that the majority of the important advances in this field of medicine have been made. Israel, where some of the first CBD research was conducted, has invested millions of dollars in research into cannabinoids and their effects.

The International Cannabinoid Research Society (www.ICRS.co) was incorporated as a scientific research society in 1992 but has organized symposia for various researchers in the field since 1970. There were fifty members in its first year, and there are now five hundred members from all over the world. We expect this trend to continue, and snowball, unless political forces push this research underground.

The role of terpenes in the body's healing response is also a fairly recent discovery (see more on terpenes in Chapter 3). Terpenes are widespread in nature, often responsible for the smell of plants, appearing in the leaves, roots, flowers, bark, and fruit. They have been used as flavorings for food, drink, and perfumes for millennia. New scientific research is showing that these smell and flavor molecules are important players in the body's healing response to plant medicines. Different strains of cannabis have different terpene profiles, and it is only in the last decade that these important molecules have been identified as players in cannabis medicine. We expect that scientific research will continue in this area and will eventually result in a doctor's ability to customize both cannabinoid and terpene profiles to a particular patient's condition, prescribing a particularly effective strain for a particular disease state, for example.

The FDA is the gatekeeper for medical treatments, and as of press time it has not approved marijuana as a safe and effective drug for any indication or condition. The agency has approved three drugs containing synthetic versions of molecules in cannabis, but no drug product containing or derived from botanical marijuana. Because it can cost anywhere from $5 to $50 million to go through the Investigational New Drug procedures, and the expensive clinical trials required for the entire drug approval process, only pharmaceutical companies can afford to apply for this designation. Pharmaceutical companies make money only by getting approval for medicines they can patent, where they have intellectual property rights, giving them total control over the manufacture, distribution, and sale of what they patent.

At this time, you cannot patent a whole plant, so no pharmaceutical company wants anything to do with cannabis. What they do want is to derive or synthesize a molecule that has the same effect as one of the molecules in cannabis and patent that. This is why Western medicine is oriented toward single-molecule medicines rather than whole-plant medicines. For example, aspirin is made from the leaves of the willow tree, which has documented use for at least 2,400 years. Yet willow-bark tincture is not available in drug stores because Bayer turned it into a refined product in 1899 and earned billions of dollars from its trademarked product until its rights ran out.

The pharmaceutical companies are aware of the healing properties of cannabis and have sponsored legislation and members of Congress to keep cannabis illegal. They simply don't want the competition for their products, especially from a plant medicine they cannot control and make money from. They are likely behind the FDA's decision at the end of 2016 to declare CBD and all other cannabinoids Schedule 1 drugs and its denial that marijuana has any medicinal use. There is a tight linkage between the FDA and the pharmaceutical industry, and neither of them are fans of state laws liberalizing policies on cannabis (see more on this in Chapter 9).

Pharmaceutical research provides an important function, performing clinical trials on specific doses and delivery methods of specific molecules. This process extends knowledge about how specific molecules function in the human body. There is a role for single-molecule medicine, and we value its contributions. But if citizens lose the ability to legally use whole-plant medicines, we feel this must be battled in the courts and the halls of the legislature until all adults are given access as a human right.

We also see an important trend in medical education. Consumers have been spreading the word about cannabis's benefits for many years, and the internet has helped to distribute information to patients and the general public. Doctors, on the other hand, are restricted from prescribing Schedule 1 drugs without specific approval and rigorous oversight by government agencies. More and more doctors have become educated (often by their patients) about the positive impact that cannabis has had on their patients' disease states, and many would be happy to prescribe it if they were allowed to do so. To get around this, states in which medicinal use of cannabis is legal require a doctor's recommendation, not a prescription. Although the stigma of cannabis is being improved in most of the United States, it is still illegal in many states, and in those states doctors' hands are tied, regardless of their desire to help their patients.

Doctors need to be educated, and most of their medical education comes from pharmaceutical company literature, government-sponsored research, and peer-reviewed journals. Fortunately, a growing number of clinical training programs and research symposia are offered throughout the United States and overseas every year. Examples include the Medical Cannabis Institute, the Society of Cannabis Clinicians, the Institute of Cannabis Research Conference, the Carolina Cannabinoid Collaborative Conference, Marijuana for Medical Professionals, the National Clinical Conference on Cannabis Therapeutics, the Cannabis-Based Therapies Summit, the International Cannabinoid Research Society, the International Association for Cannabinoid Medicines, and the National University of Natural Medicine.

We expect this clinical education trend to continue as more and more doctors learn about the incredible healing power resident within the cannabis plant. Many physicians are waiting for a sufficient number of research papers to be published, as well as government withdrawal of Schedule 1 status, before they prescribe cannabinoid medicine.

In January 2017, the National Academies of Sciences, Engineering, and Medicine released a review of studies related to the health effects of cannabis and cannabinoids. After reviewing more than ten thousand studies, they came to numerous conclusions, some positive and some negative. They found sufficient evidence to officially support treatment for three therapeutic uses: to reduce nausea and vomiting from chemotherapy, to treat chronic pain, and to reduce spasms from multiple sclerosis.[486] "Most of the therapeutic reasons people use medical marijuana aren't substantiated beneficial effects," said Sean Hennessy, a professor of epidemiology at the University of Pennsylvania, and a member of the sixteen-scientist committee (including neurologists, oncologists, epidemiologists, and child psychiatrists) that carried out the review.[487] This means that the studies are too few or not at an adequate standard for drawing scientific or medical conclusions.

As scientists, the reviewers expressed concern that the cannabis industry will evolve into something like the vitamin and nutritional supplement market, with wild claims and dubious medical benefits. They are holding medical therapeutics to the highest standards, and thus used the highest standards of medical research to look in-depth at recent research and publications.

The report called for additional funding to advance marijuana research, and they noted that cannabis researchers have had difficulty gaining access to the quantity, quality, and types of cannabis necessary. (The cannabis available to researchers is not even close to that available in the average dispensary.) The authors' most fervent calls were for much more high-caliber investigation.[488]

There are thousands of brave medical pioneers who are eager to help their patients heal faster, get off opioid medications, relieve symptoms, and fight cancer. We believe that the cannabis plant will prevail, as it has for at least five thousand years, and that as the research continues to accumulate, the majority of physicians will eventually be convinced to add cannabis medications to their pharmaceutical toolkit.

Epilogue

Exercise: Connecting to the Medicine Intuitively

By Terumi Leinow

Close your eyes, take several deep breaths, and focus to gain a sense of how everything in your body is connected. "Hip bone connected to the thigh bone," as captured in a popular song. Notice on your in-breath how your lungs are receiving the out-breath of the trees and plants that surround you, circulating oxygen throughout your body. Our entire world is an intricate network of interdependent connections.

Likewise, consider the interplay of nature and how the microorganisms in the earth, wind, water, and sun all work together for creation. The powerful forces of nature during a winter storm can also bring us to our knees when we experience travel interruptions or an extended power outage. At such times, we may experience how dependent we have become on our internet and phone lines and power sources for our appliances that provide heat and light. Mother Nature humbles us at such times. On the other hand, she fills us with awe and wonder in the presence of a waterfall, the moonrise, or an exquisite sunset, reminding us of our universal oneness.

As a user of cannabis products, you hold in your hand the end result of a long process involving many cycles. Recognize that at one time this product was a living, breathing, thriving, flowering plant—not just any plant but one that contains life force energy that can connect to your body's innate ability to restore itself to health and well-being. It is important, therefore, before you ingest any cannabis product, that you take the time to connect to the "Spirit" of the plant. As spiritual teacher Eckhart Tolle writes, "Flowers more delicate than the plants out of which they emerged become like messengers from another realm, like a bridge between the world of physical forms and the formless. . . . We could look upon flowers as the enlightenment of plants . . . temporary manifestations of the underlying One Life, one indwelling consciousness or spirit in every life form."[489]

When you take the time to feel appreciation and gratitude, you connect and tune into the divine life force essence of the plant and within yourself. Together you ignite that remembrance in you, that everything is connected and you are connected to everything. What an elegant journey to know that you are not alone, but have a powerful, healing plant ally on your path to well-being.

ENDNOTES

Introduction

1   S. Burstein, "Cannabidiol (CBD) and Its Analogs: A Review of Their Effects on Inflammation," *Bioorganic & Medicinal Chemistry* 23, no. 7 (April 2015): 1377–1385. doi:10.1016/j.bmc.2015.01.059.

2   Marcus A. Bachhuber, Brendan Saloner, Chinazo O. Cunningham, and Colleen L. Barry, "Medical Cannabis Laws and Opioid Analgesic Overdose Mortality in the United States, 1999-2010," *JAMA Internal Medicine* 174, no. 10 (2014): 1668. doi:10.1001/jamainternmed.2014.4005.

3   Ruth Galilly, Z. Yekhtin, and L. Hanuš, "Overcoming the Bell-Shaped Dose-Response of Cannabidiol by Using Cannabis Extract Enriched in Cannabidiol," *Pharmacology & Pharmacy* 6 (February 2015): 75–85. doi:10.4236/pp.2015.62010.

4   Ethan Russo, "History of Cannabis as a Medicine," in *The Medicinal Uses of Cannabis and Cannabinoid,* eds. Geoffrey W. Guy, Brian A. Whittle, and Philip J. Robson (London: Pharmaceutical Press, 2004), 1–16.

5   "Clarification of the New Drug Code (7350) for Marijuana Extract," *U.S. Department of Justice, Drug Enforcement Administration,* accessed April 10, 2017, https://www.deadiversion.usdoj.gov/schedules/marijuana/m_extract_7350.html

6   Wei-Ni Lin Curry, *Hyperemesis Gravidarum and Clinical Cannabis: To Eat or Not to Eat?* (Binghamton: Haworth Press, 2002), www.cannabis-med.org/data/pdf/2002-03-04-4.pdf.

7   John M. McPartland and Ethan B. Russo, "Cannabis and Cannabis Extracts: Greater Than the Sum of Their Parts?" *Journal of Cannabis Therapeutics* 1, no. 3/4 (2001): 132.

Part I

8   1907–1914 Materia Medica 3.148

9 James L. Butrica, "The Medical Use of Cannabis Among the Greeks and Romans," *Journal of Cannabis Therapeutics* 2, no. 2 (2002): 51–70.

10 Raphael Mechoulam, William Devane, Aviva Breuer, and J. Zahalka, "A Random Walk through a Cannabis Field," *Pharmacology Biochemistry and Behavior* 40, no. 3 (1991): 461–464.

11 Rabbi Aryeh Kaplan, *The Living Torah* (New York: Moznaim, 1981), 40–41.

12 William Brooke O'Shaughnessy, *On the Preparations of the Indian Hemp, or Gunjah,* Med. and Phy. Soc., Bengal, Calcutta, 1839; and Brit. and For. Med. Rev. July, 1840, p. 224.

13 Ibid.

14 Lester Grinspoon, *Marihuana Reconsidered* (Cambridge: Harvard University Press, 1971), 15.

15 Roger G. Pertwee, "Cannabinoid Pharmacology: The First 66 Years," *British Journal of Pharmacology* 147, suppl. 1 (2006): S163–S171. doi:10.1038/sj.bjp.0706406.

16 Miles O'Brien, "Medical Marijuana Research Comes out of the Shadows," *PBS NewsHour,* July 13, 2016, www.pbs.org/newshour/bb/medical-marijuana-research-comes-shadows/.

17 "Medical Hemp: The Story to Date," *O'Shaughnessy's,* Autumn 2011, 7, www.os-extra.cannabisclinicians.org/wp-content/uploads/2013/11/CBD-Reintroduction-Era-2011.pdf.

18 "The Re-emergence of CBD—A Brief History," *Project CBD,* www.projectcbd.org/re-emergence-cbd-brief-history.

19 David Bienenstock, "The U.S. Government Now Supplies Cannabis Extracts to Epileptic Kids," *Vice Magazine,* March 11, 2011, www.vice.com/en_us/article/the-us-government-now-supplies-cannabis-extracts-to-epileptic-kids.

20 Martin A. Lee, "The Discovery of the Endocannabinoid System," *The Prop 215 Era,* 2010, www.beyondthc.com/wp-content/uploads/2012/07/eCBSystemLee.pdf.

21 David B. Allen, MD, "Survey Shows Low Acceptance of the Science of the ECS (Endocannabinoid System) at American Medical Schools," *Outword Magazine,* accessed March 3, 2017, www.outwordmagazine.com/inside-outword/glbt-news/1266-survey-shows-low-acceptance-of-the-science-of-the-ecs-endocannabinoid-system.

22 W. A. Devane, F. A. Dysarz 3rd, M. R. Johnson, L. S. Melvin, and A. C. Howlett, "Determination and Characterization of a Cannabinoid Receptor in Rat Brain," *Molecular Pharmacology* 34 (1988): 605–613.

23 S. Munro, K. L. Thomas, and M. Abu-Shaar. "Molecular Characterization of a Peripheral Receptor for Cannabinoids," *Nature* 365 (1993): 61–65.

24 R. Mechoulam, L. O. Hanus, R. Pertwee, and A. C. Howlett, "Early Phytocannabinoid History to Endocannabinoids and Beyond: A Cannabinoid Timeline," *Nature Neuroscience Review* 15 (November 2014): 757–764.

25 R. Mechoulam, S. Ben-Shabat, L. Hanuš, M. Ligumsky, N. E. Kaminski, A. R. Schatz, A. Gopher, S. Almoq, B. R. Martin, D. R. Compton et al. "Identification of an Endogenous 2-monoglyceride, Present in Canine Gut, That Binds to Cannabinoid Receptors," *Biochemical Pharmacology* 50 (1995): 83–90.

26 T. Bisogno, F. Howell, G. Williams, A. Minassi, M. G. Cascio, A. Ligresti, I. Matias, A. Schiano-Moriello, P. Paul, E. J. Williams, U. Gangadharan, C. Hobbs, V. Di Marzo, and P. Doherty, "Cloning of the First sn1-DAG Lipases Points to the Spatial and Temporal Regulation of Endocannabinoid Signaling in the Brain," *Journal of Cell Biology* 163 (2003): 463–468.

27 P. Pacher and G. Kunos, "Modulating the Endocannabinoid System in Human Health and Diseases: Successes and Failures," *Federation of European Biochemical Society Journal* 280, no. 9 (May 2013): 1918.

28 R. Mechoulam, L. O. Hanus, R. Pertwee, and A. C. Howlett, "Early Phytocannabinoid History to Endocannabinoids and Beyond: A Cannabinoid Timeline," *Nature Neuroscience Review* 15 (November 2014): 757–764.

29 A. R. Wilson-Poe, M. M. Morgan, S. A. Aicher, and D. M. Hegarty, "Distribution of CB1 Cannabinoid Receptors and Their Relationship with Mu-opioid Receptors in the Rat Periaqueductal Gray," *Neuroscience* 213 (2012): 191–200.

30 T. Lowin and R. H. Straub, "Cannabinoid Based Drugs Targeting CB1 and TRPV-1, the Sympathetic Nervous System and Arthritis," *Arthritis Research and Therapy* 17 (2015): 226.

31 A. E. Bonnett and Y. Marchalant, "Potential Therapeutic Contribution of the Endocannabinoid System towards Aging and Alzheimer's Disease," *Aging and Disease* 6, no. 5 (October 2015): 400–405.

32 M. Fitzgibbon, D. P. Finn, and M. Roche, "High Times for Painful Blues: The Endocannabinoid System in Pain-Depression Co-morbidity," *International Journal of Neuropharmacology* (2015): 1–20.

33 S. V. Mahler, K. S. Smith, and K. C. Berridge, "Endocannabinoid Hedonic Hotspots for Sensory Pleasure: Anandamide in the Nucleus Accumbens, Shell Enhances Liking of a Sweet Reward," *Neuropharmacology* 32 (2007): 2267–2278.

34 P. Pacher and R. Mechoulam, "Is Lipid Signaling through Cannabinoid 2 Receptors Part of a Protective System?" *Progress in Lipid Research* (April 2011): 193–211.

35 N. M. Kogan, E. Melamed, E. Wasserman, B. Raphael, A. Breuer, K. S. Stok, R. Sondergaard, A. V. Escudero, S. Baraghithy, M. Attar-Namdar, S. Friedlander-Barenboim, N. Mathavan, H. Isaksson, R. Mechoulam, R. Müller, A. Bajayo, Y. Gabet, and I. Bab, "Cannabidiol, A Major Non-psychotropic Cannabis Constituent, Enhances Fracture Healing and Stimulates Lysyl Hydroxylase Activity in Osteoblasts," *Journal of Mineral and Bone Research* 30, no. 10 (October 2015): 1905–1913.

36 R. G. Pertwee, A. C. Howlett, M. E. Abood, S. P. Alexander, V. Di Marzo, M. R. Elphick, P. J. Greasley, H. S. Hansen, G. Kunos, K. Mackie, R. Mechoulam, and R. A. Ross, "International Union of Basic and Clinical Pharmacology, LXXIX: Cannabinoid Receptors and Their Ligands, Beyond CB1 and CB2," *Pharmacologic Reviews* 62, no. 4 (2010): 588–631.

37 Antonio Currais, Oswald Quehenberger, Aaron M. Armando, Daniel Daugherty, Pam Maher, and David Schubert, "Amyloid Proteotoxicity Initiates an Inflammatory Response Blocked by Cannabinoids," *Nature Partner Journals: Aging and Mechanisms of Disease* 2, no. 16012 (June 23, 2016). doi:10.1038.

38 E. Shohami, A. Cohen-Yeshurun, L. Magid, M. Algali, and R. Mechoulam, "Endocannabinoids and Traumatic Brain Injury," *British Journal of Pharmacology* 163, no. 7 (August 2011): 1402–1410.

39 Rocío Sancho, Marco A. Calzado, Vincenzo Di Marzo, Giovanni Appendino, and Eduardo Muñoz, "Anandamide Inhibits Nuclear Factor K-beta Activation through a Cannabinoid Receptor Independent Pathway," *Molecular Pharmacology* 63, no. 2 (2003): 429–438.

40 G. A. Cabral, T. J. Rogers, and A. H. Lichtman, "Turning Over a New Leaf: Cannabinoid and Endocannabinoid Modulation of Immune Function," *Journal of Neuroimmune Pharmacology* 10 (2015): 193–203.

41 F. Rossi, G. Bellini, C. Tortora, M. E. Bernardo, L. Luongo, A. Conforti, N. Starc, I. Manzo, B. Nobili, F. Locatelli, and S. Maione, "CB2 and TRPV-1 Receptors Oppositely Modulate In Vitro Human Osteoblast Activity," *Pharmacology Research* 99 (2015): 194–201.

42 T. Lowin and R. H. Straub, "Cannabinoid Based Drugs Targeting CB1 and TRPV-1, the Sympathetic Nervous System and Arthritis," *Arthritis Research and Therapy* 17 (2015): 226.

43 Vincenzo DiMarzo, "Endocannabinoid Signaling in the Brain: Biosynthesis Mechanisms in the Limelight," *Nature Neuroscience* 14, no. 1 (January 2011): 9–15.

44 K. A. Sharkey and J. W. Wiley, "The Role of the Endocannabinoid System in the Brain-Gut Axis," *Gastroenterology* 151, no. 2 (2016): 252. doi:10.1053/j. gastro.2016.04.015.

45 Mauro Maccarrone, Itai Bab, Tamás Bíró, Guy A. Cabral, Sudhansu K. Dey, Vincenzo Di Marzo, Justin C. Konje, George Kunos, Raphael Mechoulam, Pal Pacher, Keith A. Sharkey, and Andreas Zimmer, "Endocannabinoid Signaling at the Periphery, 50 Years after THC," *Cell: Trends in Pharmacological Science* 36, no. 5 (May 2015): 277–296.

46 P. Pacher and G. Kunos, "Modulating the Endocannabinoid System in Human Health and Diseases: Successes and Failures," *The FEBS Journal* 280, no. 9 (May 2013): 1918–1943.

47 Fabio Iannotti, Cristoforo Silvestri, Enrico Mazzarella, Andrea Martella, Daniela Calvigoni, Fabiana Piscitelli, Paolo Ambrosino, Stefania Petrosino, Gabriella Czifra, Tamás Biro, Tibo Harkany, Maurizio Taglialatela, and Vincenzo Di Marzo, "The Endocannabinoid 2-AG Controls Skeletal Muscle Cell Differentiation via CB1 Receptor-Dependent Inhibition of Kv7 Channels," *Proceedings of the National Academy of Science, USA* 117 (2014): 2472–2481.

48 Mauro Maccarrone, Itai Bab, Tamás Bíró, Guy A. Cabral, Sudhansu K. Dey, Vincenzo Di Marzo, Justin C. Konje, George Kunos, Raphael Mechoulam, Pal Pacher, Keith A. Sharkey, and Andreas Zimmer, "Endocannabinoid Signaling at the Periphery, 50 Years after THC," *Cell: Trends in Pharmacological Science* 36, no. 5 (May 2015): 277–296.

49 M. Karsak, E. Gaffal, R. Date, L. Wang-Eckhardt, J. Rehnelt, S. Petrosino, K. Starowicz, R. Steuder, E. Schlicker, B. Cravatt, R. Mechoulam, R. Buettner, S. Werner, V. Di Marzo, T. Tüting, and Z. Zimmer, "Attenuation of Allergic Contact Dermatitis through the Endocannabinoid System," *Science* 316 (2007): 1494–1497.

50 J. Palazuelos, T. Aguado, A. Egia, R. Mechoulam, M. Guzmán, and I. Galve-Roperh, "Non-psychoactive CB2 Cannabinoid Agonists Stimulate Neural Progenitor Proliferation," *The FASEB Journal* 20 (2006): 2405–2407.

51 J. Begbie, P. Doherty, and A. Graham, "Cannabinoid Receptor, CB1, Expression Follows Neuronal Differentiation in the Early Chick Embryo," *Journal of Anatomy* 205 (2004): 213–218.

52 T. Aguado, J. Palazuelos, K. Monory, N. Stella, B. Cravatt, B. Lutz, G. Marsicano, Z. Kokaia, M. Guzmán, and I. Galve-Roperh, "The Endocannabinoid System Promotes Astroglial Differentiation by Acting on Neural Progenitor Cells," *Journal of Neuroscience* 26 (2006): 1551–1561.

53 A. Periera Jr and F. A. Furlan, "Astrocyte and Human Cognition: Modeling Information Integration and Modulation of Neuronal Activity," *Progress in Neurology* 92 (2010): 405–420.

54 N. J. Abbott, L. Ronnback, and E. Hansson, "Astrocyte-endothelial Interactions at the Blood Brain Barrier," *Nature Reviews Neuroscience* 7 (January 2006): 41–53.

55 P. G. Haydon and G. Carmignoto, "Astrocyte Control of Synaptic Transmission and Neurovascular Coupling," *Physiology Review* 86 (July 2006): 1009–1031.

56 M. Sild and E. S. Ruthazer, "Radial Glia: Progenitor, Pathway and Partner," *The Neuroscientist* 17, no. 3 (2011): 288–302.

57 Y. Gao, D. V. Vasilyev, M. B. Goncalves, F. V. Howell, C. Hobbs, M. Reisenberg, R. Shen, M. Y. Zhang, B. W. Strassle, P. Lu, L. Mark, M. J. Piesla, K. Deng, E. V. Kouranova, R. H. Ring, G. T. Whiteside, B. Bates, F. S. Walsh, G. Williams, M. N. Pangalos, T. A. Samad, and P. Doherty, "Loss of Retrograde Endocannabinoid Signaling and Reduced Adult Neurogenesis in Diacylglycerol Lipase Knock-out Mice," *Journal of Neuroscience* 30 (2010): 2017–2024.

58 V. DiMarzo, "Endocannabinoid Signaling in the Brain: Biosynthetic Mechanisms in the Limelight," *Nature Neuroscience* 14, no. 1 (January 2011): 9–14.

59 A. Lourbopoulos, N. Grigoriadis, R. Lagoudaki, O. Touloumi, E. Polyzoidou, I. Mavromatis, N. Tascos, A. Breuer, H. Ovadia, D. Karussis, E. Shohami, R. Mechoulam, and C. Simeonidou, "Administration of 2-arachodonylglycerol Ameliorates Both Acute and Chronic Autoimmune Encephalomyelitis," *Brain Research* 1390 (May 16, 2011): 126–141.

60 F. Rossi, G. Bellini, C. Tortora, M. E. Bernardo, L. Luongo, A. Conforti, N. Starc, I. Manzo, B. Nobili, F. Locatelli, and S. Maione, "CB2 and TRPV-1 Receptors Oppositely Modulate In Vitro Human Osteoblast Activity," *Pharmacology Research* 99 (2015): 194–201.

61 A. E. Bonnet and Y. Marchalant, "Potential Therapeutical Contributions of the Endocannabinoid System towards Aging and Alzheimer's Disease," *Aging and Disease* 6, no. 5 (October 2015): 400–405.

62 Antonio Currais, Oswald Quehenberger, Aaron M. Armando, Daniel Daugherty, Pam Maher, and David Schubert, "Amyloid Proteotoxicity

Initiates an Inflammatory Response Blocked by Cannabinoids," *Nature Partner Journals: Aging and Mechanisms of Disease* 2, no. 16012 (June 23, 2016). doi:10.1038.

63 Rocío Sancho, Marco A. Calzado, Vincenzo Di Marzo, Giovanni Appendino, and Eduardo Muñoz, "Anandamide Inhibits Nuclear Factor K-beta Activation through a Cannabinoid Receptor Independent Pathway," *Molecular Pharmacology* 63, no. 2 (2003): 429–438.

64 E. Murillo-Rodriguez, C. Blanco-Centurion, C. Sanchez, D. Piomelli, and P. J. Shiromani, "Anandamide Enhances Extracellular Levels of Adenosine and Induces Sleep: An In Vivo Microdialysis Study," *Sleep* 26, no. 8 (2003): 943–947.

65 Satish Kathuria, Silvana Gaetani, Darren Fegley, Fernando Valiño, Andrea Duranti, Andrea Tontini, Marco Mor, Giorgio Tarzia, Giovanna La Rana, Antonio Calignano, Arcangela Giustino, Maria Tattoli, Maura Palmery, Vincenzo Cuomo, and Daniele Piomelli, "Modulation of Anxiety through Blockade of Anandamide Hydrolysis," *Nature Medicine* 9, no. 1 (January 2003): 76–81.

66 D. J. Hermanson and L. J. Marnet, "Cannabinoids, Endocannabinoids and Cancer," *Cancer Metastasis Review* 30, nos. 3–4 (December 2011): 599–612.

67 Luciano De Petrocellis, Dominique Melck, Antonella Palmisano, Tiziana Bisogno, Chiara Laezza, Maurizio Bifulco, and Vincenzo Di Marzo, "The Endogenous Cannabinoid Anandamide Inhibits Human Breast Cell Cancer Proliferation," *Proceedings of the National Academy of Science* 95 (July 1998): 8375–8380.

68 E. Soliman and R. V. Dross, "Anandamide-Induced Endoplasmic Reticulum Stress and Apoptosis Are Mediated by Oxidative Stress in Non-melanoma Skin Cancer: Receptor-Independent Endocannabinoid Signaling," *Molecular Carcinogenesis* 55, no. 11 (2016): 1807–1821.

69 T. Ayakannu, A. Taylor, J. Willets, T. Marczylo, L. Brown, Q. Davies, E. Moss, and J. Konje, "Effect of Anandamide on Endometrial Adenocarcinoma (Isikawa) Cell Numbers: Implications for Endometrial Cancer Therapy," *The Lancet* 385, suppl. 1 (February 26, 2015): S20.

70 D. Vara, M. Salazar, N. Olea-Herrero, M. Guzmán, G. Velasco, and I. Díaz-Laviada, "Anti-tumoral Effect of Cannabinoids on Hepatocellular Carcinoma: Role of AMPK Dependent Activation of Autophagy," *Cell Death and Differentiation* 18 (2011): 1099–1111.

71 S. Sailler, K. Schmitz, E. Jäger, N. Ferreiros, S. Wicker, K. Zschiebsch, G. Pickert, G. Geisslinger, C. Walter, I. Tegeder, and J. Lötsch, "Regulation of Circulating Endocannabinoids Associated with Cancer and Metastases in Mice and Humans," *Oncoscience* 1, no. 4 (2014): 272–282.

72 J. Guindon and A. G. Hohmann, "The Endocannabinoid System and Cancer: Therapeutic Implications," *British Journal of Pharmacology* 163, no. 7 (2011): 1447–1463.

73 M. Karsak, E. Gaffal, R. Date, L. Wang-Eckhardt, J. Rehnelt, S. Petrosino, K. Starowicz, R. Steuder, E. Schlicker, B. Cravatt, R. Mechoulam, R. Buettner, S. Werner, V. Di Marzo, T. Tüting, and Z. Zimmer, "Attenuation of Allergic Contact Dermatitis through the Endocannabinoid System," *Science* 316 (2007): 1494–1497.

74 Mauro Maccarrone, Itai Bab, Tamás Bíró, Guy A. Cabral, Sudhansu K. Dey, Vincenzo Di Marzo, Justin C. Konje, George Kunos, Raphael Mechoulam, Pal Pacher, Keith A. Sharkey, and Andreas Zimmer, "Endocannabinoid Signaling at the Periphery, 50 Years after THC," *Cell: Trends in Pharmacological Science* 36, no. 5 (May 2015): 277–296.

75 Maria Grazia Cascio and Pietro Marini, "Biosynthesis and Fate of Endocannabinoids," in *Endocannabinoids: Handbook of Experimental Pharmacology*, ed. Roger G. Pertwee (Springer International Publishing, 2015), 39–58.

76 R. Mechoulam, L. O. Hanus, R. Pertwee, and A. C. Howlett, "Early Phytocannabinoid History to Endocannabinoids and Beyond: A Cannabinoid Timeline," *Nature Neuroscience Review* 15 (November 2014): 760.

77 Marcu, Jahan, Ali S. Matthews, and Martin A. Lee, "Is CBD Really Non-Psychoactive?" *Project CBD,* May 17, 2016, www.projectcbd.org/article /cbd-really-non-psychoactive.

78 PubMed search for cannabinoids over the last ten years.

79 A. A. Izzo, F. Borrelli, R. Capasso, V. Di Marzo, and R. Mechoulam, "Non-psychotropic Plant Cannabinoids: New Therapeutic Opportunities from an Ancient Herb," *Trends in Pharmacological Sciences* 30, no. 10 (2009): 609.

80 R. Brenneisen, "Chemistry and Analysis of Phytocannabinoids and Other Cannabis Constituents," in *Forensic Science and Medicine: Marijuana and the Cannabinoids*, ed. M. A. ElSohly (Totowa: Humana Press Inc, 2007), 17–59.

81 E. M. Rock, R. L. Kopstick, C. L. Limebeer, and L. A. Parker, "Tetrahydrocannabinolic Acid Reduces Nausea-Induced Conditioned Gaping in Rats and Vomiting in *Suncus murinus*," *British Journal of Pharmacology* 70, iss. 3 (October 2013): 641–648.

82 R. Moldzio, T. Pacher, C. Krewenka, B. Kranner, J. Novak, J. C. Duvigneau, and W. D. Rausch, "Effects of Cannabinoids Δ(9)-tetrahydrocannabinol, Δ(9)-tetrahydrocannabinolic Acid and Cannabidiol in MPP+ Affected Murine Mesencephalic Cultures," *Phytomedicine* 19, nos. 8–9 (June 15, 2012): 819–824.

83 A. Willbanks, M. Leary, M. Greenshields, C. Tyminski, S. Heerboth, K. Lapinska, K. Haskins, and S. Sarkar, "The Evolution of Epigenetics: From Prokaryotes to Humans and Its Biological Consequences," *Genetics and Epigenetics* 8 (2016): 25–36.

84 R. Mechoulam, L. O. Hanus, R. Pertwee, and A. C. Howlett, "Early Phytocannabinoid History to Endocannabinoids and Beyond: A Cannabinoid Timeline," *Nature Neuroscience Review* 15 (November 2014): 757–764.

85 C. M. Andre, J. F. Hausman, and G. Guirriero, "Cannabis Sativa: The Plant of a Thousand Molecules," *Frontiers of Plant Science* 7 (February 2016): 19.

86 E. B. Russo, "Taming THC: Potential Cannabis Synergy and Phytocannabinoid-Terpinoid Entourage Effects," *The British Journal of Pharmacology* 163 (2011): 1344–1364.

87 R. Mechoulam, L. O. Hanus, R. Pertwee, and A. C. Howlett, "Early Phytocannabinoid History to Endocannabinoids and Beyond: A Cannabinoid Timeline," *Nature Neuroscience Review* 15 (November 2014): 757–764.

88 Y. Y. Syed, K. McKeage, and L. J. Scott, "Delta-9-tetrahydrocannabinol/cannabidiol (Sativex®): A Review of Its Use in Patients with Moderate to Severe Spasticity Due to Multiple Sclerosis," *Drugs* 74, no. 5 (April 2014): 563–578.

89 M. Moreno-Martet, A. Feliú, F. Espejo-Porras, M. Mecha, F. J. Carrillo-Salinas, J. Fernández-Ruiz, C. Guaza, and E. de Lago, "The Disease-Modifying Effects of a Sativex-Like Combination of Phytocannabinoids in Mice with Experimental Autoimmune Encephalomyelitis Are Preferentially Due to Δ9-tetrahydrocannabinol Acting through CB1," *Multiple Sclerosis Related Disorders* 6 (November 4, 2015): 505–511.

90 R. Gallily, Z. Yekhtin, and L. O. Hanuš, "Overcoming the Bell-Shaped Dose-Response of Cannabidiol by Using Cannabis Extract Enriched in Cannabidiol," *Pharmacology & Pharmacy* 6 (2015): 75–85.

91 J. A. Ramos and F. J. Bionco, "The Role of Cannabis in Prostate Cancer: Basic Science Perspective and Potential Clinical Applications," *Indian Journal of Urology* 28, no. 1 (January–March, 2012): 9–14.

92 C. Walter, B. G. Oertel, L. Felden, C. A. Kell, U. Nöth, J. Vermehren, J. Kaiser, R. Deichmann, and J. Lötsch, "Brain Mapping Based Model of Delta-9-Tetrahydrocannabinol Effects on Connectivity in the Pain Matrix," *Neuropsychopharmacology* 41 (2016): 1659–1669.

93 L. De Petrocellis, A. Ligresti, A. S. Moriello, M. Allarà, T. Bisogno, S. Petrosino, C. G. Stott, and V. Di Marzo, "Effects of Cannabinoids and Cannabinoid-Enriched Cannabis Extracts on TRP Channels and Endocannabinoid Metabolic Enzymes," *British Journal of Pharmacology* 163 (2011): 1479–1494.

94 Antonio Currais, Oswald Quehenberger, Aaron M Armando, Daniel Daugherty, Pam Maher, and David Schubert, "Amyloid Proteotoxicity Initiates an Inflammatory Response Blocked by Cannabinoids," *Nature Partner Journals: Aging and Mechanisms of Disease* 2, no. 16012 (June 23, 2016). doi:10.1038.

95 D. Vara, M. Salazar, N. Olea-Herrero, M. Guzmán, G. Velasco, and I. Díaz-Laviada, "Anti-tumoral Effect of Cannabinoids on Hepatocellular Carcinoma: Role of AMPK Dependent Activation of Autophagy," *Cell Death and Differentiation* 18 (2011): 1099–1111.

96 V. DiMarzo and F. Piscitelli, "The Endocannabinoid System and Its Modulation by Phytocannabinioids," *Neurotherapeutics* 12 (2015): 692–698.

97 L. R. Ruhaak, J. Felth, P. C. Karlsson, J. J. Rafter, R. Verpoorte, and L. Bohlin, "Evaluation of Cyclooxegenase Inhibiting Effects of Six Major Cannabinoids," *Biological Pharmacology Bulletin* 34, no. 5 (2011): 774–778.

98 R. Mechoulam and L. Parker, "Commentary—Toward a Better Cannabis Drug," *British Journal of Pharmacology* 170 (2013): 1363–1364.

99 N. M. Kogan, E. Melamed, E. Wasserman, B. Raphael, A. Breuer, K. S. Stok, R. Sondergaard, A. V. Escudero, S. Baraghithy, M. Attar-Namdar, S. Friedlander-Barenboim, N. Mathavan, H. Isaksson, R. Mechoulam, R. Müller, A. Bajayo, Y. Gabet, and I. Bab, "Cannabidiol, A Major Nonpsychotropic Cannabis Constituent, Enhances Fracture Healing and Stimulates Lysyl Hydroxylase Activity in Osteoblasts," *Journal of Mineral and Bone Research* 30, no. 10 (October 2015): 1905–1913.

100 H. J. Parray and J. W. Yun, "Cannabidiol Promotes Browning in 3T3-L1 Adipocytes," *Molecular and Cellular Biochemistry* 416 (2016): 131–139.

101 M. Rajesh, P. Mukhopadhyay, S. Bátkai, V. Patel, K. Saito, S. Matsumoto, Y. Kashiwaya, B. Horváth, B. Mukhopadhyay, L. Becker, G. Haskó, L.

Liaudet, D. A. Wink, A. Veves, R. Mechoulam, and P. Pacher, "Cannabidiol Attenuates Cardiac Dysfunction, Oxidative Stress, Fibrosis, Inflammatory and Cell Death Signaling Pathways in Diabetic Cardiomyopathy," *Journal of the American College of Cardiology* 56, no. 25 (December 14, 2010): 2115–2125.

102 J. Guidon and A. G. Hohmann, "The Endocannabinoid System and Cancer: Therapeutic Implications," *British Journal of Pharmacology* 163 (2011): 1447–1463.

103 L. De Petrocellis, A. Ligresti, A. Schiano Moriello, M. Iappelli, R. Verde, C. G. Stott, L. Cristino, P. Orlando, and V. Di Marzo, "Non-THC Cannabinoids Inhibit Prostate Carcinoma Growth In Vitro and In Vivo: Pro-apoptotic Effects and Underlying Mechanisms," *British Journal of Pharmacology* 168 (2013): 79–102.

104 I. Ujvary and L. Hanus, "Human Metabolites of Cannabidiol: A Review of Their Formation, Biological Activity and Relevance in Therapy," *Cannabis and Cannabinoid Research* 1, no. 1 (March 2016): 90–101.

105 J. Fernández-Ruiz, O. Sagredo, M. R. Pazos, C. García, R. Pertwee, R. Mechoulam, and J. Martínez-Orgado, "Cannabidiol for Neurodegenerative Disorders: Important New Clinical Applications for This Phytocannabinoid?" *British Journal of Clinical Pharmacology* 75, no. 2 (May 25, 2012): 323–333.

106 J. D. Wilkinson and E. M. Williamson, "Cannabinoids Inhibit Human Keratinocyte Proliferation through a Non-CB1/CB2 Mechanism and Have a Potential Therapeutic Value in the Treatment of Psoriasis," *Journal of Dermatological Science* 45 (2007): 87–92.

107 A. W. Zuardi, F. S. Guimaraes, and A. C. Moreira, "Effect of Cannabidiol on Plasma Prolactin, Growth Hormone and Cortisol in Human Volunteers," *Brazilian Journal of Medical and Biological Research* 26, no. 2 (February 1993): 213–217.

108 B. Romano, F. Borrelli, I. Fasolino, R. Capasso, F. Piscitelli, M. Cascio, R. Pertwee, D. Coppola, L. Vassallo, P. Orlando, V. Di Marzo, and A. Izzo, "The Cannabinoid TRPA1 Agonist Cannabichromene Inhibits Nitric Oxide Production in Macrophages and Ameliorates Murine Colitis," *British Journal of Pharmacology* 69 (2013): 213–229.

109 Abir T. El-Alfy, Kelly Ivey, Keisha Robinson, Safwat Ahmed, Mohamed Radwan, Desmond Slade, Ikhlas Khan, Mahmoud ElSohly, and Samir

Ross, "Antidepressant-Like Effect of Δ9-tetrahydrocannabinol and Other Cannabinoids Isolated from *Cannabis sativa*," *Journal of Pharmacology, Biochemistry and Behavior* 95, no. 4 (June 2010): 434–442.

110 L. De Petrocellis, A. Ligresti, A. S. Moriello, M. Allarà, T. Bisogno, S. Petrosino, C. G. Stott, and V. Di Marzo, "Effects of Cannabinoids and Cannabinoid-Enriched Cannabis Extracts on TRP Channels and Endocannabinoid Metabolic Enzymes," *British Journal of Pharmacology* 163 (2011):1479–1494.

111 "Introduction to Terpenes," *Medical Jane,* last modified February 27, 2017, https://www.medicaljane.com/category/cannabis-classroom/terpenes/#terpenes-in-cannabis.

112 S. Casano, G. Grassi, V. Martini, and M. Michelozzi, "Variations in Terpene Profiles of Different Strains of *Cannabis sativa L.*," *Acta Horticulturae* 925 (2011): 115–121.

113 "Introduction to Terpenes," *Medical Jane,* last modified February 27, 2017, https://www.medicaljane.com/category/cannabis-classroom/terpenes/#terpenes-in-cannabis.

114 Ibid.

115 Ibid.

116 Ibid.

117 Ibid.

118 Ibid.

119 "Limonene," *WebMD,* accessed February 27, 2017, www.webmd.com/vitamins-supplements/ingredientmono-1105-limonene.aspx?activeingredientid=1105&activeingredientname.

120 "Introduction to Terpenes," *Medical Jane,* last modified February 27, 2017, https://www.medicaljane.com/category/cannabis-classroom/terpenes/#terpenes-in-cannabis.

121 "Marijuana Terpenes and Their Effects," *Alchimiaweb,* accessed February 27, 2017, www.alchimiaweb.com/blogen/marijuana-terpenes-effects/.

122 "Introduction to Terpenes," *Medical Jane,* last modified February 27, 2017, https://www.medicaljane.com/category/cannabis-classroom/terpenes/#terpenes-in-cannabis.

123 Horváth, Béla, Partha Mukhopadhyay, Malek Kechrid, Vivek Patel, Galin Tanchian, David A. Wink, Jürg Gertsch, and Pál Pacher, "β-Caryophyllene Ameliorates Cisplatin-Induced Nephrotoxicity in a Cannabinoid 2

Receptor-Dependent Manner," *Free Radical Biology and Medicine* 52, no. 8 (2012): 1325–1333. doi:10.1016/j.freeradbiomed.2012.01.014.

124 Susan Kristiniak, Jean Harpel, Diane M. Breckenridge, and Jane Buckle, "Black Pepper Essential Oil to Enhance Intravenous Catheter Insertion in Patients with Poor Vein Visibility: A Controlled Study," *The Journal of Alternative and Complementary Medicine* 18, no. 11 (November 2012): 1003–1007. doi:10.1089/acm.2012.0106.

125 P. G. Fine and M. J. Rosenfeld, "The Endocannabinoid System, Cannabinoids, and Pain," *Rambam Maimonides Medical Journal* 4, no. 4 (2013): e0022, doi.org/10.5041/RMMJ.10129.

126 "Introduction to Terpenes," *Medical Jane*, last modified February 27, 2017, https://www.medicaljane.com/category/cannabis-classroom/terpenes/#terpenes-in-cannabis.

127 E. B. Russo, "Taming THC: Potential Cannabis Synergy and Phytocannabinoid-Terpenoid Entourage Effects," *British Journal of Pharmacology* 163 (2011): 1344–1364. doi:10.1111/j.1476-5381.2011.01238.x.

128 Annette C. Rohr, Cornelius K. Wilkins, Per A. Clausen, Maria Hammer, Gunnar D. Nielsen, Peder Wolkoff, and John D. Spengler, "Upper Airway and Pulmonary Effects of Oxidation Products of (+)- α-pinene, d-limonene, and Isoprene in Balb/ c Mice," *Inhalation Toxicology* 14, no. 7 (2002): 663–684. doi:10.1080/08958370290084575.

129 "Marijuana Terpenes and Their Effects," *Alchimiaweb*, accessed February 27, 2017, www.alchimiaweb.com/blogen/marijuana-terpenes-effects/.

130 Weiqiang Chen, Ying Liu, Ming Li, Jianwen Mao, Lirong Zhang, Rongbo Huang, Xiaobao Jin, and Lianbao Ye, "Anti-tumor Effect of α-pinene on Human Hepatoma Cell Lines through Inducing G2/M Cell Cycle Arrest," *Journal of Pharmacological Sciences* 127, iss. 3 (March 2015): 332–338, http://dx.doi.org/10.1016/j.jphs.2015.01.008.

131 "Introduction to Terpenes," *Medical Jane*, last modified February 27, 2017, https://www.medicaljane.com/category/cannabis-classroom/terpenes/#terpenes-in-cannabis.

132 "Marijuana Terpenes and Their Effects," *Alchimiaweb*, accessed February 27, 2017, www.alchimiaweb.com/blogen/marijuana-terpenes-effects/.

133 "Introduction to Terpenes," *Medical Jane*, last modified February 27, 2017, https://www.medicaljane.com/category/cannabis-classroom/terpenes/#terpenes-in-cannabis.

134 Ibid.

135 Jianqun Ma, Hai Xu, Jun Wu, Changfa Qu, Fenglin Sun, and Shidong Xu, "Linalool Inhibits Cigarette Smoke-Induced Lung Inflammation by Inhibiting NF-κB Activation," *International Immunopharmacology* 29, iss. 2 (December 2015): 708–713, http://dx.doi.org/10.1016/j.intimp.2015.09.005.

136 Sabogal-Guáqueta, Angélica Maria, Edison Osorio, and Gloria Patricia Cardona-Gómez, "Linalool Reverses Neuropathological and Behavioral Impairments in Old Triple Transgenic Alzheimer's Mice," *Neuropharmacology* 102 (2016): 111–120. doi:10.1016/j.neuropharm.2015.11.002.

137 "Introduction to Terpenes," *Medical Jane,* last modified February 27, 2017, https://www.medicaljane.com/category/cannabis-classroom/terpenes/#terpenes-in-cannabis.

138 Ibid.

139 Ibid.

140 Ken Ito and Michiho Ito, "The Sedative Effect of Inhaled Terpinolene in Mice and Its Structure-Activity Relationships," *Journal of Natural Medicines* 67, no. 4 (2013): 833–837. doi:10.1007/s11418-012-0731.

141 Naoko Okumura, Hitomi Yoshida, Yuri Nishimura, Yasuko Kitagishi, and Satoru Matsuda, "Terpinolene, a Component of Herbal Sage, Downregulates AKT1 Expression in K562 Cells," *Oncology Letters* 3, no. 2 (2011): 321–324. doi:10.3892/ol.2011.491.

142 "Introduction to Terpenes," *Medical Jane,* last modified February 27, 2017, https://www.medicaljane.com/category/cannabis-classroom/terpenes/#terpenes-in-cannabis.

143 Ibid.

144 Ibid.

145 Gallily, Ruth, Zhannah Yekhtin, and Lumír Ondřej Hanuš, "Overcoming the Bell-Shaped Dose-Response of Cannabidiol by Using *Cannabis* Extract Enriched in Cannabidiol," *Pharmacology & Pharmacy* 06, no. 02 (2015): 75–85. doi:10.4236/pp.2015.62010.

146 Edward Group, "What is Vegetable Glycerin?" *Global Healing Center,* last modified November 24, 2015, www.globalhealingcenter.com/natural-health/what-is-vegetable-glycerin/.

147 L. R. Zhang, H. Morgenstern, S. Greenland, S.-C. Chang, P. Lazarus, M. D. Teare, P. Woll, I. Orlow, B. Cox, on behalf of the Cannabis and Respiratory Disease Research Group of New Zealand, Y. Brhane, G. Liu, and R. J. Hung, "Cannabis Smoking and Lung Cancer Risk: Pooled Analysis

in the International Lung Cancer Consortium," *International Journal of Cancer* 136 (2015): 894–903. doi:10.1002/ijc.29036.

148 Nicholas V. Cozzi, "Effects of Water Filtration on Marijuana Smoke: A Literature Review," *UK Cannabis Internet Activist,* accessed February 28, 2017, www.ukcia.org/research/EffectsOfWaterFiltrationOnMarijuana-Smoke.php.

149 Mitch Earleywine and Sara Smucker Barnwell, "Decreased Respiratory Symptoms in Cannabis Users Who Vaporize," *Harm Reduction Journal* 4 (2007): 11. doi:10.1186/1477-7517-31.

150 "Can Marijuana Help COPD?" *Lung Institute,* March 23, 2015, https://lunginstitute.com/blog/can-marijuana-help-copd/.

151 "Be Careful When You Buy Your Next CBD Oil," *Ministry of Hemp,* July 27, 2016. http://ministryofhemp.com/blog/careful-buying-cbd-oil/.

152 "10 Pharmaceutical Drugs Based on Cannabis," *ProCon,* last modified November 27, 2013, http://medicalmarijuana.procon.org/view. resource.php?resourceID=000883.

153 Mateus Machado Bergamaschi, Regina Helena Costa Queiroz, Antonio Waldo Zuardi, and Jose Alexandre S. Crippa, "Safety and Side Effects of Cannabidiol, a *Cannabis sativa* Constituent," *Current Drug Safety* 6, no. 4 (2011): 237–249. doi:10.2174/157488611798280924.

154 Madeline H. Meier, Avshalom Caspi, Antony Ambler, HonaLee Harrington, Renate Houts, Richard S. E. Keefe, Kay McDonald, Aimee Ward, Richie Poulton, and Terrie E. Moffitt, "Persistent Cannabis Users Show Neuropsychological Decline from Childhood to Midlife," *Proceedings of the National Academy of Sciences* 109, no. 40 (2012): E2657–E2664. doi:10.1073/pnas.1206820109.

155 "How Safe is Cannabis? This Doctor Takes a Cold Hard Look at the Facts," *Illegally Healed,* last modified March 22, 2016, https://illegallyhealed.com/how-safe-is-cannabis-this-doctor-takes-a-cold-hard-look-at-the-facts/.

156 Paul Armentano, "Cannabis Smoke and Cancer: Assessing the Risk," *NORML Foundation,* last modified March 7, 2017, http://norml.org/component/zoo/category/cannabis-smoke-and-cancer-assessing-the-risk.

157 A. J. Budney and B. A. Moore, "Development and Consequences of Cannabis Dependence," *Journal of Clinical Pharmacology* 42, suppl. 11 (2002): 28S–33S.

158 J. A. Crippa, J. E. Hallak, J. P. Machado-de-Sousa, R. H. Queiroz, M. Bergamaschi, M. H. Chagas, and A. W. Zuardi, "Cannabidiol for the

Treatment of Cannabis Withdrawal Syndrome: A Case Report," *Journal of Clinical Pharmacy and Therapeutics* 38, no. 2 (April 2013): 162–164. doi:10.1111/jcpt.12018.

159 Michael Backes, *Cannabis Pharmacy: A Practical Guide to Medicinal Marijuana* (New York: Black Dog & Leventhal Publishers, 2014), 237.

160 P. Fried, B. Watkinson, D. James, and R. Gray, "Current and Former Marijuana Use: Preliminary Findings of a Longitudinal Study of Effects on IQ in Young Adults," *Canadian Medical Association Journal* 166, no. 7 (2002): 887–891.

161 Madeline H. Meier, Avshalom Caspi, Antony Ambler, HonaLee Harrington, Renate Houts, Richard S. E. Keefe, Kay McDonald, Aimee Ward, Richie Poulton, and Terrie E. Moffitt, "Persistent Cannabis Users Show Neuropsychological Decline from Childhood to Midlife," *Proceedings of the National Academy of Sciences USA* 109, no. 40 (2012): E2657–E2664.

162 Jodi M. Gilman, John K. Kuster, Sang Lee, Myung Joo Lee, Byoung Woo Kim, Nikos Makris, Andre van der Kouwe, Anne J. Blood, and Hans C. Breiter, "Cannabis Use Is Quantitatively Associated with Nucleus Accumbens and Amygdala Abnormalities in Young Adult Recreational Users," *Journal of Neuroscience* 34 (2014): 5529–5538.

163 Barbara J. Weiland, Rachel E. Thayer, Brendan E. Depue, Amithrupa Sabbineni, Angela D. Bryan, and Kent E. Hutchison, "Daily Marijuana Use Is Not Associated with Brain Morphometric Measures in Adolescents and Adults," *The Journal of Neuroscience* 35, no. 4 (January 28, 2015): 1505–1512.

164 P. Silva and W. Standton, *From Child to Adult: The Dunedin Multidisciplinary Health and Development Study* (Oxford University Press, 1996).

165 G. C. Patton, C. Coffey, J. B. Carlin, L. Degenhardt, M. Lynskey, and W. Hall, "Cannabis Use and Mental Health in Young People: Cohort Study," *British Medical Journal* 325, no. 7374 (2002): 1195–1198.

166 Yvette Brazier, "Teens who use cannabis at risk of schizophrenia," *Medical News Today* (January 17, 2016): 1

167 Adrian Devitt-Lee, "CBD-Drug Interactions: Role of Cytochrome P450," *Project CBD*, last modified September 8, 2015, www.projectcbd.org /article/cbd-drug-interactions-role-cytochrome-p450.

168 Alexandra L. Geffrey, Sarah F. Pollack, Patricia L. Bruno, and Elizabeth A. Thiele, "Drug-Drug Interaction between Clobazam and Cannabidiol

in Children with Refractory Epilepsy," *Epilepsia* 56, no. 8 (2015): 1246–1251. doi:10.1111/epi.13060.

169   K. Watanabe, S. Yamaori, T. Funahashi, T. Kimura, and I. Yamamoto, "Cytochrome P450 Enzymes Involved in the Metabolism of Tetrahydrocannabinols and Cannabinol by Human Hepatic Microsomes," *Life Sciences* 80, no. 15 (2007): 1415–1419.

170   Adrian Devitt-Lee, "CBD-Drug Interactions: Role of Cytochrome P450," *Project CBD*, last modified September 8, 2015, www.projectcbd.org/article /cbd-drug-interactions-role-cytochrome-p450.

171   Ibid.

172   D. A. Flockhart, "Drug Interactions: Cytochrome P450 Drug Interaction Table," *Indiana University School of Medicine* (2007), last modified March 7, 2017.

173   Uwe Blesching, *The Cannabis Health Index* (Berkeley: North Atlantic Books, 2013), 20.

Part II

174   Zachary Wilmer Reichenbach and Ron Schey, "Cannabinoids and GI Disorders: Endogenous and Exogenous," *Current Treatment Options in Gastroenterology* 14, no. 4 (2016): 461–477. doi:10.1007/s11938-016-0110.

175   Bradley E. Alger, "Getting High on the Endocannabinoid System," *Cerebrum: The Dana Forum on Brain Science* (2013): 14.

176   Yann LeStrat and Bernard Le Foll, "Obesity and Cannabis Use: Results From 2 Representative National Surveys," *American Journal of Epidemiology* 174, no. 8 (2011): 929–933. doi:10.1093/aje/kwr200.

177   L. Weiss, M. Zeira, S. Reich, M. Har-Noy, R. Mechoulam, S. Slavin, and R. Gallily, "Cannabidiol Lowers Incidence of Diabetes in Non-obese Diabetic Mice," *Autoimmunity* 39, no. 2 (2006): 143–151.

178   Abigail Klein Leichman, "Cannabis Extract to Be Used to Treat Diabetes," *Israel 21c*, April 21, 2015, www.israel21c.org/cannabis-extract -to-be-used-to-treat-diabetes/.

179   H. J. Parray and J. W. Yun, "Cannabidiol Promotes Browning in 3T3-L1 Adipocytes," *Molecular and Cellular Biochemistry* 416 (2016): 131–139.

180   E. A. Penner, H. Buettner, and M. A. Mittleman, "Marijuana Use on Glucose, Insulin, and Insulin Resistance among US Adults," *American Journal of Medicine* 126 (2013): 583–589.

181 Sabine Steffens, Niels R. Veillard, Claire Arnaud, Graziano Pelli, Fabienne Burger, Christian Staub, Andreas Zimmer, Jean-Louis Frossard, and François Mach, "Low Dose Oral Cannabinoid Therapy Reduces Progression of Atherosclerosis in Mice," *Nature* 434 (2005): 782–786.

182 Francois Mach and Sabine Steffens, "The Role of the Endocannabinoid System in Atherosclerosis," *Journal of Neuroendocrinology* 20, no. S1 (2008): 53–57. doi:10.1111/j.1365-2826.2008.01685.x.

183 Mauro Maccarrone, Itai Bab, Tamás Bíró, Guy A. Cabral, Sudhansu K. Dey, Vincenzo Di Marzo, Justin C. Konje, George Kunos, Raphael Mechoulam, Pal Pacher, Keith A. Sharkey, and Andreas Zimmer, "Endocannabinoid Signaling at the Periphery, 50 Years after THC," *Cell: Trends in Pharmacological Science* 36, no. 5 (May 2015): 277–296.

184 Sabine Steffens and Francois Mach, "Cannabinoid Receptors in Atherosclerosis," *Current Opinion in Lipidology* 17, no. 5 (2006): 519–526. doi:10.1097/01.mol.0000245257.17764.b2.

185 Ronen Durst, Haim Danenberg, Ruth Gallily, Raphael Mechoulam, Keren Meir, Etty Grad, Ronen Beeri, Thea Pugatsch, Elizabet Tarsish, and Chaim Lotan, "Cannabidiol, A Nonpsychoactive Cannabis Constituent, Protects against Myocardial Ischemic Reperfusion Injury," *American Journal of Physiology – Heart and Circulatory Physiology* 293, no. 6 (2007): H3602–H3607. doi:10.1152/ajpheart.00098.2007.

186 John C. Ashton and Paul F. Smith, "Cannabinoids and Cardiovascular Disease: The Outlook for Clinical Treatments," *Current Vascular Pharmacology* 5, no. 3 (2007): 175–184. doi:10.2174/157016107781024109.

187 Gabriella Aviello, Barbara Romano, Francesca Borrelli, Raffaele Capasso, Laura Gallo, Fabiana Piscitelli, Vincenzo Di Marzo, and Angelo A. Izzo, "Chemopreventive Effect of the Non-psychotropic Phytocannabinoid Cannabidiol on Experimental Colon Cancer," *Journal of Molecular Medicine* 90, no. 8 (2012): 925–934. doi:10.1007/s00109-011-0856-x.

188 "NTP Toxicology and Carcinogenesis Studies of 1-Trans-Delta(9)-Tetrahydrocannabinol (CAS No. 1972-08-3) in F344 Rats and B6C3F1 Mice (Gavage Studies)," *National Toxicology Program Technical Report Series* 446 (1996): 1–317.

189 A. A. Thomas, L. P. Wallner, V. P. Quinn, J. Slezak, S. K. Van Den Eeden, G. W. Chien, and S. J. Jacobsen, "Association between Cannabis Use and the Risk of Bladder Cancer: Results from the California Men's Health Study," *Urology* 85, iss. 2 (2015): 388–393.

190 Andras Bilkei-Gorzo, "The Endocannabinoid System in Normal and Pathological Brain Ageing," *Philosophical Transactions of the Royal Society of London* 367, no. 1607 (2012): 3326–3341. doi:10.1098/rstb.2011.0388.

191 J. Fernández-Ruiz, O. Sagredo, M. R. Pazos, C. García, R. Pertwee, R. Mechoulam, and J. Martínez-Orgado, "Cannabidiol for Neurodegenerative Disorders: Important New Clinical Applications for This Phytocannabinoid?" *British Journal of Clinical Pharmacology* 75, no. 2 (May 25, 2012): 323–333.

192 Gary L. Wenk, "Animal Models of Alzheimer's Disease," *Animal Models of Neurological Disease* I (1992): 29–64, doi:10.1385/0-89603-208-6:29.

193 N. M. Kogan, E. Melamed, E. Wasserman, B. Raphael, A. Breuer, K. S. Stok, R. Sondergaard, A. V. Escudero, S. Baraghithy, M. Attar-Namdar, S. Friedlander-Barenboim, N. Mathavan, H. Isaksson, R. Mechoulam, R. Müller, A. Bajayo, Y. Gabet, and I. Bab, "Cannabidiol, A Major Nonpsychotropic Cannabis Constituent, Enhances Fracture Healing and Stimulates Lysyl Hydroxylase Activity in Osteoblasts," *Journal of Mineral and Bone Research* 30, no. 10 (October 2015): 1905–1913.

194 A. J. Hampson, M. Grimaldi, J. Axelrod, and D. Wink, "Cannabidiol and (−)Δ9-Tetrahydrocannabinol Are Neuroprotective Antioxidants," *Proceedings of the National Academy of Sciences of the United States of America* 95, no. 14 (1998): 8268–8273.

195 N. Dobrosi, B. I. Toth, G. Nagy, A. Dozsa, T. Geczy, L. Nagy, C. C. Zouboulis, R. Paus, L. Kovacs, and T. Biro, "Endocannabinoids Enhance Lipid Synthesis and Apoptosis of Human Sebocytes via Cannabinoid Receptor-2-Mediated Signaling," *The FASEB Journal* 22, no. 10 (2008): 3685–3695. doi:10.1096/fj.0604877.

196 P. Nagarkatti, R. Pandey, S. A. Rieder, V. L. Hegde, and M. Nagarkatti, "Cannabinoids as Novel Anti-inflammatory Drugs," *Future Medicinal Chemistry* 1, no. 7 (2009): 1333–1349, http://doi.org/10.4155/fmc.09.93.

197 S. S. Lee, K. L. Humphreys, K. Flory, R. Liu, and K. Glass, "Prospective Association of Childhood Attention-Deficit/Hyperactivity Disorder (ADHD) and Substance Use and Abuse/Dependence: A Meta-Analytic Review," *Clinical Psychology Review* 31, no. 3 (2011): 328–341, http://doi.org/10.1016/j.cpr.2011.01.006.

198 Peter Strohbeck-Kuehner, Gisela Skopp, and Rainer Mattern, "Case Report: Cannabis Improves Symptoms of ADHD," *Cannabinoids* 3, no. 1 (2008): 1–3.

199 Heather Won Tesoreiro, "Doctor of the Day: David Bearman, Cannabi-noidologist," *Wall Street Journal*, December 20, 2007.

200 Michael Backes, *Cannabis Pharmacy: A Practical Guide to Medicinal Mari-juana* (New York: Black Dog & Leventhal Publishers, 2014).

201 Anand Gururajan, David A. Taylor, and Daniel T. Malone, "Cannabidiol and Clozapine Reverse MK-801-Induced Deficits in Social Interaction and Hyperactivity in Sprague–Dawley Rats," *Journal of Psychopharmacology* 26, no. 10 (2012): 1317–1332. doi:10.1177/0269881112441865.

202 Mallory Loflin, Mitch Earleywine, Joseph De Leo, and Andrea Hobkirk, "Subtypes of Attention Deficit-Hyperactivity Disorder (ADHD) and Can-nabis Use," *Substance Use & Misuse* 49, no. 4 (2013): 427–434. doi:10.310 9/10826084.2013.841251.

203 Didier Jutras-Aswad, Mélissa Prud'Homme, and Romulus Cata, "Canna-bidiol as an Intervention for Addictive Behaviors: A Systematic Review of the Evidence," *Substance Abuse: Research and Treatment* 33, no. 9 (2015): 33–38. doi:10.4137/sart.s25081.

204 Marcus A. Bachhuber, Brendan Saloner, Chinazo O. Cunningham, and Colleen L. Barry, "Medical Cannabis Laws and Opioid Analgesic Over-dose Mortality in the United States, 1999-2010," *JAMA Internal Medicine* 174, no. 10 (2014): 1668. doi:10.1001/jamainternmed.2014.4005.

205 Dr. Michael Moskowitz, personal communication with authors, October 2016.

206 Vicky Katsidoni, Ilektra Anagnostou, and George Panagis, "Cannabidiol Inhibits the Reward-Facilitating Effect of Morphine: Involvement of 5-HT 1A Receptors in the Dorsal Raphe Nucleus," *Addiction Biology* 18, no. 2 (2012): 286–296. doi:10.1111/j.1368600.2012.00483.x.

207 J. A. S. Crippa, J. E. C. Hallak, J. P. Machado-De-Sousa, R. H. C. Que-iroz, M. Bergamaschi, M. H. N. Chagas, and A. W. Zuardi, "Cannabidiol for the Treatment of Cannabis Withdrawal Syndrome: A Case Report," *Journal of Clinical Pharmacy and Therapeutics* 38, no. 2 (2012): 162–164. doi:10.1111/jcpt.12018.

208 Kenneth Stoller, MD, personal communication with authors, January 2017.

209 Y. Ren, J. Whittard, A. Higuera-Matas, C. V. Morris, and Y. L. Hurd, "Cannabidiol, a Nonpsychotropic Component of Cannabis, Inhib-its Cue-Induced Heroin-Seeking and Normalizes Discrete Mesolim-bic Neuronal Disturbances," *The Journal of Neuroscience: The Official*

Journal of the Society for Neuroscience 29, no. 47 (2009): 14764. doi:10.1523/JNEUROSCI.4291-09.2009.

210 Celia J. A. Morgan, Ravi K. Das, Alyssa Joye, H. Valerie Curran, and Sunjeev K. Kamboj, "Cannabidiol Reduces Cigarette Consumption in Tobacco Smokers: Preliminary Findings," *Addictive Behaviors* 38, no. 9 (2013): 2433–2436. doi:10.1016/j.addbeh.2013.03.011.

211 Homa Zarrabi, Mohammadrasoul Khalkhali, Azam Hamidi, Reza Ahmadi, and Maryam Zavarmousavi, "Clinical Features, Course and Treatment of Methamphetamine-Induced Psychosis in Psychiatric Inpatients," *BMC Psychiatry* 16, no. 1 (2016). doi:10.1186/s12888-016-0745-5.

212 "What is ALS?" *ALS Therapy Development Institute,* last modified March 7, 2017, www.als.net/what-is-als/.

213 Gregory T. Carter and Bill S. Rosen, "Marijuana in the Management of Amyotrophic Lateral Sclerosis," *American Journal of Hospice and Palliative Medicine* 18, iss. 4 (2016): 264–270. doi:10.1177/104990910101800411.

214 "ALS and Cannabis," *My Chronic Relief,* September 8, 2014, http://mychronicrelief.com/als-cannabis/.

215 "Keeping ALS at Bay with Cannabis," *Illegally Healed,* April 7, 2015, http://illegallyhealed.com/keeping-als-at-bay-with-cannabis/.

216 G. T. Carter, M. E. Abood, S. K. Aggarwal, and M. D. Weiss, "Cannabis and Amyotrophic Lateral Sclerosis: Hypothetical and Practical Applications, and a Call for Clinical Trials," *American Journal of Hospice and Palliative Medicine* 27, no. 5 (2010): 347. doi:10.1177/1049909110369531.

217 Ethan Russo and Geoffrey W. Guy, "A Tale of Two Cannabinoids: The Therapeutic Rationale for Combining Tetrahydrocannabinol and Cannabidiol," *Medical Hypotheses* 66, no. 2 (2006): 234–246. doi:10.1016/j.mehy.2005.08.026.

218 G. T. Carter, M. E. Abood, S. K. Aggarwal, and M. D. Weiss, "Cannabis and Amyotrophic Lateral Sclerosis: Hypothetical and Practical Applications, and a Call for Clinical Trials," *American Journal of Hospice and Palliative Medicine* 27, no. 5 (2010): 347–356. doi:10.1177/1049909110369531.

219 T. H. Ferreira-Vieira, C. P. Bastos, G. S. Pereira, F. A. Moreira, and A. R. Massensini, "A Role for the Endocannabinoid System in Exercise-Induced Spatial Memory Enhancement in Mice," *Hippocampus* 24 (2014): 86. doi:10.1002/hipo.22206.

220 Antonio Currais, Oswald Quehenberger, Aaron M. Armando, Daniel Daugherty, Pam Maher, and David Schubert, "Amyloid Proteotoxicity

Initiates an Inflammatory Response Blocked by Cannabinoids," *Nature Partner Journals: Aging and Mechanisms of Disease* 2, no. 16012 (June 23, 2016). doi:10.1038.

221 T. Iuvone, G. Esposito, R. Esposito, R. Santamaria, M. Di Rosa, and A. A. Izzo, "Neuroprotective Effect of Cannabidiol, a Non-psychoactive Component from *Cannabis sativa,* on β-amyloid-induced Toxicity in PC12 Cells," *Journal of Neurochemistry* 89 (2004): 134–141. doi:10.1111/j.1471-4159.2003.02327.x.

222 Teresa Iuvone, Giuseppe Esposito, Daniele De Filippis, Caterina Scuderi, and Luca Steardo, "Cannabidiol: A Promising Drug for Neurodegenerative Disorders?" *CNS Neuroscience & Therapeutics* 15, no. 1 (2009): 65–75. doi:10.1111/j.1755-5949.2008.00065.x.

223 Lisa M. Eubanks, C. J. Rogers, A. E. Beuscher, G. F. Koob, A. J. Olson, T. J. Dickerson, and K. D. Janda, "A Molecular Link Between the Active Component of Marijuana and Alzheimer's Disease Pathology," *Molecular Pharmaceutics* 3, no. 6 (2006): 773–777, http://doi.org/10.1021/mp060066m.

224 C. Cao, Y. Li, H. Liu, G. Bai, J. Mayl, X. Lin, K. Sutherland, N. Nabar, and J. Cai, "The Potential Therapeutic Effects of THC on Alzheimer's Disease," *Journal of Alzheimer's Disease* 42, no. 3 (2014): 973–984. doi:10.3233/JAD-140093.

225 Antonio Currais, Oswald Quehenberger, Aaron M. Armando, Daniel Daugherty, Pam Maher, and David Schubert, "Amyloid Proteotoxicity Initiates an Inflammatory Response Blocked by Cannabinoids," *Nature Partner Journals: Aging and Mechanisms of Disease* 2, no. 16012 (June 23, 2016). doi:10.1038.

226 Antonio Currais, Oswald Quehenberger, Aaron M. Armando, Daniel Daugherty, Pam Maher, and David Schubert, "Amyloid Proteotoxicity Initiates an Inflammatory Response Blocked by Cannabinoids," *Nature Partner Journals: Aging and Mechanisms of Disease* 2, no. 16012 (June 23, 2016): 6. doi:10.1038.

227 G. Esposito, C. Scuderi, M. Valenza, G. I. Togna, V. Latina, D. De Filippis, M. Cipriano, M. R. Carratù, T. Iuvone, and L. Steardo, "Cannabidiol Reduces Aβ-induced Neuroinflammation and Promotes Hippocampal Neurogenesis through PPARγ Involvement," *PLoS One* 6, no. 12 (2011): e28668. doi:10.1371/journal.pone.0028668.

228 V. A. Campbell and A. Gowran, "Alzheimer's Disease; Taking the Edge Off with Cannabinoids?" *British Journal of Pharmacology*, 152 (2007): 655–662. doi:10.1038/sj.bjp.0707446.

229 E. Aso and I. Ferrer, "Cannabinoids for Treatment of Alzheimer's Disease: Moving toward the Clinic," *Frontiers in Pharmacology* 5 (2014): 37. doi:10.3389/fphar.2014.00037.

230 D. Cheng, J. K. Low, W. Logge, B. Garner, and T. Karl, "Chronic Cannabidiol Treatment Improves Social and Object Recognition in Double Transgenic APPswe/PS1ΔE9 Mice," *Psychopharmacology* 231 (2014): 3009. doi:10.1007/s00213-014-3478-5.

231 G. Esposito, C. Scuderi, M. Valenza, G. I. Togna, V. Latina, D. De Filippis, M. Cipriano, M. R. Carratù, T. Iuvone, and L. Steardo, "Cannabidiol Reduces Aβ-induced Neuroinflammation and Promotes Hippocampal Neurogenesis through PPARγ Involvement," *PLoS One* 6, no. 12 (2011): e28668. doi:10.1371/journal.pone.0028668.

232 A. Shelef, Y. Barak, U. Berger, D. Paleacu, S. Tadger, I. Plopsky, and Y. Baruch, "Safety and Efficacy of Medical Cannabis Oil for Behavioral and Psychological Symptoms of Dementia: An-Open Label, Add-On, Pilot Study," *Journal of Alzheimer's Disease* 51, no. 1 (2016): 15–19. doi:10.3233/JAD-150915.

233 B. Van Klingeren and M. Ten Ham, "Antibacterial Activity of Delta-9-tetrahydrocannabinol and Cannabidiol," *Antonie van Leeuwenhoek* 42 (1976): 9–12.

234 Giovanni Appendino, Simon Gibbons, Anna Giana, Alberto Pagani, Gianpaolo Grassi, Michael Stavri, Eileen Smith, and M. Mukhlesur Rahman, "Antibacterial Cannabinoids from *Cannabis sativa*: A Structure–Activity Study," *Journal of Natural Products* 71, no. 8 (**2008**):1427–1430. doi:10.1021/np8002673.

235 A. C. Rivas da Silva, P. M. Lopes, M. M. Barros de Azevedo, D. C. Costa, C. S. Alviano, and D. S. Alviano, "Biological Activities of α-pinene and β-pinene Enantiomers," *Molecules* 17, no. 6 (2012): 6305–6316. doi:10.3390/molecules17066305.

236 Nora Schultz, "A New MRSA Defense," *MIT Technology Review* (September 12, 2008) https://www.technologyreview.com/s/410815/a-new-mrsa-defense/

237 Z. B. Zhao, D. W. Guan, W. W. Liu, T. Wang, Y. Y. Fan, Z. H. Cheng, J. L. Zheng, and G. Y. Hu, "Expression of Cannabinoid Receptor I during Mice Skin Incised Wound Healing Course," *Fa Yi Xue Za Zhi* 26, no. 4 (2010): 241–245. PubMed PMID: 20967946.

238 G. A. Grierson, "The Hemp Plant in Sanskrit and Hindi Literature," *Indian Antiquary* (September 1894): 260–262.

239 A. R. Schier, N. P. Ribeiro, A. C. Silva, J. E. Hallak, J. A. Crippa, A. E. Nardi, and A. W. Zuardi, "Cannabidiol, a *Cannabis sativa* Constituent, As an Anxiolytic Drug," *Revista Brasileira de Psiquiatri* 34, suppl. 1 (2012): S104–S110. PubMed PMID: 22729452.

240 R. J. Bluett, J. C. Gamble-George, D. J. Hermanson, N. D. Hartley, L. J. Marnett, and S. Patel, "Central Anandamide Deficiency Predicts Stress-Induced Anxiety: Behavioral Reversal through Endocannabinoid Augmentation," *Translational Psychiatry* 8, no. 4 (2014): e408. doi:10.1038/tp.2014.53.

241 A. C. Campos, Z. Ortega, J. Palazuelos, M. V. Fogaça, D. C. Aguiar, J. Díaz-Alonso, S. Ortega-Gutiérrez, H. Vázquez-Villa, F. A. Moreira, M. Guzmán, I. Galve-Roperh, and F. S. Guimarães, "The Anxiolytic Effect of Cannabidiol on Chronically Stressed Mice Depends on Hippocampal Neurogenesis: Involvement of the Endocannabinoid System," *International Journal of Neuropsychopharmacology* 16, no. 6 (2013): 1407–1419. doi:10.1017/S1461145712001502.

242 N. Schuelert and J. J. McDougall, "The Abnormal Cannabidiol Analogue O-1602 Reduces Nociception in a Rat Model of Acute Arthritis via the Putative Cannabinoid Receptor GPR55," *Neuroscience Letters* 500, no. 1 (2011): 72. doi:10.1016/j.neulet.2011.06.004.

243 Michael Backes, *Cannabis Pharmacy: A Practical Guide to Medicinal Marijuana* (New York: Black Dog & Leventhal Publishers, 2014).

244 D. C. Hammell, L. P. Zhang, F. Ma, S. M. Abshire, S. L. McIlwrath, A. L. Stinchcomb, and K. N. Westlund, "Transdermal Cannabidiol Reduces Inflammation and Pain-Related Behaviours in a Rat Model of Arthritis," *European Journal of Pain* 20, no. 6 (2016): 936–948. doi:10.1002/ejp.818.

245 A. M. Malfait, R. Gallily, P. F. Sumariwalla, A. S. Malik, E. Andreakos, R. Mechoulam, and M. Feldmann, "The Nonpsychoactive Cannabis Constituent Cannabidiol Is an Oral Anti-arthritic Therapeutic in Murine Collagen-Induced Arthritis," *Proceedings of the National Academy of Science* 97, no. 17 (2000): 9561–9566.

246 D. R. Blake, P. Robson, M. Ho, R. W. Jubb, and C. S. McCabe, "Preliminary Assessment of the Efficacy, Tolerability and Safety of a Cannabis-Based Medicine (Sativex) in the Treatment of Pain Caused by Rheumatoid Arthritis," *Rheumatology* 45, no. 1 (2006): 50.

247 S. H. Burstein and R. B. Zurier, "Cannabinoids, Endocannabinoids, and Related Analogs in Inflammation," *The AAPS Journal* 11, no. 1 (March 2009): 109–119.

248 A. Pini, G. Mannaioni, D. Pellegrini-Giampietro, M. B. Passani, R. Mastroianni, D. Bani, and E. Masini, "The Role of Cannabinoids in Inflammatory Modulation of Allergic Respiratory Disorders, Inflammatory Pain and Ischemic Stroke," *Current Drug Targets* 13, no. 7 (2012): 984–993.

249 L. Giannini, S. Nistri, R. Mastroianni, L. Cinci, A. Vannacci, C. Mariottini, M. B. Passani, P. F. Mannaioni, D. Bani, and E. Masini, "Activation of Cannabinoid Receptors Prevents Antigen-Induced Asthma-Like Reaction in Guinea Pigs," *Journal of Cellular and Molecular Medicine* 12, no. 6A (2008): 2381–2394. doi:10.1111/j.1582-4934.2008.00258.x.

250 Louis Vachon, Muiris X. Fitzgerald, Norman H. Solliday, Ira A. Gould, and Edward A. Gaensler, "Single-Dose Effect of Marihuana Smoke," *New England Journal of Medicine* 288, no. 19 (1973): 985–989. doi:10.1056/nejm197305102881902.

251 Donald P. Tashkin, Bertrand J. Shapiro, and Ira M. Frank, "Acute Effects of Smoked Marijuana and Oral Delta-9-tetrahydrocannabinol on Specific Airway Conductance in Asthmatic Subjects," *American Review of Respiratory Disease* 109 (1974): 420–428.

252 J. P. Hartley, S. G. Nogrady, and A. Seaton, "Bronchodilator Effect of Delta1-tetrahydrocannabinol," *British Journal of Clinical Pharmacology* 5, no. 6 (1978): 523–525.

253 Francieli Vuolo, Fabricia Petronilho, Beatriz Sonai, Cristiane Ritter, Jaime E. C. Hallak, Antonio Waldo Zuardi, José A. Crippa, and Felipe Dal-Pizzol, "Evaluation of Serum Cytokines Levels and the Role of Cannabidiol Treatment in Animal Model of Asthma," *Mediators of Inflammation* (2015). doi:10.1155/2015/538670.

254 D. Siniscalco, A. Sapone, C. Giordano, A. Cirillo, L. de Magistris, F. Rossi, A. Fasano, J. J. Bradstreet, S. Maione, and N. Antonucci, "Cannabinoid Receptor Type 2, But Not Type 1, Is Up-regulated in Peripheral Blood Mononuclear Cells of Children Affected by Autistic Disorders," *Journal of Autism and Developmental Disorders* 43, no. 11 (2013): 2686–2695. doi:10.1007/s10803-012824-9.

255 Cell Press. "Mutations found in individuals with autism interfere with endocannabinoid signaling in the brain." ScienceDaily. ScienceDaily, 11 April 2013. www.sciencedaily.com/releases/2013/04/130411123852.htm

256 Ido Efrati, "Israeli Doctors to Use Cannabis to Treat Autism in First-of-its-kind Study," *Haaretz,* August 29, 2016, www.haaretz.com/israel-news/science/1.739199.

257 Debra Borchardt, "Desperate Parents of Autistic Children Trying Cannabis Despite Lack of Studies," *Forbes,* June 10, 2015, www.forbes.com/sites/debraborchardt/2015/06/10/desperate-parents-of-autistic-children-trying-cannabis-despite-lack-of-studies/#7fe3128f2c94.

258 E. Onaivi, R. Benno, T. Halpern, M. Mehanovic, N. Schanz, C. Sanders, X. Yan, H. Ishiguro, Q. R. Liu, A. L. Berzal, M. P. Viveros, and S. F. Ali, "Consequences of Cannabinoid and Monoaminergic System Disruption in a Mouse Model of Autism Spectrum Disorders," *Current Neuropharmacology* 9, no. 1 (2011): 214. doi:10.2174/157015911795017047.

259 Chakrabarti, A. Persico, N. Battista, M. Maccarrone, "Endocannabinoid Signaling in Autism," Neurotherapeutics 12, no. 4 (2015): 842.

260 G. W. Booz, "Cannabidiol As an Emergent Therapeutic Strategy for Lessening the Impact of Inflammation on Oxidative Stress," *Free Radical Biology and Medicine* 51, no. 5 (2011): 1054–1061. doi:10.1016/j.freeradbiomed.2011.01.007.

261 Jessica Assaf, "Constance and Me," *Beauty Lies Truth,* January 31, 2015, www.beautyliestruth.com/blog/2015/1/constance-and-me.

262 Jasenna Elikkottil, P. Gupta, and K. Gupta, "The Analgesic Potential of Cannabinoids," *Journal of Opioid Management* 5, no. 6 (2009): 341–357.

263 X. Yang, V. L. Hegde, R. Rao, J. Zhang, P. S. Nagarkatti, and M. Nagarkatti, "Histone Modifications Are Associated with 9-Tetrahydrocannabinol-mediated Alterations in Antigen-specific T Cell Responses," *Journal of Biological Chemistry* 289, no. 27 (2014): 18707–18718. doi:10.1074/jbc.m113.545210.

264 V. Maida and P. J. Daeninck, "A User's Guide to Cannabinoid Therapies in Oncology," *Current Oncology* 23.6 (2016): 398.

265 P. Massi, M. Solinas, V. Cinquina, and D. Parolaro, "Cannabidiol as Potential Anticancer Drug," *British Journal of Clinical Pharmacology* 75, no. 2 (2013): 303. doi:10.1111/j.1365-2125.2012.04298.x.

266 Jun'ichi Nakajima, Department of Pharmaceutical and Environmental Sciences, Tokyo Metropolitan Institute of Public Health, 3-23, Hyakunin-cho, Sinjuku-ku, Tokyo 169-0073, Japan.

267 Satoshi Yamaori, Yoshimi Okushima, Kazufumi Masuda, Mika Kushihara, Takashi Katsu, Shizuo Narimatsu, Ikuo Yamamoto, and Kazuhito

Watanabe, "Structural Requirements for Potent Direct Inhibition of Human Cytochrome P450 1A1 by Cannabidiol: Role of Pentylresorcinol Moiety," *Biological and Pharmaceutical Bulletin* 36, no. 7 (2013): 1197–11203. doi:10.1248/bpb.b13-00183.

268 D. Vara, M. Salazar, N. Olea-Herrero, M. Guzmán, G. Velasco, and I. Díaz-Laviada, "Anti-tumoral Effect of Cannabinoids on Hepatocellular Carcinoma: Role of AMPK Dependent Activation of Autophagy," *Cell Death and Differentiation* 18 (2011): 1099–1111.

269 P. Massi, M. Solinas, V. Cinquina, and D. Parolaro, "Cannabidiol as Potential Anticancer Drug," *British Journal of Clinical Pharmacology* 75, no. 2 (2013): 303–312. doi:10.1111/j.1365-2125.2012.04298.x.

270 Ido Efrati, "Israeli Doctors to Use Cannabis to Treat Autism in First-of-its-kind Study," *Haaretz*, August 29, 2016, www.haaretz.com/israel-news/science/1.739199.

271 Michael Backes, *Cannabis Pharmacy: A Practical Guide to Medicinal Marijuana* (New York: Black Dog & Leventhal Publishers, 2014).

272 Katherine Ann Scott, S. Shah, A.G. Dalgleish, and Wai Man Liu, "The Combination of Cannabidiol and {Delta}9-Tetrahydrocannabinol Enhances the Anticancer Effects of Radiation in an Orthotopic Murine Glioma Model," *Molecular Cancer Therapeutics* 13, no. 12 (2014): 2955–2967.

273 David Meiri, "Profiling Cannabis Spp anti-tumor effects in cancer," last modified July 31, 2016, http://dmeiri.net.technion.ac.il/research/cancer1/.

274 T. Yamada, T. Ueda, Y. Shibata, Y. Ikegami, M. Saito, Y. Ishida, S. Ugawa, K. Kohri, and S. Shimada, "TRPV2 Activation Induces Apoptotic Cell Death in Human T24 Bladder Cancer Cells: A Potential Therapeutic Target for Bladder Cancer," *Urology* 76, no. 2 (2010): 509.e1-7. doi:10.1016/j.urology.2010.03.029.

275 P. Massi, A. Vaccani, S. Ceruti, A. Colombo, M. P. Abbracchio, and D. Parolaro, "Antitumor Effects of Cannabidiol, A Nonpsychoactive Cannabinoid, on Human Glioma Cell Lines," *Journal of Pharmacology and Experimental Therapeutics* 308, no. 3 (2004): 838–845.

276 J. P. Marcu, R. T. Christian, D. Lau, A. J. Zielinski, M. P. Horowitz, J. Lee, A. Pakdel, J. Allison, C. Limbad, D. H. Moore, G. L. Yount, P. Y. Desprez, and S. D. McAllister, "Cannabidiol Enhances the Inhibitory Effects of Delta9-tetrahydrocannabinol on Human Glioblastoma Cell

Proliferation and Survival," *Molecular Cancer Therapeutics* 9, no. 1 (2010): 180. doi:10.1158/1535-7163.MCT-09-0407.

277 J. P. Marcu, R. T. Christian, D. Lau, A. J. Zielinski, M. P. Horowitz, J. Lee, A. Pakdel, J. Allison, C. Limbad, D. H. Moore, G. L. Yount, P. Y. Desprez, and S. D. McAllister, "Cannabidiol Enhances the Inhibitory Effects of Delta9-tetrahydrocannabinol on Human Glioblastoma Cell Proliferation and Survival," *Molecular Cancer Therapeutics* 9, no. 1 (2010): 17989. doi:10.1158/1535-7163.MCT-09-0407.

278 "GW Pharmaceuticals Achieves Positive Results in Phase 2 Proof of Concept Study in Glioma," GW Pharmeceuticals, Press Release, February 7, 2017, www.gwpharm.com/about-us/news/gw-pharmaceuticals-achieves -positive-results-phase-2-proof-concept-study-glioma.

279 F. C. Rocha, J. G. Dos Santos Júnior, S. C. Stefano, and D. X. da Silveira, "Systematic Review of the Literature on Clinical and Experimental Trials on the Antitumor Effects of Cannabinoids in Gliomas," *Journal of Neurooncology* 116, no. 1 (2014): 11–24. doi:10.1007/s11060-012276.

280 MedicalMarijuana.com.au, "Dr Cristina Sanchez PhD Cannabis and Cancer,"August3,2015,www.youtube.com/watch?v=rnVisZVZfHc&t=17s.

281 A. Ligresti, A. S. Moriello, K. Starowicz, I. Matias, S. Pisanti, L. De Petrocellis, C. Laezza, G. Portella, M. Bifulco, and V. Di Marzo, "Antitumor Activity of Plant Cannabinoids with Emphasis on the Effect of Cannabidiol on Human Breast Carcinoma," *Journal of Pharmacology and Experimental Therapeutics* 318, no. 3 (2006): 1375–1387.

282 María M. Caffarel, Clara Andradas, Emilia Mira, Eduardo Pérez-Gómez, Camilla Cerutti, Gema Moreno-Bueno, Juana M. Flores, Isabel García-Real, José Palacios, Santos Mañes, Manuel Guzmán, and Cristina Sánchez, "Cannabinoids Reduce ErbB2-Driven Breast Cancer Progression through Akt Inhibition," *Molecular Cancer* 9, no. 1 (2010): 196. doi:10.1186/1476-4598-896.

283 M. Elbaz, M. W. Nasser, J. Ravi, N. A. Wani, D. K. Ahirwar, H. Zhao, S. Oghumu, A. R. Satoskar, K. Shilo, W. E. Carson, and R. K. Ganju, "Modulation of the Tumor Microenvironment and Inhibition of EGF/ EGFR Pathway; Novel Anti-tumor Mechanisms of Cannabidiol in Breast Cancer," *Molecular Oncology* 9, no. 4 (2015): 906. doi:10.1016/j. molonc.2014.12.010.

284 MedicalMarijuana.com.au, "Dr Cristina Sanchez PhD Cannabis and Cancer,"August3,2015,www.youtube.com/watch?v=rnVisZVZfHc&t=17s.

285 David Gorski, "Medical Marijuana as the New Herbalism Part 3: A 'Cannabis Cures Cancer Testimonial,'" *Science-Based Medicine,* March 16, 2015, https://sciencebasedmedicine.org/medical-marijuana-as-the-new -herbalism-part-3-a-cannabis-cures-cancer-testimonial/.

286 Gabriella Aviello, Barbara Romano, Francesca Borrelli, Raffaele Capasso, Laura Gallo, Fabiana Piscitelli, Vincenzo Di Marzo, and Angelo A. Izzo, "Chemopreventive Effect of the Non-psychotropic Phytocannabinoid Cannabidiol on Experimental Colon Cancer," *Journal of Molecular Medicine* 90, no. 8 (2012): 925. doi:10.1007/s00109-011-0856-x.

287 Luke Sumpter, "Man Cures Colon Cancer with Cannabis Oil," *Reset. me,* July 10, 2015, http://reset.me/story/man-cures-colon-cancer-with -cannabis-oil/.

288 M. Bifulco, A. M. Malfitano, S. Pisanti, and C. Laezza, "Endocannabinoids in Endocrine and Related Tumours," *Endocrine-Related Cancer* 15, no. 2 (2008): 391. doi:10.1677/ERC-07-0258.

289 Y. Maor, J. Yu, P. M. Kuzontkoski, B. J. Dezube, X. Zhang, and J. E. Groopman, "Cannabidiol Inhibits Growth and Induces Programmed Cell Death in Kaposi Sarcoma-Associated Herpesvirus-Infected Endothelium," *Genes Cancer* 3, no. 7–8 (2012): 512. doi:10.1177/1947601912466556.

290 Katherine Ann Scott, S. Shah, A.G. Dalgleish, and Wai Man Liu, "The Combination of Cannabidiol and {Delta}9-Tetrahydrocannabinol Enhances the Anticancer Effects of Radiation in an Orthotopic Murine Glioma Model," *Molecular Cancer Therapeutics* 13, no. 12 (2014): 2955–2967.

291 R. Ramer, K. Heinemann, J. Merkord, H. Rohde, A. Salamon, M. Linnebacher, and B. Hinz, "COX-2 and PPAR-▨ Confer Cannabidiol-Induced Apoptosis of Human Lung Cancer Cells," *Molecular Cancer Therapeutics* 12, no. 1 (2013): 69–82. doi:10.1158/1535-7163.MCT-12-0335.

292 Lincoln Horsley, "The Sharon Kelly Story: How She Beat Her Lung Cancer with Cannabis," *Cure Your Own Cancer,* last modified January 8, 2015, www.cureyourowncancer.org/the-sharon-kelly-story-how-she-beat -her-lung-cancer-with-cannabis-oil.html#sthash.pPXwJz61.dpuf.

293 P. Pacher, "Towards the Use of Non-psychoactive Cannabinoids for Prostate Cancer," *British Journal of Pharmacology* 168, no. 1 (2013): 76–78. doi: 10.1111/j.1476-5381.2012.02121.x.

294 M. Sharma, J. Hudson, H. Adomat, E. Guns, and M. Cox, "In Vitro Anti-cancer Activity of Plant-Derived Cannabidiol on Prostate Cancer

Cell Lines," *Pharmacology & Pharmacy* 5 (2014): 806. doi:10.4236/pp.2014.58091.

295 Dennis Hill, "Dennis Hill's Story: Beating Prostate Cancer with Cannabis Oil," *Cure Your Own Cancer,* last modified October 20, 2013, www.cureyourowncancer.org/dennis-hills-story-beating-prostate-cancer-with-cannabis-oil.html.

296 "Is Cannabis Oil a Viable Treatment for Skin Cancer?" *United Patients Group,* last modified July 15, 2014, https://unitedpatientsgroup.com/blog/2014/07/15/is-cannabis-oil-a-viable-treatment-for-skin-cancer.

297 B. Adinolfi, A. Romanini, A. Vanni, E. Martinotti, A. Chicca, S. Fogli, and P. Nieri, "Anticancer Activity of Anandamide in Human Cutaneous Melanoma Cells," European *Journal of Pharmacology* 718, no. 1–3 (2013): 154–159. doi:10.1016/j.ejphar.2013.08.039.

298 "Is Cannabis Oil a Viable Treatment for Skin Cancer?" *United Patients Group,* last modified July 15, 2014, https://unitedpatientsgroup.com/blog/2014/07/15/is-cannabis-oil-a-viable-treatment-for-skin-cancer.

299 "Cannabis and Cannabinoids," *National Cancer Institute,* last modified July 15, 2015, www.cancer.gov/about-cancer/treatment/cam/patient/cannabis-pdq.

300 L. A. Parker, E. M. Rock, and C. L. Limbeer, "Regulation of Nausea and Vomiting by Cannabinoids," *British Journal of Pharmacology* 163, no. 7 (August 2011): 1411–1422.

301 F. C. Machado Rocha, S. C. Stefano, R. De Cassia Haiek, L. M. Rosa Oliveira, and D. X. Da Silveira, "Therapeutic Use of *Cannabis sativa* on Chemotherapy-Induced Nausea and Vomiting among Cancer Patients: Systematic Review and Meta-analysis," *European Journal of Cancer Care* 17, no. 5 (September 2008): 431–443.

302 J. R. Johnson, M. Burnell-Nugent, D. Lossignol, E. D. Ganae-Motan, R. Potts, and M. T. Fallon, "Multicenter, Double-Blind, Randomized, Placebo-Controlled, Parallel-Group Study of the Efficacy, Safety, and Tolerability of THC:CBD Extract and THC Extract in Patients with Intractable Cancer-Related Pain," *Journal of Pain and Symptom Management* 39, no. 2 (February 2010): 167–179.

303 T. D. Brisbois, I. H. de Kock, S. M. Watanabe, M. Mirhosseini, D. C. Lamoureux, M. Chasen, N. MacDonald, V. E. Baracos, and W. V. Wismer, "Delta-9-tetrahydrocannabinol May Palliate Altered Chemosensory Perception in Cancer Patients: Results of a Randomized-Double-Blind,

Placebo-Controlled Pilot Trial," *Annals of Oncology* 22 (February 2011): 2086–2093.

304 S. H. Burstein and R. B. Zurier, "Cannabinoids, Endocannabinoids, and Related Analogs in Inflammation," *The AAPS Journal* 11, no. 1 (March 2009): 109–119.

305 G. Bar-Sela, M. Vorobeichik, S. Drawsheh, A. Omer, V. Goldberg, and E. Muller, "The Medical Necessity for Medicinal Cannabis: Prospective, Observational Study Evaluating the Treatment in Cancer Patients on Supportive or Palliative Care," *Evidence-Based Complementary and Alternative Medicine* 2013 (2013): 510392, www.hindawi.com/journals/ecam/2013/510392/.

306 T. D. Brisbois, I. H. de Kock, S. M. Watanabe, M. Mirhosseini, D. C. Lamoureux, M. Chasen, N. MacDonald, V. E. Baracos, and W. V. Wismer, "Delta-9-tetrahydrocannabinol May Palliate Altered Chemosensory Perception in Cancer Patients: Results of a Randomized-Double-Blind, Placebo-Controlled Pilot Trial," *Annals of Oncology* 22 (February 2011): 2086–2093.

307 Derick T. Wade, Philip Robson, Heather House, Petra Makela, and Julia Aram, "A Preliminary Controlled Study to Determine Whether Whole-Plant Cannabis Extracts Can Improve Intractable Neurogenic Symptoms," *Clinical Rehabilitation* 17, no. 1 (2003): 21–29. doi:10.1191/0269215503cr581oa.

308 M. Kwiatkoski, F. S. Guimarães, and E. Del-Bel, "Cannabidiol-Treated Rats Exhibited Higher Motor Score after Cryogenic Spinal Cord Injury," *Neurotoxicity Research* 21, no. 3 (2012): 271–280. doi:10.1007/s12640-011-9273-8.

309 D. Fernández-López, I. Lizasoain, M. A. Moro, and J. Martínez-Orgado, "Cannabinoids: Well-Suited Candidates for the Treatment of Perinatal Brain Injury," *Brain Sciences* 3, no. 3 (2013): 1043.

310 Jack Kaskey, "NFL Marijuana Policy in Spotlight as Former Players Push for Opioid Alternative," February 3, 2017, www.thecannabist.co/2017/02/03/nfl-marijuana-policy-alternative-to-opiods/73040/.

311 B. Wilsey, T. D. Marcotte, R. Deutsch, H. Zhao, H. Prasad, and A. Phan, "An Exploratory Human Laboratory Experiment Evaluating Vaporized Cannabis in the Treatment of Neuropathic Pain from Spinal Cord Injury and Disease," *Journal of Pain* 17, no. 9 (2016): 982. doi:10.1016/j.jpain.2016.05.010.

312 McGill University, "Cannabis: Potent Anti-depressant In Low Doses, Worsens Depression At High Doses," *ScienceDaily*, October 24, 2007.

313 M. N. Hill, C. J. Hillard, F. R. Bambico, S. Patel, B. B. Gorzalka, and G. Gobbi, "The Therapeutic Potential of the Endocannabinoid System for the Development of a Novel Class of Antidepressants," *Trends in Pharmacological Sciences* 30, no. 9 (2009): 484–493. doi:10.1016/j.tips.2009.06.006.

314 R. Linge, L. Jiménez-Sánchez, L. Campa, F. Pilar-Cuéllar, R. Vidal, A. Pazos, and A. Adell Díaz, "Cannabidiol Induces Rapid-Acting Antidepressant-Like Effects and Enhances Cortical 5-HT/Glutamate Neurotransmission: Role of 5-HT1A Receptors," *Neuropharmacology* 103 (2016): 16. doi:10.1016/j.neuropharm.2015.12.017.

315 Samir Haj-Dahmane and Roh-Yu Shen, "Endocannabinoid Signaling and the Regulation of the Serotonin System," in *Endocannabinoid Regulation of Monoamines in Psychiatric and Neurological Disorders,* ed. Elisabeth J. Van Bockstaele (New York: Springer, 2013), 239–254. doi:10.1007/977-4614-7940-6_11.

316 M. N. Hill, C. J. Hillard, F. R. Bambico, S. Patel, B. B. Gorzalka, and G. Gobbi, "The Therapeutic Potential of the Endocannabinoid System for the Development of a Novel Class of Antidepressants," *Trends in Pharmacological Sciences* 30, no. 9 (2009): 484–493. doi:10.1016/j.tips.2009.06.006.

317 C. H. Ashton, P. B. Moore, P. Gallagher, and A. H. Young, "Cannabinoids in Bipolar Affective Disorder: A Review and Discussion of Their Therapeutic Potential," *Journal of Psychopharmacology* 19, no. 3 (2005): 293–300.

318 A. Zuardi, J. Crippa, S. Dursun, S. Morais, J. Vilela, R. Sanches, and J. Hallak, "Cannabidiol Was Ineffective for Manic Episode of Bipolar Affective Disorder," *Journal of Psychopharmacology* 24, no. 1 (2010): 135–137. doi:10.1177/0269881108096521.

319 Abir T. El-Alfy, Kelly Ivey, Keisha Robinson, Safwat Ahmed, Mohamed Radwan, Desmond Slade, Ikhlas Khan, Mahmoud ElSohly, and Samir Ross, "Antidepressant-Like Effect of Δ9-tetrahydrocannabinol and Other Cannabinoids Isolated from *Cannabis sativa*," *Journal of Pharmacology, Biochemistry and Behavior* 95, no. 4 (June 2010): 434–442.

320 A. R. de Mello Schier, N. P. de Oliveira Ribeiro, D. S. Coutinho, S. Machado, O. Arias-Carrión, J. A. Crippa, A. W. Zuardi, A. E. Nardi, and A. C. Silva, "Antidepressant-Like and Anxiolytic-Like Effects of Cannabidiol:

A Chemical Compound of *Cannabis sativa*," *CNS Neurol Disorders – Drug Targets* 13, no. 6 (2014): 953–960.

321 Michael Moskowitz MD, personal communication with the authors, February 2, 2017.

322 V. Di Marzo, F. Piscitelli, and R. Mechoulam, "Cannabinoids and Endocannabinoids in Metabolic Disorders with Focus on Diabetes," in *Handbook of Experimental Pharmacology* (New York: Springer, 2011), 75. doi:10.1007/978-3-6417214-4_4.

323 E. A. Penner, H. Buettner, and M. A. Mittleman, "The Impact of Marijuana Use on Glucose, Insulin, and Insulin Resistance among US Adults," *The American Journal of Medicine* 126, iss. 7 (2013): 583–589.

324 "CBD Compound in Cannabis Could Treat Diabetes, Researchers Suggest," *Diabetes News,* April 24, 2015, www.diabetes.co.uk/news/2015 /apr/cbd-compound-in-cannabis-could-treat-diabetes,-researchers -suggest-95335970.html.

325 V. Di Marzo, "The Endocannabinoid System in Obesity and Type 2 Diabetes," *Diabetologia* 51, no. 8 (2008): 1356–1367. doi:10.1007/s00125-007048-2.

326 L. Weiss, M. Zeira, S. Reich, M. Har-Noy, R. Mechoulam, S. Slavin, and R. Gallily. "Cannabidiol Lowers Incidence of Diabetes in Non-obese Diabetic Mice," *Autoimmunity* 39.2 (2006): 143–151.

327 M. Rajesh, P. Mukhopadhyay, S. Bátkai, V. Patel, K. Saito, S. Matsumoto, Y. Kashiwaya, B. Horváth, B. Mukhopadhyay, L. Becker, G. Haskó, L. Liaudet, D. A. Wink, A. Veves, R. Mechoulam, and P. Pacher, "Cannabidiol Attenuates Cardiac Dysfunction, Oxidative Stress, Fibrosis, Inflammatory and Cell Death Signaling Pathways in Diabetic Cardiomyopathy," *Journal of the American College of Cardiology* 56, no. 25 (December 14, 2010): 2115.

328 Natasha Devon, "Obesity is an Eating Disorder Just like Anorexia and It's Time We Started Treating It That Way," *The Independent,* last modified February 23, 2016, www.independent.co.uk/voices/obesity-is-an-eating -disorder-just-like-anorexia-and-its-time-we-started-treating-it-that-way -a6891166.html.

329 M. Scherma, L. Fattore, M. P. Castelli, W. Fratta, and P. Fadda, "The Role of the Endocannabinoid System in Eating Disorders: Neurochemical and Behavioural Preclinical Evidence," *Current Pharmaceutical Design* 20, no. 13 (2014): 2089–2099.

330 J. A. Farrimond, B. J. Whalley, and C. M. Williams, "Cannabinol and Cannabidiol Exert Opposing Effects on Rat Feeding

Patterns," *Psychopharmacology* 223, no. 1 (2012): 117–129. doi:10.1007/s00213-012-2697-x.

331 H. J. Parray and J. W. Yun, "Cannabidiol Promotes Browning in 3T3-L1 Adipocytes," *Molecular and Cellular Biochemistry* 416 (2016): 131.

332 R. W. Gorter, "Cancer Cachexia and Cannabinoids," *Forsch Komplementarmed* 6, suppl. 3 (1991): 21–22.

333 A. Andries, J. Frystyk, A. Flyvbjerg, and R. K. Støving, "Dronabinol in Severe, Enduring Anorexia Nervosa: A Randomized Controlled Trial," *International Journal of Eating Disorders* 47 (2014): 18–23. doi:10.1002/eat.22173.

334 Kelly Mickle, "Can Marijuana Really Help Treat Anorexia?" *Cosmopolitan,* June 23, 2015, www.cosmopolitan.com/health-fitness/news/a42398/marijuana-anorexia/.

335 Michael Backes, *Cannabis Pharmacy: A Practical Guide to Medicinal Marijuana* (New York: Black Dog & Leventhal Publishers, 2014).

336 P. Monteleone, M. Bifulco, C. Di Filippo, P. Gazzerro, B. Canestrelli, F. Monteleone, M. C. Proto, M. Di Genio, C. Grimaldi, and M. Maj, "Association of CNR1 and FAAH Endocannabinoid Gene Polymorphisms with Anorexia Nervosa and Bulimia Nervosa: Evidence for Synergistic Effects," *Genes, Brain and Behavior* 8 (2009): 728–732. doi:10.1111/j.160083X.2009.00518.x.

337 F. Borrelli, G. Aviello, B. Romano, P. Orlando, R. Capasso, F. Maiello, F. Guadagno, S. Petrosino, F. Capasso, V. Di Marzo, and A. A. Izzo, "Cannabidiol, a Safe and Non-psychotropic Ingredient of the Marijuana Plant *Cannabis sativa,* Is Protective in a Murine Model of Colitis," *Journal of Molecular Medicine* 87, no. 11 (2009): 1111–1121. doi:10.1007/s00109-009-0512-x.

338 H. Shamran, N. P. Singh, E. E. Zumbrun, A. Murphy, D. D. Taub, M. K. Mishra, R. L. Price, S. Chatterjee, M. Nagarkatti, P. S. Nagarkatti, and U. P. Singh, "Fatty Acid Amide Hydrolase (FAAH) Blockade Ameliorates Experimental Colitis by Altering MicroRNA Expression and Suppressing Inflammation," *Brain, Behavior, and Immunity* 59 (2017):10–20. doi:10.1016/j.bbi.2016.06.008.

339 Ibid.

340 K. A. Sharkey and J. W. Wiley, "The Role of the Endocannabinoid System in the Brain-Gut Axis," *Gastroenterology* 151, no. 2 (2016): 252–266. doi:10.1053/j.gastro.2016.04.015.

341 Michael Backes, *Cannabis Pharmacy: A Practical Guide to Medicinal Marijuana* (New York: Black Dog & Leventhal Publishers, 2014).

342 Michael Backes, *Cannabis Pharmacy: A Practical Guide to Medicinal Marijuana* (New York: Black Dog & Leventhal Publishers, 2014).

343 R. Schicho and M. Storr, "Topical and Systemic Cannabidiol Improves Trinitrobenzene Sulfonic Acid Colitis in Mice," *Pharmacology* 89, no. 3–4 (2012): 149–155. doi:10.1159/000336871.

344 G. Esposito, D. D. Filippis, C. Cirillo, T. Iuvone, E. Capoccia, C. Scuderi, A. Steardo, R. Cuomo, and L. Steardo, "Cannabidiol in Inflammatory Bowel Diseases: A Brief Overview," *Phytotherapy Research* 27, no. 5 (2013): 633–636. doi:10.1002/ptr.4781.

345 Ibid.

346 Migraine Research Foundation, "Migraine Facts," last modified March 3, 2017, https://migraineresearchfoundation.org/about-migraine/migraine -facts/.

347 Headache Classification Subcommittee of the International Headache Society, "The International Classification of Headache Disorders: 2nd edition," *Cephalalgia* 24, suppl. 1 (2004): 9–160. doi:10.1111/j.1468-2982.2004.00653.x.

348 Ibid.

349 J. D. Bartleson and F. M. Cutrer, "Migraine Update. Diagnosis and Treatment," *Minnesota Medical* 93, no. 5 (May 2010): 36–41.

350 Migraine Research Foundation, "Migraine Facts," last modified March 3, 2017. https://migraineresearchfoundation.org/about-migraine/migraine-facts/.

351 Allan Frankel, MD, "Treating Migraines with Cannabidiol," *Frankelly Speaking*, last modified February 26, 2016, www.greenbridgemed.com /treating-migraines-with-cannabidiol/.

352 Ibid.

353 Headache Classification Subcommittee of the International Headache Society, "The International Classification of Headache Disorders: 2nd edition," *Cephalalgia* 24, suppl. 1 (2004): 9–160. doi:10.1111 /j.1468-2982.2004.00653.x.

354 David Baker, Gareth Pryce, Samuel J. Jackson, Chris Bolton, and Gavin Giovannoni, "The Biology That Underpins the Therapeutic Potential of Cannabis-Based Medicines for the Control of Spasticity in Multiple Sclerosis," *Multiple Sclerosis and Related Disorders* 1, iss. 2 (2012): 64.

355 C. Perras, "Sativex for the Management of Multiple Sclerosis Symptoms," *Issues in Emerging Health Technologies* 72 (2005): 1–4.

356 J. Sastre-Garriga, C. Vila, S. Clissold, and X. Montalban, "THC and CBD Oromucosal Spray (Sativex®) in the Management of Spasticity Associated with Multiple Sclerosis," *Expert Review of Neurotherapeutics* 11, no. 5 (2011): 627–637. doi:10.1586/ern.11.47.

357 "Seven Things You Need to Know About Sativex," *Leaf Science*, March 8, 2014, www.leafscience.com/2014/03/08/7-things-need-know-sativex/.

358 Linda A. Parker, Erin M. Rock, and Cheryl L. Limebeer, "Regulation of Nausea and Vomiting by Cannabinoids," *British Journal of Pharmacology* 163, no. 7 (2011): 1411–1422, http://doi.org/10.1111/j.1476-5381.2010.01176.x.

359 L. A. Parker, R. Mechoulam, and C. Schlievert, "Cannabidiol, a Non-psychoactive Component of Cannabis and Its Synthetic Dimethylheptyl Homolog Suppress Nausea in an Experimental Model with Rats," *NeuroReport* 13, no. 5 (2002): 567–570.

360 Linda A. Parker, Erin M. Rock, and Cheryl L. Limebeer, "Regulation of Nausea and Vomiting by Cannabinoids," *British Journal of Pharmacology* 163, no. 7 (2011): 1411–1422, http://doi.org/10.1111/j.1476-5381.2010.01176.x.

361 Ibid.

362 Megan B. May and Ashley E. Glode, "Dronabinol for Chemotherapy-Induced Nausea and Vomiting Unresponsive to Antiemetics," *Cancer Management and Research* 8 (2016): 49–55. doi:10.2147/CMAR.S81425.

363 Linda A. Parker, Erin M. Rock, and Cheryl L. Limebeer, "Regulation of Nausea and Vomiting by Cannabinoids," *British Journal of Pharmacology* 163, no. 7 (2011): 1411–1422, http://doi.org/10.1111/j.1476-5381.2010.01176.x.

364 S. V. More and D. K. Choi, "Promising Cannabinoid-Based Therapies for Parkinson's Disease: Motor Symptoms to Neuroprotection," *Molecular Neurodegeneration* 10 (April 2015): 17.

365 V. K. da Silva, B. S. de Freitas, A. da Silva Dornelles, L. R. Nery, L. Falavigna, R. D. Ferreira, M. R. Bogo, J. E. Hallak, A. W. Zuardi, J. A. Crippa, and N. Schroder, "Cannabidiol Normalizes Caspase 3, Synaptophysin, and Mitochondrial Fission Protein DNM1L Expression Levels in Rats with Brain Iron Overload: Implications for Neuroprotection," *Molecular Neurobiology* 49, no. 1 (February 2014): 222–233.

366 S. V. More and D. K. Choi, "Promising Cannabinoid-Based Therapies for Parkinson's Disease: Motor Symptoms to Neuroprotection," *Molecular Neurodegeneration* 10 (April 2015): 17.

367 A. W. Zuardi, J. A. Crippa, J. E. Hallak, J. P. Pinto, M. H. Chagas, G. G. Rodrigues, S. M. Dursun, and V. Tumas, "Cannabidiol for the Treatment

of Psychosis in Parkinson's Disease," *Journal of Psychopharmacology* 23, no. 8 (November 2009): 979–983.

368 M. L. Zeissler, J. Eastwood, C. O. Hanemann, J. Zajicek, and C. Carroll, "9-tetrahydrocannabinol Is Protective through PPARy Dependent Mitochondrial Biogenesis in a Cell Culture Model of Parkinson's Disease," *Journal of Neurology, Neurosurgery and Psychiatry,* 84, no. 11 (2013): e2.

369 I. Lotan, T. A. Treves, Y. Roditi, and R. Djaldetti, "Cannabis (Medical Marijuana) Treatment for Motor and Non-motor Symptoms of Parkinson Disease: An Open-Label Observational Study," *Clinical Neuropharmacology* 37, no. 2 (March–April 2014): 41–44.

370 M. Garcia-Arencibia, C. Garcia, and J. Fernandez-Ruiz, "Cannabinoids and Parkinson's Disease," *CNS & Neurological Disorders Drug Targets* 8, no. 6 (December 2009): 432–439.

371 I. Lastres-Becker and J. Fernandez-Ruiz, "An Overview of Parkinson's Disease and the Cannabinoid System and Possible Benefits of Cannabinoid-Based Treatments," *Current Medicinal Chemistry* 13, no. 30 (2006): 3705–3718.

372 M. H. Chagas, A. W. Zuardi, V. Tumas, M. A. Pena-Pereira, E. T. Sobreira, M. M. Bergamaschi, A. C. dos Santos, A. L. Teixeira, J. E. Hallak, and J. A. Crippa, "Effects of Cannabidiol in the Treatment of Patients with Parkinson's Disease: An Exploratory Double-Blind Trial," *Journal of Psychopharmacology* 29, no. 11 (November 2014): 1088–1098.

373 J. A. S. Crippa, J. E. C. Hallak, J. P. Machado-De-Sousa, R. H. C. Queiroz, M. Bergamaschi, M. H. N. Chagas, and A. W. Zuardi, "Cannabidiol for the Treatment of Cannabis Withdrawal Syndrome: A Case Report," *Journal of Clinical Pharmacy and Therapeutics* 38, no. 2 (2012): 162–164. doi:10.1111/jcpt.12018.

374 Onintza Sagredo, M. Ruth Pazos, Valentina Satta, José A. Ramos, Roger G. Pertwee, and Javier Fernández-Ruiz, "Neuroprotective Effects of Phytocannabinoid-Based Medicines in Experimental Models of Huntington's Disease," *Journal of Neuroscience Research* 89, no. 9 (2011): 1509–1518. doi:10.1002/jnr.22682.

375 Ibid.

376 Sara Valdeolivas, Carmen Navarrete, Irene Cantarero, María L. Bellido, Eduardo Muñoz, and Onintza Sagredo, "Neuroprotective Properties of Cannabigerol in Huntington's Disease: Studies in R6/2 Mice and 3-Nitropropionate-lesioned Mice," *Neurotherapeutics* 12, no. 1 (2014): 185–199. doi:10.1007/s13311-014-0304-z.

377 Carey Wedler, "Former Cop Tries Cannabis as Last Resort to Treat Par-
     kinson's Disease," *Antimedia.org*, December 1, 2016, http://theantimedia
     .org/former-cop-cannabis-parkinsons-disease/.

378 A. W. Zuardi, J. A. Crippa, J. E. Hallak, J. P. Pinto, M. H. Chagas, G. G.
     Rodrigues, S. M. Dursun, and V. Tumas, "Cannabidiol for the Treatment
     of Psychosis in Parkinson's Disease," *Journal of Psychopharmacology* 23, no.
     8 (November 2009): 979–983.

379 C. García, C. Palomo-Garo, M. García-Arencibia, J. Ramos, R. Pert-
     wee, and J. Fernández-Ruiz, "Symptom-Relieving and Neuroprotective
     Effects of the Phytocannabinoid Δ9-THCV in Animal Models of Parkin-
     son's Disease," *British Journal of Pharmacology* 163, no. 7 (2011): 1495.
     doi:10.1111/j.1476-5381.2011.01278.x.

380 J. Fernández-Ruiz, M. Moreno-Martet, C. Rodríguez-Cueto, C. Palomo-
     Garo, M. Gómez-Cañas, S. Valdeolivas, C. Guaza, J. Romero, M. Guzmán,
     R. Mechoulam, and J. A. Ramos, "Prospects for Cannabinoid Therapies
     in Basal Ganglia Disorders," *British Journal of Pharmacology* 163, no. 7
     (2011): 1365–1378. doi:10.1111/j.1476-5381.2011.01365.x.

381 H. Javed, S. Azimullah, M. E. Haque, and S. K. Ojha, "Cannabinoid Type
     2 (CB2) Receptors Activation Protects against Oxidative Stress and Neu-
     roinflammation Associated Dopaminergic Neurodegeneration in Rote-
     none Model of Parkinson's Disease," *Frontiers in Neuroscience* 10 (2016):
     321. doi:10.3389/fnins.2016.00321.

382 J. Russell Reynolds, "On Some of the Therapeutical Uses of Indian
     Hemp," in *Archives of Medicine,* vol. 2 (London, 1859), 154.

383 R. Greco, V. Gasperi, M. Maccarrone, and C. Tassorelli, "The Endocannabi-
     noid System and Migraine," *Experimental Neurololgy* 224, no. 1 (2010): 85–91.
     doi:10.1016/j.expneurol.2010.03.029.

384 Ethan Russo and Andrea Hohmann, "Role of Cannabinoids in Pain
     Management," in *Comprehensive Treatment of Chronic Pain by Medical, Inter-
     ventional and Integrative Approaches,* ed. Timothy R. Deer et al. (New York:
     Springer, 2013), 181–197.

385 "Testimonials," *No High CBD Oil,* last modified March 8, 2017, http://
     nohighcbdoil.weebly.com/testimonials.html.

386 E. B. Russo, "Cannabinoids in the Management of Difficult to Treat
     Pain," *Journal of Therapeutics and Clinical Risk Management* 4, no. 1 (2008):
     245–259.

387 S. Maione, F. Piscitelli, L. Gatta, D. Vita, L. De Petrocellis, E. Palazzo,
     V. de Novellis, and V. Di Marzo, "Non-psychoactive Cannabinoids

Modulate the Descending Pathway of Antinociception in Anaesthetized Rats through Several Mechanisms of Action," *British Journal of Phramacology* 162, no. 3 (2011): 584. doi:10.1111/j.1476-5381.2010.01063.x.

388 W. Xiong, T. Cui, K. Cheng, F. Yang, S. R. Chen, D. Willenbring, Y. Guan, H. L. Pan, K. Ren, Y. Xu, and L. Zhang, "Cannabinoids Suppress Inflammatory and Neuropathic Pain by Targeting α3 Glycine Receptors," *Journal of Experimental Medicine* 209, no. 6 (2012): 1121–1134. doi:10.1084/jem.20120242.

389 M. DeGeorge, E. Dawson, P. Woster, L. Burke, and K. Bronstein, *An Analysis of the Association between Marijuana Use and Potential Nonadherence in Patients Prescribed Hydrocodon* (Baltimore: Ameritox, 2013), www.ameritox.com/wp-content/uploads/Ananalysisoftheassociationbetweenmarijuanauseandpotentialnonadherence_AAPM2013.pdf.

390 M. N. Hill, L. M. Bierer, I. Makotkine, J. A. Golier, S. Galea, B. S. McEwen, C. J. Hillard, and R. Yehuda, "Reductions in Circulating Endocannabinoid Levels in Individuals with Post-traumatic Stress Disorder Following Exposure to the World Trade Center Attacks," *Psychoneuroendocrinology* 38, no. 12 (2013): 2952. doi:10.1016/j.psyneuen.2013.08.004.

391 Elizabeth Limbach, *Cannabis Saved My Life: Stories of Hope and Healing* (Whitman Publishing, 2016), 116.

392 J. Renard, M. Loureiro, L. G. Rosen, J. Zunder, C. de Oliveira, S. Schmid, W. J. Rushlow, and S. R. Laviolette, "Cannabidiol Counteracts Amphetamine-Induced Neuronal and Behavioral Sensitization of the Mesolimbic Dopamine Pathway through a Novel mTOR/p70S6 Kinase Signaling Pathway," *Journal of Neuroscience* 36, no. 18 (2016): 5160. doi:10.1523/JNEUROSCI.33865.2016.

393 Maia Szalavitz, "Marijuana Compound Treats Schizophrenia with Few Side Effets: Clinical Trial," *Time*, May 30, 2012, http://healthland.time.com/2012/05/30/marijuana-compound-treats-schizophrenia-with-few-side-effects-clinical-trial/.

394 Ibid.

395 F. M. Leweke, D. Piomelli, F. Pahlisch, D. Muhl, C. W. Gerth, C. Hoyer, J. Klosterkötter, M. Hellmich, and D. Koethe, "Cannabidiol Enhances Anandamide Signaling and Alleviates Psychotic Symptoms of Schizophrenia," *Translational Psychiatry* 2 (2012): e94. doi:10.1038/tp.2012.15.

396 J. Renard, M. Loureiro, L. G. Rosen, J. Zunder, C. de Oliveira, S. Schmid, W. J. Rushlow, and S. R. Laviolette, "Cannabidiol Counteracts

Amphetamine-Induced Neuronal and Behavioral Sensitization of the Mesolimbic Dopamine Pathway through a Novel mTOR/p70S6 Kinase Signaling Pathway," *Journal of Neuroscience* 36, no. 18 (2016): 5160. doi:10.1523/JNEUROSCI.33865.2016.

397 C. D. Schubart, I. E. Sommer, W. A. van Gastel, R. L. Goetgebuer, R. S. Kahn, and M. P. Boks, "Cannabis with High Cannabidiol Content Is Associated with Fewer Psychotic Experiences," *Schizophrenia Research* 130, no. 1–3 (2011): 216–221. doi:10.1016/j.schres.2011.04.017.

398 A. W. Zuardi, J. A. Crippa, J. E. Hallak, S. Bhattacharyya, Z. Atakan, R. Martin-Santos, P. K. McGuire, and F. S. Guimarães, "A Critical Review of the Antipsychotic Effects of Cannabidiol: 30 Years of a Translational Investigation," *Current Pharmaceutical Design* 18, no. 32 (2012): 5131.

399 Selina McKee, "GW Pharma's Cannabinoid Shows Schizophrenia Promise," *PharmaTimes* online, September 15, 2015, www.pharmatimes.com/news /gw_pharmas_cannabinoid_shows_schizophrenia_promise_971897.

400 Elizabeth Limbach, *Cannabis Saved My Life: Stories of Hope and Healing* (Whitman Publishing, 2016), 142.

401 Indalecio Lozano, "The Therapeutic Use of Cannabis Sativa in Arabic Medicine," *Journal of Cannabis Therapeutics* 1, no. 1 (2001): 63–70.

402 Shyanshree S. Manna and Sudhir N. Umathe, "Involvement of Transient Receptor Potential Vanilloid Type 1 Channels in the Pro-convulsant Effect of Anandamide in Pentylenetetrazole-Induced Seizures," *Epilepsy Research* 100, no. 1 (2012): 113–124.

403 Michael Backes, *Cannabis Pharmacy: A Practical Guide to Medicinal Marijuana* (New York: Black Dog & Leventhal Publishers, 2014).

404 Bonni Goldstein, *Medical Cannabis: Practical Treatment of Pediatric Patients for Epilepsy, Autism, Cancer, and Psychiatric Disorders* (presentation, CannMed Harvard Conference, 2016), www.medicinalgenomics.com/wp -content/uploads/2016/05/Bonni-Goldstein-CannMed2016.pdf.

405 M. Tzadok, S. Uliel-Siboni, I. Linder, U. Kramer, O. Epstein, S. Menascu, A. Nissenkorn, O. B. Yosef, E. Hyman, D. Granot, M. Dor, T. Lerman-Sagie, and B. Ben-Zeev, "CBD-Enriched Medical Cannabis for Intractable Pediatric Epilepsy: The Current Israeli Experience," *Seizure* 35 (2016): 41–44. doi:10.1016/j.seizure.2016.01.004.

406 "GW Pharmaceuticals Announces Second Positive Phase 3 Pivotal Trial for Epidiolex (cannabidiol) in the Treatment of Lennox-Gastaut Syndrome,"

Globe Newswire, September 26, 2016, https://globenewswire.com /news-release/2016/09/26/874464/0/en/GW-Pharmaceuticals -Announces-Second-Positive-Phase-3-Pivotal-Trial-for-Epidiolex -cannabidiol-in-the-Treatment-of-Lennox-Gastaut-Syndrome.html.

407 T. Bíró, B. I. Tóth, G. Haskó, R. Paus, and P. Pacher, "The Endocannabinoid System of the Skin in Health and Disease: Novel Perspectives and Therapeutic Opportunities," *Trends in Pharmacological Science* 30, no. 8 (2009): 411–420. doi:10.1016/j.tips.2009.05.004.

408 S. Ständer, H. W. Reinhardt, and T. A. Luger, "Topical Cannabinoid Agonists. An Effective New Possibility for Treating Chronic Pruritus," *Hautarzt* 57, no. 9 (2006): 801–807.

409 M. Karsak, E. Gaffal, R. Date, L. Wang-Eckhardt, J. Rehnelt, S. Petrosino, K. Starowicz, R. Steuder, E. Schlicker, B. Cravatt, R. Mechoulam, R. Buettner, S. Werner, V. Di Marzo, T. Tüting, and Z. Zimmer, "Attenuation of Allergic Contact Dermatitis through the Endocannabinoid System," *Science* 316 (2007): 1494–1497.

410 J. D. Wilkinson and E. M. Williamson, "Cannabinoids Inhibit Human Keratinocyte Proliferation through a Non-CB1/CB2 Mechanism and Have a Potential Therapeutic Value in the Treatment of Psoriasis," *Journal of Dermatological Science* 45 (2007): 92.

411 Gooey Rabinski, "Treating Psoriasis with Topical Cannabis," *Whaxy,* last modified February 22, 2016.

412 A. Oláh, B. I. Tóth, I. Borbíró, K. Sugawara, A. G. Szöllõsi, G. Czifra, B. Pál, L. Ambrus, J. Kloepper, E. Camera, M. Ludovici, M. Picardo, T. Voets, C. C. Zouboulis, R. Paus, and T. Bíró, "Cannabidiol Exerts Sebostatic and Antiinflammatory Effects on Human Sebocytes," *Journal of Clinical Investigation* 124, no. 9 (2014): 3713. doi:10.1172/JCI64628.

413 J. D. Wilkinson and E. M. Williamson, "Cannabinoids Inhibit Human Keratinocyte Proliferation through a Non-CB1/CB2 Mechanism and Have a Potential Therapeutic Value in the Treatment of Psoriasis," *Journal of Dermatological Science* 45 (2007): 92.

414 M. Pucci, C. Rapino, A. Di Francesco, E. Dainese, C. D'Addario, and M. Maccarrone, "Epigenetic Control of Skin Differentiation Genes by Phytocannabinoids," *British Journal of Pharmacology* 170, no. 3 (2013): 581. doi:10.1111/bph.12309.

415 Charmie Gholson, "Michael McShane's Story: Beating Squamous Cell Carcinoma Skin Cancer," *Cure Your Own Cancer,* last modified October 1, 2012, www.cureyourowncancer.org/michael-mcshanes-story-beating -squamous-cell-carcinoma-skin-cancer-with-cannabis-oil.html.

416 A. N. Nicholson, C. Turner, B. M. Stone, and P. J. Robson, "Effect of Delta-9-tetrahydrocannabinol and Cannabidiol on Nocturnal Sleep and Early-Morning Behavior in Young Adults," *Journal of Clinical Psychopharmacology* 24, no. 3 (2004): 305–313.

417 E. Murillo-Rodríguez, D. Millán-Aldaco, M. Palomero-Rivero, R. Mechoulam, and R. Drucker-Colín, "The Nonpsychoactive Cannabis Constituent Cannabidiol Is a Wake-Inducing Agent," *Behavioral Neuroscience* 122, no. 6 (2008): 1378–1382.

418 Dr. Michael Moskowitz, personal communication with authors, October 2016

419 D. W. Carley, S. Paviovic, M. Janelidze, and M. Radulovacki, "Functional Role for Cannabinoids in Respiratory Stability during Sleep," *Sleep* 25, no. 4 (2002): 391–398. PubMed PMID: 12071539.

420 Bharati Prasad, Miodrag G. Radulovacki, and David W. Carley, "Proof of Concept Trial of Dronabinol in Obstructive Sleep Apnea," *Frontiers in Psychiatry* 4 (2013): 1.

421 E. B. Russo, G. W. Guy, and P. J. Robson, "Cannabis, Pain, and Sleep: Lessons from Therapeutic Clinical Trials of Sativex, a Cannabis-Based Medicine," *Chemistry and Biodiversity* 4, no. 8 (2007): 1729–1743.

422 M. H. N. Chagas, A. L. Eckeli, A. W. Zuardi, M. A. Pena-Pereira, M. A. Sobreira-Neto, E. T. Sobreira, M. R. Camilo, M. M. Bergamaschi, C. H. Schenck, J. E. C. Hallak, V. Tumas, and J. A. S. Crippa, "Cannabidiol Can Improve Complex Sleep-Related Behaviours Associated with Rapid Eye Movement Sleep Behaviour Disorder in Parkinson's Disease Patients: A Case Series," *Journal of Clinical Pharmacy and Therapeutics* 39 (2014): 564–566. doi:10.1111/jcpt.12179.

423 "Cannabis and Perimenopause: Help Through 'The Transition,'" *United Patients Group,* last modified March 10, 2016, https://unitedpatientsgroup.com/blog/2016/03/10/cannabis-and-peri-menopause -help-through-the-transition.

424 J. M. Riddle, *Eve's Herbs: A History of Contraception and Abortion in the West* (Cambridge, MA: Harvard University, 1997).

425 L. S. Thompson, *The Assyrian Herbal* (London: Luzac and Co., 1972).

426 V. Crawford, "A Homelie Herbe: Medicinal Cannabis in Early England," *Journal of Cannabis Therapeutics* 2, no. 2 (2002): 71–79.

427 Ethan Russo, "Cannabis Treatments in Obstetrics and Gynecology: A Historical Review," *Journal of Cannabis Therapeutics* 2 (2002): 5–35.

428 J. M. Scudder, *Specific Medication and Specific Medicines* (Cincinnati: Wilstach, Baldwin & Co., 1875).

429 J. W. Farlow, "On the Use of Belladonna and *Cannabis indica* by the Rectum in Gynecological Practice," *Boston Medical and Surgical Journal* 120 (1889): 508.

430 Seshata, "Top Five Ways That Cannabis Can Affect the Menstrual Cycle," https://sensiseeds.com/en/blog/top-5-ways-that-cannabis-can-affect -the-menstrual-cycle/.

431 Ramona G. Almirez, Carol Grace Smith, and Ricardo H. Asch, "The Effects of Marijuana Extract and Δ9-tetrahydrocannabinol on Luteal Function in the Rhesus Monkey," *Fertility and Sterility* 39, no. 2 (1983): 212–217. doi:10.1016/s0015-0282(16)46821-4.

432 M. Ranganathan, G. Braley, B. Pittman, T. Cooper, E. Perry, J. Krystal, and D. C. D'Souza, "The Effects of Cannabinoids on Serum Cortisol and Prolactin in Humans," *Psychopharmacology* 203, no. 4 (2009): 737–744, http://doi.org/10.1007/s00213-007422-2.

433 "I think hash oil cured my infertility and healed endometriosis," *Grass City Forums*, last modified March 28, 2012, https://forum.grasscity .com/threads/i-think-hash-oil-cured-my-infertility-and-healed -endometriosis.1024345/.

434 Natalia Dmitrieva, H. Nagabukuro, D. Resuehr, G. Zhang, S. L. McAllister, K. A. McGinty, K. Mackie, and K. J. Berkley, "Endocannabinoid Involvement in Endometriosis," *Pain* 151.3 (2010): 703–710.

435 Delilah Butterfield, "Marijuana and Pregnancy #2: Does Marijuana Have an Impact on Fertility?" *Herb*, March 21, 2016, http://herb .co/2016/03/21/fertility-does-marijuana-have-an-impact/.

436 M. Maccarone, H. Valensise, M. Bari, N. Lazzarin, C. Romanini, and A. Finazzi-Agrò, "Relation between Decreased Anandamide Hydrolase Concentrations in Human Lymphocytes and Miscarriage," *The Lancet* 355, no. 9212 (2000): 1326–1329. doi:10.1016/S0140-6736(00)02115-2.

437 S. K. Das, B. C. Paria, I. Chakraborty, and S. K. Dey, "Cannabinoid Ligand-Receptor Signaling in the Mouse Uterus," *Proceedings of the National Academy of Sciences* 92, no. 10 (1995): 4332–4336. doi:10.1073/pnas.92.10.4332.

438 B. C. Paria, S. K. Das, and S. K. Dey, "The Preimplantation Mouse Embryo Is a Target for Cannabinoid Ligand-Receptor Signaling," *Proceedings of the National Academy of Sciences* 92, no. 21 (1995): 9460–9464. doi:10.1073/pnas.92.21.9460.

439 Ethan Russo, Geoffrey Guy, and Phillip Rodson, "Cannabis, Pain, and Sleep: Lessons from Therapeutic Clinical Trials of Sativex®, a Cannabis-Based Medicine," *Chemistry and Biodiversity* 4, no. 8 (2007): 1729–1743. doi:10.1002/cbdv.200790150.

440 "How Cannabis Helps Menopause," *Impact Network,* last modified March 2, 2017, http://www.impactcannabis.org/medical-marijuana-menopause/.

441 Ibid.

442 A. I. Idris, A. Sophocleous, E. Landao-Bassonga, M. Canals, G. Milligan, D. Baker, R. J. van't Hof, and S. H. Ralston, "Cannabinoid Receptor Type 1 Protects against Age-Related Osteoporosis by Regulating Osteoblast and Adipocyte Differentiation in Marrow Stromal Cells," *Cell Metabolism* 10 (2009): 139–147.

443 "How Cannabis Helps Menopause," *Impact Network,* last modified March 2, 2017, http://www.impactcannabis.org/medical-marijuana-menopause/.

444 National Academies of Sciences, Engineering, and Medicine, *The Health Effects of Cannabis and Cannabinoids: The Current State of Evidence and Recommendations for Research* (Washington, DC: The National Academies Press, 2017).

445 D. M. Fergusson, L. J. Horwood, K. Northstone, and ALSPAC Study Team, "Maternal Use of Cannabis and Pregnancy Outcome," *BLOG: An International Journal of Obstetrics and Gynaecology* 109 (2002): 21–27.

446 Paul Armentano, "Breathe, Push, Puff? Pot Use and Pregnancy: A Review of the Literature," *Heads* magazine, June 2007.

447 J. S. Hayes, R. Lampart, M. C. Dreher, and L. Morgan, "Five-Year Follow-up of Rural Jamaican Children Whose Mothers Used Marijuana during Pregnancy," *West Indian Medical Journal* 40, no. 3 (1991): 120–123.

448 Melanie C. Dreher, Kevin Nugent, and Rebekah Hudgins, "Prenatal Marijuana Exposure and Neonatal Outcomes in Jamaica: An Ethnographic Study," *Pediatrics* 93, iss. 2 (1994): 254–260.

449 Peter A. Fried, "The Consequences of Marijuana Use During Pregnancy: A Review of the Human Literature," *Journal of Cannabis Therapeutics* 2 (2002): 85–104.

450 Giuseppe Tortoriello, Claudia V. Morris, Alan Alpar, Janos Fuzik, Sally L. Shirran, Daniela Calvigioni, Erik Keimpema, Catherine H. Botting, Kirstin Reinecke, Thomas Herdegen, Michael Courtney, Yasmin L. Hurd, and Tibor Harkany, "Miswiring the Brain Delta-9-tetra-hydro-cannabinol Disrupts Cortical Development by Inducing an SCG10/stathmin-2 Degradation Pathway," *EMBO Journal* 33, no. 7 (January 27, 2014): 668–685.

451 Ethan Russo, "Cannabis Treatments in Obstetrics and Gynecology: A Historical Review," *Journal of Cannabis Therapeutics* 2 (2002): 5–35.

452 Yvan Ruetsch, Thomas Boni, and Alain Borgeat, "From Cocaine to Ropivacaine: The History of Local Anesthetic Drugs," *Current Topics in Medicinal Chemistry* 1, no. 3 (2001): 175–182. doi:10.2174/1568026013395335.

453 Shayna N Conner, Victoria Bedell, Kim Lipsey, George A. Macones, Alison G. Cahill, and Methodius G. Tuuli, "Maternal Marijuana Use and Adverse Neonatal Outcomes," *Obstetrics & Gynecology* 128, no. 4 (2016): 713–723. doi:10.1097/aog.0000000000001649.

454 Lidush Goldschmidt, Nancy L. Day, and Gale A. Richardson, "Effects of Prenatal Marijuana Exposure on Child Behavior Problems at Age 10," *Neurotoxicology and Teratology* 22, iss. 3 (2000): 325–336, http://dx.doi.org/10.1016/S0892-0362(00)00066-0.

Part III

455 James L. Butrica, "The Medical Use of Cannabis Among the Greeks and Romans," *Journal of Cannabis Therapeutics* 2, no. 2 (2002): 51–70.

456 W. E. Dixon, "The Pharmacology of *Cannabis indica*," *British Medical Journal* 2 (1899): 1354–1357.

457 Claudia Bensimoun, "Medical Marijuana for Dogs," *Animal Wellness Magazine,* https://animalwellnessmagazine.com/medical-marijuana-for-dogs/.

458 Ray Wright, personal communication with the authors, January 15, 2017.

459 Ibid.

Part IV

460 Michael Backes, *Cannabis Pharmacy: A Practical Guide to Medicinal Marijuana* (New York: Black Dog & Leventhal Publishers, 2014).

461 R. Clarke, "Naming Cannabis: The 'Indica' versus 'Sativa' Debate," *Sensi Seeds* (blog), March 9, 2015, https://sensiseeds.com/en/blog/naming-cannabis-the-indica-versus-sativa-debate/.

462 Robert C. Clarke and Mark D. Merlin, *Cannabis-Evolution and Ethnobotany* (Berkeley: University of California Press, 2013).

463 Michael Backes, *Cannabis Pharmacy: A Practical Guide to Medicinal Marijuana* (New York: Black Dog & Leventhal Publishers, 2014), 52.

464 D. Butterfield, "Cannabis Ruderalis: The Overlooked Middle Child of the Cannabis Family," *Herb*, August 18, 2016, http://herb.co/2016/08/18/cannabis-ruderalis/.

465 Drake Dorm, "Cannabinol (CBN): The Cannabinoid That Makes You Sleepy," *Medical Jane,* 2013, www.medicaljane.com/2013/08/19/cannabinol-cbn-will-put-you-to-bed/.

466 "2016 Warning Letters and Test Results for Cannabidiol-Related Products," *U.S. Food and Drug Administration,* last modified August 31, 2016, www.fda.gov/NewsEvents/PublicHealthFocus/ucm484109.htm.

467 CNN, *Weed: Dr. Sanjay Gupta Reports,* August 11, 2013.

Part V

468 "Sour Tsunami Stabilized," *O'Shaughnessy's,* Autumn 2011, 11, www.os-extra.cannabisclinicians.org/wp-content/uploads/2013/11/CBD-Reintroduction-Era-2011.pdf.

469 Alexandra Sifferlin, "Can Medical Marijuana Help End the Opioid Epidemic?" *Time Magazine* (July 2016), http://time.com/4419003/can-medical-marijuana-help-end-the-opioid-epidemic/

470 Ibid.

471 Ibid.

472 Marcus A. Bachhuber, Brendan Saloner, Chinazo O. Cunningham, and Colleen L. Barry, "Medical Cannabis Laws and Opioid Analgesic Overdose Mortality in the United States, 1999-2010," *JAMA Internal Medicine* 174, no. 10 (2014): 1668. doi:10.1001/jamainternmed.2014.4005.

473 Kevin F. Boehnke, Evangelos Litinas, and Daniel J. Clauw, "Medical Cannabis Use Is Associated with Decreased Opiate Medication Use in a Retrospective Cross-Sectional Survey of Patients with Chronic Pain," *The Journal of Pain* 17, iss. 6 (2016): 739–744.

474 Ashley C. Bradford and W. David Bradford, "Medical Marijuana Laws Reduce Prescription Medication Use in Medicare Part D," *Health Affairs* 35, no. 7 (2016): 1230–1236. doi:10.1377/hlthaff.2015.1661.

475 Lee Fang, "Leading Anti-Marijuana Academics Are Paid by Painkiller Drug Companies," *Vice Magazine,* August 27, 2014, https://news.vice .com/article/leading-anti-marijuana-academics-are-paid-by-painkiller-drug-companies.

476 Philip Ross, "Marijuana Legalization: Pharmaceuticals, Alcohol Industry among Biggest Opponents of Legal Weed," *International Business Times* (August 6, 2014), http://www.ibtimes.com/marijuana-legalization-pharmaceuticals-alcohol-industry-among-biggest-opponents-legal-weed-1651166.

477 Lee Fang, "The Real Reason Pot Is Still Illegal," *The Nation* (July 21–28, 2014), http://www.thenation.com/article/180493/anti-pot-lobbys-big-bankroll?page=0,0.

478 Corrections Corporation of America, *Annual Report 2014. http://www .annualreports.com/HostedData/AnnualReportArchive/c/NYSE_CXW_2014.pdf*

479 Lee Fang, "The Real Reason Pot Is Still Illegal," *The Nation,* July 21–28, 2014, www .thenation.com/article/180493/anti-pot-lobbys-big-bankroll?page=0,0.

480 Kendall Bentsen, "Money, Not Morals, Drives Marijuana Prohibition Movement," *Center for Responsive Politics,* August 5, 2014, www.opensecrets .org/news/2014/08/money-not-morals-drives-marijuana-prohibition -movement/.

480 Marcus A. Bachhuber, Brendan Saloner, Chinazo O. Cunningham, and Colleen L. Barry. "Medical Cannabis Laws and Opioid Analgesic Overdose Mortality in the United States, 1999-2010," *JAMA Internal Medicine* 174, no. 10 (2014): 1668. doi:10.1001/jamainternmed.2014.4005.

482 James M. Cole, *Memorandum for all United States Attorneys* (Washington, DC: U.S. Department of Justice, August 29, 2013).

483 Sarah Boseley and Jessica Glenza, "Medical Experts Call for Global Drug Decriminalization," *The Guardian,* March 24, 2016.

484 Jessica Glenza, "UN Backs Prohibitionist Drug Policies Despite Call for More 'Humane Solution,'" *The Guardian,* April 19, 2016.

485 For specific information, country by country, see https://en.wikipedia .org/wiki/Legality_of_cannabis_by_country.

486 National Academies of Sciences, Engineering, and Medicine, *The Health Effects of Cannabis and Cannabinoids: The Current State of Evidence and Recommendations for Research* (Washington, DC: The National Academies Press, 2017).

487 Jessica Glenza, "Most marijuana medicinal benefits are inconclusive, wide-ranging study finds,'" *The Guardian,* January 12, 2017.

488 Ibid.

489 Eckhart Tolle, *A New Earth: Awakening to Your Life's Purpose* (New York: Dutton/Penguin Group, 2005), 1–2.

RESOURCE LIST

The following is a list of useful websites for updated information on research and access related to medicinal cannabis.

CBD4Health.com

SynergyCBD.com

HealingEssenceCBD.com

ProjectCBD.org

CannabisHealthIndex.com

Norml.org

MedicalMarijuana.ProCon.org

BeyondTHC.com

MedicalCannabis.com

UnitedPatientsGroup.com

NOTE *For the latest updates on scientific and medical research and literature, legal issues, and expert opinions, visit www.CBD-book.com/Updates.*

GLOSSARY OF TERMS
AND ABBREVIATIONS

2-AG (2-arachidonoyl glycerol): One of two endogenous cannabinoids currently identified, known to be abundant in the central nervous system.

AEA: Arachidonoyl ethanolamide, or anandamide, the first of the two endogenous cannabinoid molecules discovered by the scientific team led by Raphael Mechoulam in the early 1990s; involved in regulating numerous functions in the body, including sleep, pain, and digestion.

anandamide: Another name for the endocannabinoid-signaling molecule AEA, combining the Sanskrit word meaning bliss *(ananda)* and the chemical name for a key part of the molecular structure of this compound (amide).

beta-caryophyllene: A terpene found in some cannabis varieties.

bidirectional: Medical effects that can produce opposite results on different people, i.e., stimulating for one person and sedating for another.

bioavailability: The portion of a substance, once ingested, that can be absorbed into the bloodstream.

biphasic: When determining a dose via titration, after a certain point increasing the dose may cause a decrease in result—more is not necessarily better.

BLD (broad-leaf drug): Cannabis variety that is THC-dominant, with wide leaflets, and commonly referred to as indica.

cannabinoids: Compounds that activate cannabinoid receptors, including endocannabinoids, phytocannabinoids, and synthetic cannabinoids.

cannabis hyperemesis syndrome: A rare form of cannabinoid toxicity that develops in chronic users, characterized by cyclic episodes of nausea and vomiting.

CB1 (cannabinoid-1) receptor: A receptor believed to be located primarily in the central and peripheral nervous system, activated by all types of cannabinoids and largely responsible for the efficacy of THC.

CB2 (cannabinoid-2) receptor: A receptor believed to be located primarily in the peripheral tissues of the immune system, the gastrointestinal system, the peripheral nervous system, and to a lesser degree in the central nervous system.

CBC (cannabichromene): A phytocannabinoid that may be anti-inflammatory.

CBD (cannabidiol): A major phytocannabinoid, accounting for up to 40 percent of the cannabis plant's extract, with a wide scope of potential medical applications especially linked to the lack of psychoactivity and side effects.

CBDA (cannabidiolic acid): The raw acidic form of CBD found in the fresh plant.

CBDVA (cannabidivarin): A propyl variant of CBD, found in some Himalayan varieties.

CBG (cannabigerol): A phytocannabinoid that is the precursor used by the plant's enzymes to produce THC and CBD.

chemotype: A term for a plant type that produces a distinct combination of chemical compounds.

cytochrome P450: A family of liver enzymes.

decarboxylation: Also called "activating" or "decarbing," typically by the application of heat, describing a chemical reaction in cannabis in which acidic cannabinoids are converted into their more bioavailable form by removing a carboxyl group from the molecule.

endocannabinoid: An endogenous cannabinoid, or naturally occurring, neuromodulatory lipid in the body involved in the regulation of numerous physical systems.

endocannabinoid system: A system of endogeonous neuromodulator chemicals and their receptors found in the mammalian brain and throughout the body.

endogenous: Naturally occurring in the body.

entourage effect: The synergy of pharmacological effects that occur through the interaction of cannabinoids, terpenoids and other compounds found in the whole cannabis plant.

first-pass metabolism: A phenomenon of metabolism whereby the concentration of active ingredients in a medication or other substance is greatly reduced before it reaches the bloodstream.

indica: A term commonly used to describe broad-leaf cannabis varieties with generally more sedating properties.

industrial hemp: Low-THC, high-CBD content cannabis used for producing fiber or other industrial use.

Kush: A term broadly applied to high-potency THC-rich varieties of cannabis, usually indica strains, some of which originated in the Hindu Kush mountains of central Asia.

leaflet: A leaflike part of a compound leaf, not borne by a branch or stem.

limonene: A terpene with a citrus aroma, known for having antibacterial and stimulating properties.

linalool: A terpene with a floral aroma, known for having calming properties.

marijuana: A slang term for cannabis originating from Mexico and popularized in the United States by anti-drug crusaders attempting to associate it with minorities.

myrcene: A terpene known for having sedative properties.

NLD (narrow-leaf drug): Cannabis variety that is THC-dominant, with narrow leaflets, and commonly referred to as sativa.

oromucosal delivery: Administration of a compound by mouth spray, intended to be absorbed through the buccal mucosa lining the mouth.

peripheral body: Referring to areas away from the center, closer to the outer areas of the body.

phenotype: The distinct, observable traits of an individual plant or organism based on genetic and environmental influences.

phytocannabinoid: A cannabinoid found uniquely in the cannabis plant.

pinene: A terpene with a pine aroma, known for having uplifting properties.

psychoactivity: A property of a substance that causes a profound or significant effect on mental processes, mood, or consciousness.

sativa: A term commonly used to describe narrow-leaf cannabis varieties with stimulating properties.

sensimilla: Seedless, unpollinated female cannabis flowers, from Spanish for "without seed."

synthetic cannabinoid: A cannabinoid produced in a laboratory.

terpene, terpenoid: Volatile hydrocarbons found in the essential oils produced by many plants, including cannabis.

terpinolene: A terpene known for its anti-anxiety and anti-cancer properties.

THC (tetrahydrocannabinol/Δ^9 tetrahydrocannabinol): The principal psychoactive constituent of cannabis

THCA (tetrahydrocannabinolic acid): The raw acidic form of THC found in the fresh plant, which is non-psychoactive but converts to THC as it breaks down over time or through decarboxylation.

THCV (tetrahydrocannabivarin): A propyl variant of THC, with antagonistic effects on cannabinoid receptors and effects contrary to THC.

tincture: An ethyl alcohol extraction of a plant.

tolerance: A reaction to dose whereby effects of a medicine are progressively reduced.

trichome: Referring in cannabis to the three types of tiny, specialized, crystalline epidermal hairs present in the buds, leaves, and stalks of late-stage cannabis plants that produce the cannabinoid-rich resin responsible for the medicinal effects.

TRPV1 (transient receptor potential vanilloid receptor): A receptor that initiates inflammatory pain and response in the body.

INDEX

Triple negative breast cancer (TNBC), 121
TRPV1, 22
Turpentine, carene as component of, 34
2-AG, 16, 17, 17f, 18, 295
2-arachidonoyl glycerol (2-AG), 16

U

United States, CBD in, 10, 11
United States Drug Enforcement Administration (DEA), Schedule I drug of, xxv
U.S. Drug Enforcement Agency, 5
Uwe Blesching, 85

V

Valeant Pharmaceuticals, 56
Valencene, 35
Valentine X, 225–226, 226f
Vancouver Island Seed Company (VISC), 218
Vape pens, 50
Vaporized cannabis
    for eating disorders, 135
    for relief of degenerative diseases symptoms, 149

for restless legs syndrome, 132
for treating skin conditions, 165
Vaporizers. *see also* Herbal vaporizers
    effective, 110, 137, 142
    heating elements of, 50
Vaporizing process, 49–52
Vegetable glycerin, 43
Vomiting, nabilone for, 56

W

"War on drugs," 8
Water pipe (bongs), as smoking method, 48–49
Wax, 51
Weed (documentary), 11, 160, 213
Weight loss, cannabis and, 126
Women's health issues
    cannabis and monthly cycle, 172–174
    historical view, 172
Wright, Ray, 190

Y

Youth and adolescence, THC products and, 71

ABOUT THE AUTHORS

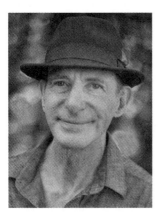

Leonard Leinow has three decades of experience cultivating and studying medicinal cannabis. He founded Synergy Wellness in 2008, a not-for-profit medical cannabis collective in Northern California with more than four thousand patient members. Synergy is dedicated to handcrafting artisanal, organic, and all-natural products made from the whole plant. Synergy Wellness specializes in products rich in CBD, the non-psychoactive molecule with healing properties. He calls cannabidiol the "get-well molecule," in contrast to THC, the "get-high molecule."

Known as an early pioneer in CBD-rich cannabis products, Leinow creates proprietary blends that are recommended by doctors throughout California for their patients with cancer, pain, epilepsy, multiple sclerosis, and many other conditions. For his seemingly magical ability to recommend the right product for each individual patient, he has been called "The Wizard of Woodacre."

He lived in India for five years while on a spiritual quest, studying the religious and cultural aspects of ancient civilizations. He has traveled to thirty-five countries around the world in search of knowledge and wisdom. His studies include more than three decades of practice in shamanic, tantric, and martial arts. For five years, he was a professional deep-tissue body worker, which began his focus on the healing arts.

Leinow earned his bachelor's degree from UCLA in engineering, with a minor in art. He applied his engineering background to his early career as an executive search consultant, recruiting technical experts for corporations nationwide. Throughout his life, he has also been dedicated to artistic expression. His bronze sculpture, ceramics, and paintings have been exhibited and sold in fine art galleries around the world.

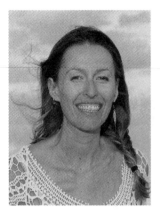 Trained as a cultural anthropologist and skilled in four languages, **Juliana Birnbaum** has lived and worked in the United States, Europe, Japan, Nepal, Costa Rica, and Brazil. In 2005 she founded Voices in Solidarity, an initiative that partnered with Ashaninka indigenous tribal leaders from the Brazilian Amazon to support the development of the Yorenka Ãtame community-led environmental educational center featured in her first book, *Sustainable [R]evolution: Permaculture in Ecovillages, Urban Farms, and Communities Worldwide,* published in February 2014 by North Atlantic Books. Birnbaum was also the first graduate of the Cornerstone school in Oakland, a rigorous training program for doulas and midwives in the United States, focusing on a holistic model of care for mothers and babies.

She has written about ecovillages, native rights, and social justice issues in a variety of newspapers, indigenous journals, blogs, and anthologies, including *Zester Daily, E-The Environmental Magazine, Bridges, El Reportero, The Rising Nepal, World Rainforest Movement Bulletin, Quechua Network,* and *Cultural Survival Quarterly.* Birnbaum is engaged variously as writer, editor, teacher, midwife assistant, and mother when not attempting yoga poses or gardening.

ABOUT THE CONTRIBUTORS

Heather Dunbar is a cannabis health educator with over a decade of experience in various aspects of the cannabis industry, including cultivation, sales, edibles production, and education. Dunbar has also worked extensively in the natural-products industry, conducting product development and community outreach for several pioneering businesses in that space. Inspired by her travels and interest in holistic health, Dunbar spent several years managing massage and wellness programs at retreat centers around the world. She is a natural leader with a passion for improving the world through holistic healing, sustainability, and community development. Dunbar holds a degree in Human Development and Health Psychology and is an MBA candidate at Presidio Graduate School, focused on sustainable business strategy and leadership.

Lion Goodman is CEO of Healing Essence, a company dedicated to all aspects of healing, including physical, psychological, emotional, relational, and spiritual. He is a Professional Certified Coach, and he coaches leaders of businesses and organizations to become whole and healthy. He is the creator of Clear Your Beliefs, a methodology for transforming beliefs at the core of the psyche, which he has taught to hundreds of coaches, therapists and healers around the world.

Goodman has studied and practiced psychology, neurology, spirituality, philosophy, and the principles of success for more than forty years. His early career was in executive search and executive coaching, where he served hundreds of CEOs and senior managers in a wide variety of companies, from early stage start-ups to Fortune 500 corporations.

He is the author of *The CBD Primer, Clear Your Beliefs, Menlightenment—A Book for Awakening Men,* and coauthor of *Creating On Purpose.*

Websites: www.HealingEssenceCBD.com, www.ClearYourBeliefs.com, and www.ClearBeliefs.com.

Michael H. Moskowitz, MD, MPH, practices in Sausalito, California, at Bay Area Pain Medical Associates and is board certified in both psychiatry and pain medicine. He graduated from Louisiana State University Medical Center in 1977, having earned a master's in public health in 1972 from Tulane University. He completed his psychiatric residency and psychosomatic fellowship training at St. Mary's Hospital in San Francisco in 1982. That same year, Dr. Moskowitz entered private psychiatric and psychosomatic practice and served as the Medical Director of the Adult Locked Psychiatric Inpatient Teaching Unit at St. Mary's from 1982 to 1987.

He was a member of the Board of Directors of SpineCare Medical Group for four years from 1988 to 1992. The practice he helped found in 1981, Psychiatric Associates of San Francisco, changed its name in 2000 to Bay Area Pain Medical Associates, reflecting the predominant practice of pain medicine in this group. Dr. Moskowitz is a member of the Educational Council of the National Initiative on Pain Control, a group of the top pain physicians in the country.

Dr. Moskowitz has published several peer-reviewed journal articles and textbook chapters with a focus on the role that brain changes play in perpetuating persistent pain states. He served as a member of the Examination Council for the American Board of Pain Medicine from 2006 to 2010 and as the former chairman of the Educational Committee of the American Academy of Pain Medicine. He has also served on the American Academy of Pain Medicine's Continuing Education Committee and the Enduring Materials Committee and chaired the Academy's website redesign committee. He has pioneered the development and use of animations to teach and understand principles of pain medicine and has designed and developed the most popular website for pain animations in the world, since 1999: www.bayareapainmedical.com. Dr. Moskowitz has been an Assistant Clinical Professor for the Department of Anesthesiology and Pain Medicine at the University of California, Davis since 2006, teaching the psychiatric and neuroplastic aspects of pain medicine.

Gary Richter, MS, DVM, has been practicing veterinary medicine in the San Francisco Bay Area since 1998. In addition to conventional veterinary medical training, Dr. Richter is certified in veterinary acupuncture as well as veterinary chiropractic. As owner and medical director of Montclair Veterinary Hospital and Holistic Veterinary Care in Oakland, California, Richter understands the benefits of both conventional and holistic treatment methods for the preventative and therapeutic care of pets. By integrating medical cannabis with other conventional and alternative therapies, Richter has been able to improve the quality of life of pets living with medical conditions ranging from arthritis to inflammatory bowel disease to cancer.

Dr. Richter and his two hospitals have been the recipients of more than twenty local and national awards including Best Veterinary Hospital, Best Veterinarian, Best Canine Therapy Facility, and Best Alternative Medicine Provider. PetPlan named Richter as one of the top ten veterinarians in the United States for 2011, and Dr. Richter was awarded the title America's Favorite Veterinarian by the American Veterinary Medical Foundation.

ALSO BY JULIA BIRNBAUM

available from North Atlantic Books

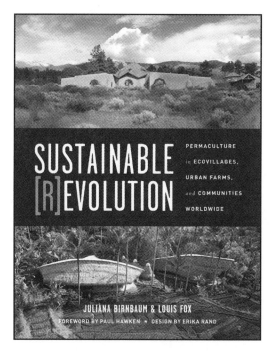

Sustainable Revolution
978-1-58394-648-0

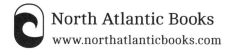

North Atlantic Books
www.northatlanticbooks.com

North Atlantic Books is an independent, nonprofit publisher committed to a bold exploration of the relationships between mind, body, spirit, and nature.

About North Atlantic Books

North Atlantic Books (NAB) is an independent, nonprofit publisher committed to a bold exploration of the relationships between mind, body, spirit, and nature. Founded in 1974, NAB aims to nurture a holistic view of the arts, sciences, humanities, and healing. To make a donation or to learn more about our books, authors, events, and newsletter, please visit www.northatlanticbooks.com.

For more information on books, authors, events, and to sign up for our newsletter, please visit www.northatlanticbooks.com.

North Atlantic Books is the publishing arm of the Society for the Study of Native Arts and Sciences, a 501(c)(3) nonprofit educational organization that promotes cross-cultural perspectives linking scientific, social, and artistic fields. To learn how you can support us, please visit our website.